Ginseng and Ginseng Products 101

What are You Buying?

Ginseng and Ginseng Products 101

What are You Buying?

Koh Hwee Ling
Wee Hai Ning
Tan Chay Hoon

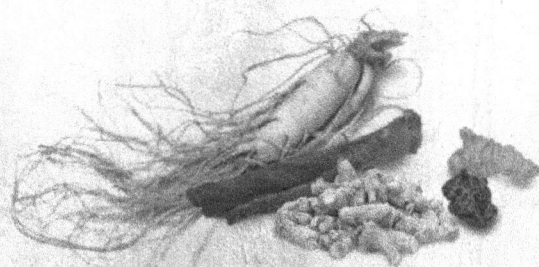

World Scientific

NEW JERSEY · LONDON · SINGAPORE · BEIJING · SHANGHAI · HONG KONG · TAIPEI · CHENNAI · TOKYO

Published by

World Scientific Publishing Co. Pte. Ltd.

5 Toh Tuck Link, Singapore 596224

USA office: 27 Warren Street, Suite 401-402, Hackensack, NJ 07601

UK office: 57 Shelton Street, Covent Garden, London WC2H 9HE

Library of Congress Control Number: 2015024789

British Library Cataloguing-in-Publication Data
A catalogue record for this book is available from the British Library.

GINSENG AND GINSENG PRODUCTS 101
What are You Buying?

ISBN 978-981-4667-30-2
ISBN 978-981-4667-31-9 (pbk)

Typeset by Stallion Press
Email: enquiries@stallionpress.com

Authors and Contributors

Associate Professor Hwee-Ling Koh obtained a BSc (Pharmacy) (Hons) and MSc (Pharmacy) from the National University of Singapore, as well as a PhD from the University of Cambridge. She is a registered pharmacist with the Singapore Pharmacy Council. A/P Koh has been teaching and carrying out research on Traditional Chinese Medicine and medicinal plants at the National University of Singapore for more than 15 years. Her research areas include quality control and safety of botanicals and the study of natural products/ medicinal plants as potential sources of lead compounds of novel therapeutics. She reviews for various international journals and grant-awarding bodies, and publishes in various international peer-reviewed journals including the *Journal of Ethnopharmacology*, *Drug Discovery Today*, *Journal of Chromatography A*, *Drug Safety*, *Journal of Pharmaceutical and Biomedical Analysis*, *Journal of Agricultural and Food Chemistry* and *Food Additives and Contaminants*. She has also published a book entitled *A Guide to Medicinal Plants: An Illustrated, Scientific and Medicinal Approach*, Singapore: World Scientific. Her long-term research objective is to apply scientific methods in the study of medicinal plants to achieve a positive impact on society and to help the general public to achieve optimal health outcomes.

Associate Professor Chay-Hoon Tan is an Associate Professor in Pharmacology, Yong Loo Lin School of Medicine of the National University of Singapore and Consultant Psychiatrist, National University Hospital. She obtained her MBBS in 1980, Master of

Medicine (Psychiatry) in 1986, PhD (Pharmacology) in 1997 and Master in Medical Education in 2011. She represented Singapore in the "Technical Review of Antidepressant Medication" Task Force to review the international use of antidepressants. She was also chairperson of the World Psychiatric Association Consensus Statement on the usefulness of second generation Antipsychotic Medications in Singapore. Currently, she is the coordinator for Research in Asia Psychotropic Drug Prescription. A/P Tan is also appointed by the Ministry of Health as member of the Chinese Proprietary Medicine Advisory Committee and National Medication Network Committee. She serves on the editorial board of the *International Journal of Mental Health* and helps review manuscripts for various international Neuroscience and Psychiatric journals. A/P Tan has been active in undergraduate and postgraduate teaching and examinations. She is also contributing to the curriculum development in the National University Health Services Residency Committee.

Mr Hai-Ning Wee is a registered TCM physician. He graduated with a double degree in Biomedical Sciences (Nanyang Technological University) and Traditional Chinese Medicine (Beijing University of Chinese Medicine), having completed his clinical internship in Dong Fang Hospital, Beijing. During his undergraduate years, he participated in the Undergraduate Research Experience on Campus (URECA) programme and presented his TCM research findings in the 7th International Postgraduate Symposium on Chinese Medicine, Hong Kong, China in 2011. Currently, he is pursuing a higher degree at NUS.

Other Contributors

Ms Klara Hess, Dr Mehdy Ghaemina and Ms Goh Sok-Hiang Goh collated and analysed the data. **Mr Jia-Jun Liew** further analysed the data and provided editorial assistance while **Ms Hui-Chuing Yew** provided editorial assistance. Photographs are taken by Mr Jia-Jun Liew, Ms Klara Hess, Dr Mehdy Ghaemina and A/P Hwee-Ling Koh.

Disclaimer

The contents of this book are intended to educate anyone who has an interest in achieving and maintaining good health through healthy food and herbs, in particular, those associated with the word "ginseng". This general, medical and scientific information should not be used to self-medicate without consulting a qualified practitioner. Readers are reminded that the information presented is subject to change as research is on-going and there are inter-individual variations.

The resources are not vetted and it is the reader's responsibility to ensure the accuracy of the information cited. Neither the authors nor publisher can be held responsible for the accuracy of the information cited and presented or the consequences from the use or misuse of the information in this book.

While every effort is made to minimise errors, there may be inadvertent omissions or errors in compiling the information. We would love to hear from you regarding any feedback and experiences that you may have with this book. Your feedback is important to us and there is always room for improvement. Please feel free to drop us an email at ginsengproducts101@gmail.com. We look forward to hearing from you.

This book is dedicated to all who want to improve their health and who strive to maintain good health, and also to those who help others to do so!

Foreword

This book is a gem! As someone who has been interested in Chinese medicine, herbal medicine and integrative health, I have longed for a source of reliable information to clarify the confusing picture of the ginseng scene. I am so delighted that Professor Koh Hwee Ling, who had completed a sabbatical at UCLA East-West Medicine in the summer of 2014, has asked me to write a foreword on a very important topic. I want to commend her leadership and dedication in working with a unique team of scientists and clinicians of both Eastern and Western tradition to complete this text.

This book is a good entry point to understand the research behind ginseng and helps address the most commonly misunderstood concepts of ginseng. I highly recommended this guide to (1) laymen who's looking for a good source to understand the Singaporean ginseng market, (2) laymen who's interested in taking a herbal supplement, such as ginseng, to enhance health and (3) physicians/scientists of western biomedical background who's looking for an introductory reference of the fundamental science of Ginseng products.

With a compilation of authoritative references, original literature and thorough market survey, this book is one of the most credible biomedical rendition of a Traditional Chinese medicine herbal text on ginseng that provides a useful reference on ginseng science and ginseng products available in the Singapore market. I hope to see more text like this to help both practitioners and consumers to understand the latest research on herbal efficacy and safety and to improve consumer's understanding of commonly used supplemental herbal products for health. A must-have reference for any practitioners recommending ginseng.

Ka-Kit Hui, MD, FACP
Founder and Director of UCLA Center
for East-West Medicine

Preface

This is an easy-to-read guide to the various herbs and products related to "ginseng". This book introduces the reader to the traditional uses and latest scientific research regarding Chinese/Korean ginseng, Notoginseng, American ginseng, Siberian ginseng and five-leaf ginseng (Jiao Gu Lan), including their names, pharmacological activities, phytoconstituents, indications, dosage, safety considerations (e.g. side effects and herb–drug interactions). It is suitable for the general public, including those who are new to ginseng related herbs, as well as well-read and informed consumers who want to find out more about the latest developments in ginseng and ginseng products. For healthcare professionals and scientists who are curious about the herbs and products that patients may be using, or for those who are exploring complementary methods and integrative health, this book will be an invaluable resource to help them understand the subject matter and to help their patients or themselves achieve optimal health outcomes and to maintain good health. Instructors and students of Traditional Chinese Medicine, Complementary and Alternative Medicine, as well as Integrative Medicine will find the comprehensive and consolidated information useful. Our team has delved into the local market and surveyed over 300 ginseng and ginseng products. Glossary of terms, explanations of Traditional Chinese Medicine terminologies, pharmacological activities, drug–herb interactions and a list of major chemical components from five herbs and their respective pharmacological activities, and products information are presented clearly in the appendices.

Chay Hoon first mooted the idea to publish a book to educate the general public about the many different types of herbs and products related to "ginseng" that are available in the local market. As health-care professionals as well as scientists, we attempt to educate ourselves first and with the support of a dedicated team of graduate students (Klara, Mehdy and Hai Ning), an undergraduate student (Sok Hiang), as well as research staff (Jia Jun and Hui Chuing), this book finally becomes a reality.

Happy reading!

Guide to Using This Book

This book is intended to educate the general public as well as health-care professionals about "ginseng". Very often, the word "ginseng" is indicated as an ingredient in herbal products. As such, five medicinal herbs which are commonly associated with the term "ginseng" have been reviewed. The five plants are *Panax ginseng* (Chinese and Korean ginseng), American ginseng (*Panax quinquefolius*), Sanqi (*Panax notoginseng*), Siberian ginseng (*Eleuthercoccus senticocus*) and five-leaf ginseng (Jiao Gu Lan or *Gynostemma pentaphyllum*). Yes, Chinese and Korean ginseng are the same plant! They are referred to as "ginseng root" (common name) in this book and are available as both the white and red forms (red ginseng). As the processing (often by steaming) may change the chemical constituents, resulting in different activities, we have chosen to have a separate section called "red ginseng" which includes information wherever the red form is clearly specified.

It is also common practice for *Panax ginseng* to be written as *P. ginseng*. Likewise, *Panax notoginseng* is *P. notoginseng* and *Eleutherococcus senticosus* is *E. senticosus*.

Published information (where available) are presented as introduction, phytoconstituents, pharmacological activities, actions, indications, administration and dosage and finally safety considerations.

The introductory section gives the scientific name, pharmaceutical name, common names, origin as well as photographs of the herb. A scale of 1 cm is included for comparisons. In the pharmaceutical names, radix means "root", rhizoma means "rhizome" (underground stem) and caulis means "stem" or "stalk".

The section "Phytoconstituents" refers to the chemicals found in the plant. This is not meant to be an exhaustive list, but to highlight what is known about the phytochemicals present in the plant, especially those that may be responsible for the health benefits and and/or are unique to the plant.

The section "Pharmacological activities" is a collation of published literature of the biological activities of the plant. These are typically reported in scientific publications as a result of laboratory tests done *in vitro* or *in vivo*, and less often, in clinical trials.

The information presented in the section "Actions" refers to the information obtained from the Chinese Pharmacopoeia, the official book on TCM herbs, preparations and western drugs used in China as well as from other sources. As most readers may not have easy access to such information, we have decided to include the information wherever it is available. As you will soon see, TCM terminologies are used and it is beyond the scope of this book to translate and explain in full details as a separate book on TCM will be required for that purpose. A word of caution: please do not take the information at face value and try to self-medicate, especially for serious conditions. The diagnosis by a qualified TCM practitioner is warranted.

The section "Indications" (i.e. uses) contains information from reliable sources only, namely, the Chinese Pharmacopoeia and the German Commission E. Similarly, the administration and dosage are obtained from these sources.

The section "Safety Considerations" include information (where available) on side effects, precautions, use during pregnancy and lactation, interactions with other herbs and interaction with drugs. Such information will be useful for the safe use of the herbs. Earlier criticisms of *Panax ginseng* causing "Ginseng Abuse Syndrome" has fallen out of favour as it was realized that the authors did not consider the dosage and whether the undesirable effects (e.g.

insomnia, hypertension, palpitation) were really due to *Panax ginseng* and hence not quoted to avoid misleading readers. The subsection 'Interactions with drugs' collates published information on the effects of the relevant herb or some of its components on drug therapy. Most of the information is related to warfarin therapy as poor control of blood coagulation can lead to excessive bleeding (because the blood is too "thin") or thrombosis (because the blood is too "thick" and coagulates too readily). Do be aware that such information should be used only as a guide as there is great interindividual variation and the presence of other components in a commercial product may have a great impact on the outcome measured.

The survey of 309 products include Chinese Proprietary Medicines (CPMs), health supplements and food supplements. CPMs are finished products in the final dosage form and are produced according to a TCM method. Health supplements are meant to supplement the health and hence may contain vitamins and minerals. Finally, food supplements are meant to supplement our diet. As they are food, they are considered to be generally safe. There is more regulatory control by the Health Sciences Authority (HSA) on the labelling requirements for CPMs and hence in this book, the information provided on the products is collated. By highlighting what is labelled, the consumers will be more aware of the information available to them and be more mindful of the many products associated with the terms "ginseng" or "Panax".

Acknowledgements

The authors would like to express our heartfelt gratitude to:

Professor Chong-Ren Yang for his kind sharing of his expert knowledge of *P. notoginseng*

Professor Zhong-Zhen Zhao for his professional advice

Managements of Fairprice 24 hours at HDB Clementi Branch, GNC Lot 1 Shopper's Mall Branch (GNC), Guardian Health and Beauty Lot 1 Shopper's Mall Branch (Guardian), Sinchong Meheco and Unity Pharmacy, NTUC Healthcare Hougang Mall Branch

Lee Foundation for the financial support (R-184-000-200-720)

Staff of World Scientific Publishing for their editorial expertise

Our families for their kind moral support and understanding

And all who have helped in one way or another

Contents

List of Figures

List of Tables

Introduction

"Ginseng is good for you." Many of us have heard or seen this statement at one time or another. What is "ginseng"? What does it do? Do you know that there are many products that are known as "ginseng"? Do you know what you are buying or have bought? The most commonly encountered herb known as "ginseng" is likely to be the Chinese ginseng (Ren Shen). That's the humanoid shape root in your herbal soup. It is the root of a herb known as *Panax ginseng*. In the world of plant taxonomy, the word "Panax" is the genus, while the word "ginseng" indicates the species. Some of us may have travelled to Korea and been brought to the specialty shops selling Korean ginseng and may have bought some. The Korean ginseng orginates from the same plant as the Chinese ginseng. Both the Chinese and Korean ginseng are available as the white or red (processed) form. Both forms have slightly different constituents and hence slightly different properties. Another commonly encountered "ginseng" is the American ginseng. It is also known as Xi Yang Shen, Hua Qi Shen and Pao Shen. It is also in the genus Panax, but is of another species known as *Panax quinquefolius*. Another Panax species is *Panax notoginseng*. It is also known as San Qi or Tian Qi. It looks different from Chinese ginseng or American ginseng roots as it appears like a hard rock which is beige in colour when uncoated, or is dark and smooth when it is coated with insect wax. Other herbs which do not belong to the genus Panax may also have the word "ginseng" in their common names. This book is a useful and quick reference to these herbs.

Our approach is two-pronged:

(1) Official and reliable information is painstakingly collated. The sources include the Chinese Pharmacopoeia, Korean Pharmacopoeia, National Center for Complementary and Integrative Health, German Commission E monographs, World Health Organisation and various scientific papers.
(2) The research team surveyed 309 products available in the local market with the words "ginseng" or "Panax" on the packaging or label.

The intention of this book is to educate the general public about the different herbs associated with the name "ginseng" as well as related products in the local market.

The fact that you are reading this book suggests that

(1) You are interested in "ginseng".
(2) You have heard that "ginseng" is good that you want to know more.
(3) You are interested in becoming and staying healthy.
(4) You are concerned about your health or your family's health (everyone should be!).
(5) Someone cares about you and has given you this book.
(6) You want to learn and improve yourself.
(7) You are bored and have nothing better to read (ha ha ha).
(8) You have insomnia and you need something to make you sleepy.
(9) You know one or more of the authors ☺.
(10) None of the above (please email and share with us, whatever the reason may be)

No matter what is the reason, we congratulate you for picking up this book.

You may be wondering what is in this book for you. Through this book, you will learn:

a) What are the different common Panax species?
b) What are the key differences and official uses of the different "ginseng"?
c) What are the different products available in the local market?
d) How to carry out a decent conversation with regards to "ginseng"?
e) Which type of "ginseng" may be more suitable for you?
f) What are you buying and what are you drinking in your herbal soup?
g) What are additional ways to stay healthy and happy?

Chapter 1 gives a general introduction to the book. Chapter 2 reviews the various herbs associated with the name "ginseng" and in the genus Panax, namely, Chinese and Korean ginseng (*Panax ginseng*), American ginseng (*Panax quinquefolius*), Notoginseng, also known as San Qi or Tian Qi (*Panax notoginseng*). Chapter 3 reviews two other plants that are also referred to as ginseng, namely, Siberian ginseng (*Eleutherococcus senticosus*) and five-leaf ginseng (*Gynostemma pentaphyllum*).

Many plants that have been referred to as "ginseng" are listed together with their common names in Chapter 4. Besides carrying out extensive literature review to know the background of five herbs of interest, the team surveyed 309 ginseng and ginseng products available in the local market, namely, health shops, pharmacies and supermarkets. Chapter 4 details the information obtained from these 309 products. Such products range from the raw herbs to final dosage forms (capsules, tablets, powder, syrup etc.) containing one or more herbal or non-herbal components. The information is collated from three stores selling herbal/health products and two pharmacies. For each product, information on name, brand, batch no., manufacturer info, expiry date, listed ingredients, dosage, indication, side effects, contraindications, caution and interactions is collated and presented. Final thoughts are presented in Chapter 5.

You may skip to any section of your interest.

It is important to note that the information presented in this book is not meant to diagnose or treat any medical condition. Consultation with qualified practitioners (e.g. clinicians, TCM practitioners) is advisable and important for anyone who would like to try herbal medicine as everybody's constitution may be different. What is suitable for one person may not be suitable for another even if the symptoms are similar. A qualified practitioner will be in a better position to evaluate what is the underlying problem (if any) and what will be suitable for health maintenance or therapeutic purposes.

As can be seen from the award of a 2015 Nobel Prize in Medicine to pharmaceutical scientist Youyou Tu for her contributions in the isolation and identification of artemisinin, an anti-malarial drug, from the TCM herb *Artemisia annua*, there are clearly valuable lessons to be learnt from TCM and other treasures that remain to be discovered and developed.

We sincerely wish that each and every one of us will take ownership of our health, learn as much as we can through various means and stay healthy and happy!

Panax Species

The term "ginseng" has been loosely used to refer to *Panax ginseng* (Chinese ginseng and Korean ginseng), *Panax quinquefolius* (American ginseng, Pao Shen, Hua Qi Shen), *Panax notoginseng* (San Qi, Tian Qi) and *Eleutherococcus senticosus* (Siberian ginseng). While the first three species belong to the Panax genus, each is distinct in its pharmacological activities, indications/traditional uses and chemical compositions. Some may be grown in the wild (very rare, e.g. wild ginseng), while others may be semi-wild (i.e. cultivated beneath natural forest canopy needing limited tending), woods-cultivated (i.e. more densely planted in the forest with more human interventions than semi-wild type, e.g. cultivated ginseng) and some are artificial shade-cultivated (i.e. grown in open field plantations beneath wooden or plastic shading materials) (Hankins A, 2009; Viana VM *et al.*, 1996). The price variations among the different types are great and in decreasing order of price: wild, followed by semi-wild, woods-cultivated and finally artificial shade-cultivated.

In this chapter, we give an overview for the three important Panax species. Figure 2.1 shows illustrated diagrams of the morphological features of the herbs (Li YC, 1999; Song XG, 2009; Wang XJ, 2009; Viana VM *et al.*, 1996; Zhang GJ, 2004). Note that cultivated roots tend to be smoother, larger, heavier and lighter in colour and with a shorter neck than ginseng roots grown in the wild. The latter also have more horizontal/concentric growth rings, a

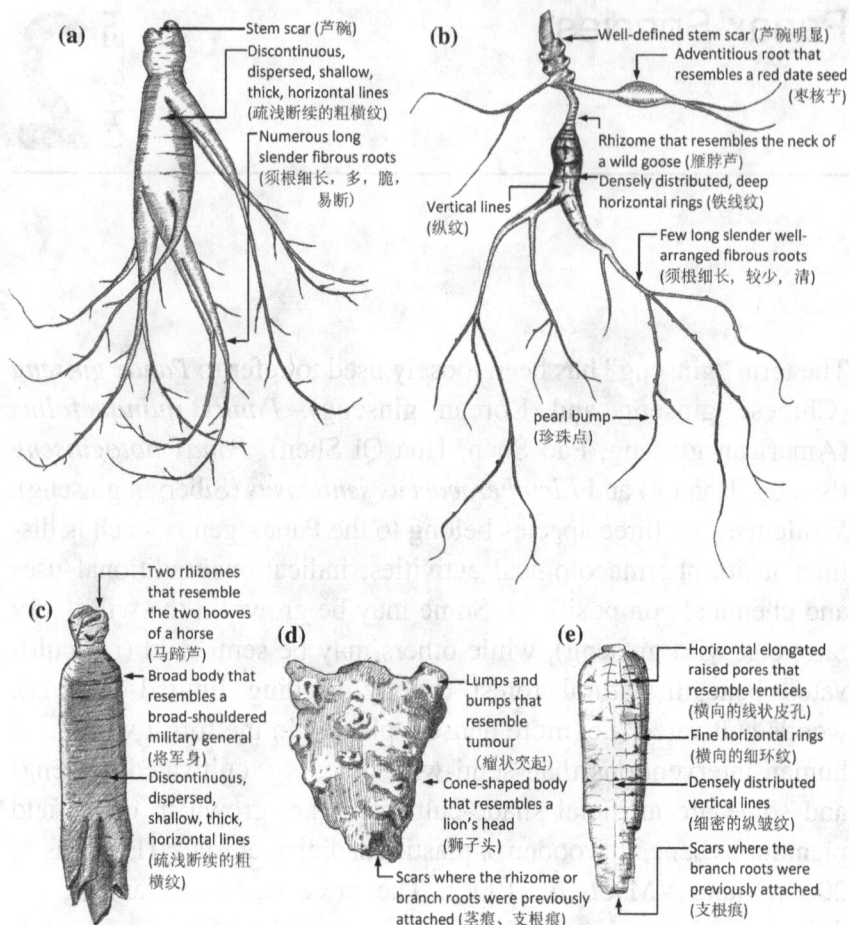

(a)
- Stem scar (芦碗)
- Discontinuous, dispersed, shallow, thick, horizontal lines (疏浅断续的粗横纹)
- Numerous long slender fibrous roots (须根细长，多，脆，易断)

(b)
- Well-defined stem scar (芦碗明显)
- Adventitious root that resembles a red date seed (枣核艼)
- Rhizome that resembles the neck of a wild goose (雁脖芦)
- Densely distributed, deep horizontal rings (铁线纹)
- Few long slender well-arranged fibrous roots (须根细长，较少，清)
- Vertical lines (纵纹)
- pearl bump (珍珠点)

(c)
- Two rhizomes that resemble the two hooves of a horse (马蹄芦)
- Broad body that resembles a broad-shouldered military general (将军身)
- Discontinuous, dispersed, shallow, thick, horizontal lines (疏浅断续的粗横纹)

(d)
- Lumps and bumps that resemble tumour (瘤状突起)
- Cone-shaped body that resembles a lion's head (狮子头)
- Scars where the rhizome or branch roots were previously attached (茎痕、支根痕)

(e)
- Horizontal elongated raised pores that resemble lenticels (横向的线状皮孔)
- Fine horizontal rings (横向的细环纹)
- Densely distributed vertical lines (细密的纵皱纹)
- Scars where the branch roots were previously attached (支根痕)

Figure 2.1   Diagrams showing the morphological features of various important herbs from the genus Panax **(a)** Cultivated ginseng, **(b)** Wild ginseng, **(c)** Korean ginseng, **(d)** San Qi, and **(e)** American ginseng.

longer neck and well-defined stem scars. The presence of the pearl bumps are indicative of wild or semi-wild ginseng roots. The Korean red ginseng is often much darker (reddish black) than the Chinese ginseng. Commercially available *P. notoginseng* root looks morphologically different from the other roots as it feels and looks like a lumpy, heavy and slightly elongated rock. American ginseng root has both horizontal rings and vertical lines.

2.1 Ginseng Root

2.1.1 *Introduction*

Latin Name/Botanical Name: *Panax ginseng* C.A. Mey. (Araliaceae family)

Pharmaceutical Name: Radix et Rhizoma Ginseng

Other Names: 人参 (Ren Shen), Asian ginseng, Chinese ginseng, Korean ginseng, true ginseng. (For local names, please refer to Table 4.2)

Origin: Eastern Siberia, Japan, North Korea, Northeast China

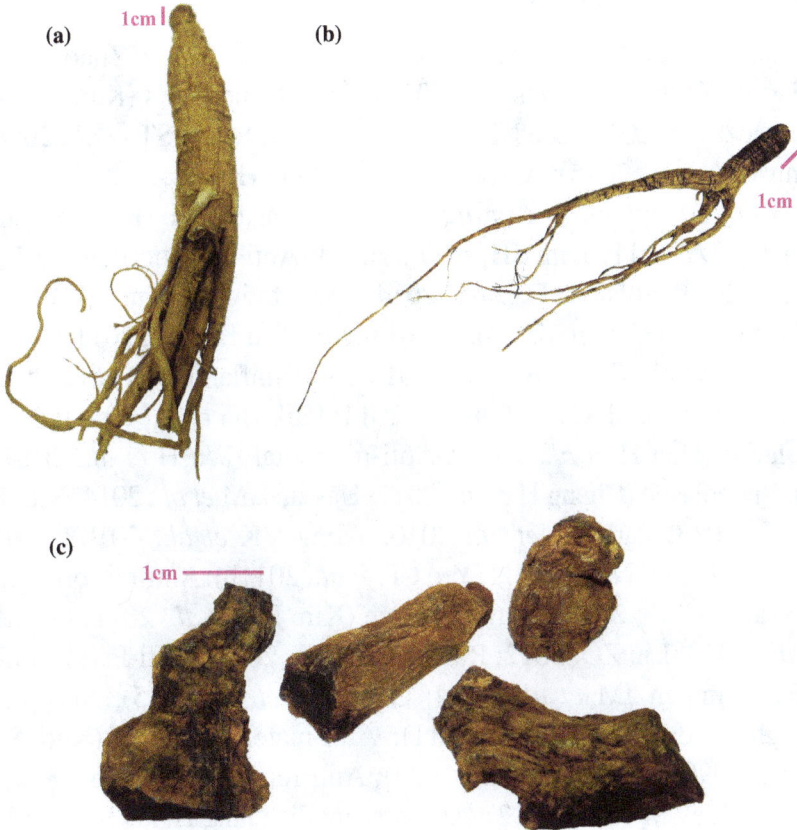

Figure 2.2 Photographs of *Panax ginseng* showing (**a**) Chinese cultivated ginseng, (**b**) Wild ginseng, and (**c**) Korean ginseng.

2.1.2 *Phytoconstituents*

P. ginseng contains saponins, polysaccharides, polyynes, flavonoids and volatile oils (Jia L and Zhao Y, 2009; Yang WZ *et al.*, 2014). The saponins in *P. ginseng* are also known as ginsenosides and are considered the main active components of ginseng. More than 100 ginsenosides have been found and isolated. Examples of the phyto-constituents in *P. ginseng* include ginsenosides, e.g. Re, Rg1, Rb1, Rc, Rb2, Rd, Rf (Guo N *et al.*, 2013; Ong WY *et al.*, 2015) and oleanolic acid (Yang WZ *et al.*, 2014).

2.1.3 *Pharmacological activities*

General reviews (Jia L *et al.*, 2009; Lü JM *et al.*, 2009; Zhao Z and Xiao P, 2009; Ong WY *et al.*, 2015); Anti-Alzheimer's (Kurz A and Perneczky R, 2011; Lee NH and Son CG, 2011; Lee ST *et al.*, 2008; Ong WY *et al.*, 2015); Anti-depressant (Dang H *et al.*, 2009; Yamada N *et al.*, 2011; Ong WY *et al.*, 2015); Anti-asthmatic (Kim DY and Yang WM, 2011; Kim JH *et al.*, 2011); Anti-diabetic (Chung SH *et al.*, 2001; Shishtar E *et al.*, 2014); Anti-fatigue (Kim HG *et al.*, 2013; Lobina C *et al.*, 2014); Anti-fouling (Wu H *et al.*, 2011); Anti-hyperlipidemic (Lee LS *et al.*, 2013); Anti-inflammatory (Choi IY *et al.*, 2010; Lee DC and Lau AS, 2011; Park BG *et al.*, 2013); Anti-malarial (Han H *et al.*, 2011); Anti-microbial (Wu H *et al.*, 2014); Anti-neoplastic (Cheng H *et al.*, 2011; Hassan AM *et al.*, 2014, Kim H *et al.*, 2013; Park HJ *et al.*, 2010; Wong VK *et al.*, 2010); Anti-obesity (Kim HJ *et al.*, 2011; Yeo CR *et al.*, 2011b); Anti-osteoporotic (Avsar U *et al.*, 2013); Anti-oxidative (Kim HG *et al.*, 2011; Lee LS *et al.*, 2013; Liu ZQ, 2012; Ramesh T *et al.*, 2012); Anti-Parkinson's (Van Kampen JM *et al.*, 2014; Ong WY *et al.*, 2015); Anti-pica (Raghavendran HR *et al.*, 2011); Anti-platelet activity (Kuo SC *et al.*, 1990; Teng CM *et al.*, 1989); Anti-remodeling (Guo J *et al.*, 2011; Moey M *et al.*, 2012); Anti-spasmodic (Jang HA *et al.*, 2012); Anti-trypanosomal (Herrmann F *et al.*, 2013); Anti-ulcer (Jeong CS, 2002); Anti-viral (Lee JS *et al.*, 2014); Cardioprotective (Karmazyn M *et al.*, 2011; Kim JH, 2012; Pei L *et al.*, 2013; Zheng SD *et al.*, 2012; Zhou H *et al.*, 2011); Chemoprotective (Raghavendran HR *et al.*, 2012); Fertility-enhancing (Park EH *et al.*, 2014; Yang WM *et al.*, 2011); Hepatoprotective (Fu YQ *et al.*, 2013; Karakus E *et al.*, 2011); Immunomodulatory (Jang HI and Shin HM, 2010; Kang S and Min H, 2012); Memory-enhancing (Geng J *et al.*, 2010); Neuroprotective (Aryal B *et al.*, 2011; Cho IH, 2012; Kim HJ *et al.*, 2013; Lee B *et al.*, 2010; Nah SY, 2014; Suleymanova E *et al.*, 2014; Rastogi *et al.*, 2015); Radioprotective (Hwang E *et al.*, 2014; Verma P *et al.*, 2011; Park E *et al.*, 2011); Renoprotective (Kalkan Y *et al.*, 2012; Qadir MI *et al.*, 2011); Wound healing (Kim YS *et al.*, 2011).

In addition, *P. ginseng* exhibits potential therapeutic effects for the following conditions: Chronic Obstructive Pulmonary Diseases (COPD) (An X *et al.*, 2011); Erectile Dysfunction (ED) (Ho CC and Tan HM, 2011; Kim TH *et al.*, 2009); Menopausal symptoms (Xu Y *et al.*, 2014); Morphine-withdrawal symptoms (Lee B *et al.*, 2011a; Lee B *et al.*, 2011b); Multiple Sclerosis (Hwang I *et al.*, 2011). Furthermore, it is shown to enhance mammary involution (Dallard BE *et al.*, 2011) and physical performance (Bahrke MS and Morgan WR, 2000; Oliynyk S and Oh S, 2013; Wang CH and Lee T, 1998).

2.1.4 *Actions*

To tonify the original qi greatly, resume pulse and secure collapse, tonify spleen and replenish kidney, engender fluid and nourish blood, tranquilize the mind and replenish wisdom (The State Pharmacopoeia Commission of P.R. China, 2010a).

In TCM, *P. ginseng* has been used for a wide range of ailments. According to the Pharmacopoeia of the People's Republic of China, it is used to reinforce the vital energy, revive a person from collapse,[1]

---

[1]Although it is documented in ancient Chinese text that *P. ginseng* has the property to revive a person from collapse, this is NOT to be followed in a real-life situation. In the case of collapse, one must seek medical help immediately. For these medical emergencies, delays in treatment can often lead to serious consequences.

restore the normal pulse, promote the production of Body Fluid, calm the mind, and tonify Spleen and Lung. The most reported neurologic actions for *P. ginseng* in TCM include tranquilizing the mind and replenishing wisdom (which may refer to its anxiolytic and memory-enhancing activities respectively). Its other reported traditional neurologic indications include vexation (which may refer to mild anxiety), restlessness (which may refer to hyperactivity), and mental confusion (which may refer to cognition problems or attention deficit) (The State Pharmacopoeia Commission of P.R. China 2010a). It has also been used for many conditions in folk medicine such as cough, fever, tuberculosis, rheumatism, vomiting of pregnancy, hypothermia, dyspnea and nervous disorders (World Health Organization, 2002).

2.1.5 *Indications*

The German Commission E approved *P. ginseng* as a "tonic for invigoration and fortification in times of fatigue and debility or declining capacity for work and concentration". *P. ginseng* was also approved for use during convalescence (Blumenthal M *et al.*, 2000). According to the Pharmacopoeia of the People's Republic of China, the indications of *P. ginseng* in TCM include "being just going to collapse caused by body deficiency, cold limbs and faint pulse, low appetite caused by spleen deficiency, dyspnea and cough caused by lung deficiency, thirsty caused by fluid damage, interior heat and wasting-thirst, deficiency of qi and blood, frail caused by long-term illness, fright palpitations and insomnia, impotence and uterine coldness" (The State Pharmacopoeia Commission of P.R. China, 2010a).

2.1.6 *Administration and dosage*

a) Three to 9 g a day, decocted separately and added into a compound decoction to be taken orally.
b) For sun-dried wild ginseng, grind into powder for oral administration, 2 g twice a day (a and b: The State Pharmacopoeia Commission of P.R. China, 2010a).

c) Unless otherwise prescribed, 1 to 2 g of root per day for up to three months; a repeated course is feasible.
d) Decoction: 1 to 2 g in 150 ml of water
e) Standardised extract (4% total ginsenosides): 100 mg twice daily. (c to e: Blumenthal M *et al.*, 2000).

2.1.7 *Safety considerations*

2.1.7.1 *Side effects and interactions with other herbs*

P. ginseng is generally a well-tolerated herb when it is taken at its recommended dosage. It is reported to have no known side effects in the Expanded Commission E (Blumenthal *et al.*, 2000). While short-term use of ginseng at recommended doses appears to be safe for most people, some sources suggest that prolonged use may result in certain side effects. According to the National Center for Complementary and Integrative Health (NCCIH), the most common side effects are headaches and sleep and gastrointestinal problems. It can cause allergic reactions. *P. ginseng* may also lower levels of blood sugar and this effect may be seen more in people with diabetes. Therefore, people with diabetes should exercise caution, especially if they are on antidiabetic drugs to lower blood sugar or are taking other herbs, such as bitter melon and fenugreek, which are also thought to lower blood sugar (National Center for Complementary and Integrative Health, 2012). There have been reports of breast tenderness, menstrual irregularities, and high blood pressure associated with use of *P. ginseng* products, but these products' components were not analysed, so the effects may have been due to another herb or drug in the product (National Center for Complementary and Integrative Health, 2012). Nevertheless, *P. ginseng* is contraindicated in patients with hypertension, possibly due to the variable effects it has on blood pressure (Blumenthal M *et al.*, 2000). Cases of patient risk associated with inappropriate use of *P. ginseng* have also been reviewed (Doo JP and Chang HL, 2015).

In TCM, *P. ginseng* is considered incompatible with Veratrum Root and Rhizome and *Trogopterori* faeces (faeces of Flying squirrel) (The State Pharmacopoeia Commission of P.R. China, 2010a) and they should not be used together.

2.1.7.2 *Use during pregnancy and lactation*

Pregnant women are strongly advised to refrain from taking *P. ginseng*, especially during the first few months of pregnancy. In a study by the Chinese University of Hong Kong, teratogenicity was observed in *in vitro* rat embryo culture models exposed to ginsenoside Rb1 at a concentration of ≥30 µg/ml (Chan LY *et al.*, 2003). Admittedly, the concentration of ginsenoside Rb1 used in this particular study exceeds possible human consumption, considering the fact that the C_{max} of plasma ginsenoside Rb1 is only 3.94 ± 1.97 ng/ml in human subjects (Kim HK, 2013). However, until further studies are carried out, women are cautioned against the use of *P. ginseng* during pregnancy.

2.1.7.3 *Interactions with drugs*

P. ginseng may alter the activity of certain drugs when they are taken together. *P. ginseng* may enhance the effects of anti-cancer drugs such as 5-fluorouracil (an antimetabolite), irinotecan (a plant alkaloid), mitomycin C (an antibiotics), docetaxel (a taxane agent belonging to a plant alkaloid), cisplatin (an alkylating agent) (Chen S *et al.*, 2014; Wang CZ *et al.*, 2012). Despite demonstrating inherent anti-platelet activity (refer to Section 2.1.3), *P. ginseng* appears to decrease the anti-coagulant effect of warfarin in one widely-cited case study (Janetzky K and Morreale AP, 1997; Spolarich AE *et al.*, 2007). The International Normalised Ratio (INR) of the patient who has been receiving warfarin for nine months was stabilised at 3.9–4.0 initially. When he began taking ginseng, his INR fell to 1.5 within two weeks. His INR subsequently returned to therapeutic level two weeks after he stopped using ginseng (Rosado MF *et al.*, 2003). A study found that coadministration of warfarin with ginseng moderately increases the ratio of S-warfarin apparent clearance (CL/F) compared to control (Jiang X *et al.*, 2006). *P. ginseng* did not alter the steady state pharmacokinetics of lopinavir and ritonavir in healthy human volunteers (Calderón MM *et al.*, 2014). The potential interaction of "ginseng" with warfarin has been reviewed by Shao J and Jia L (2013). Despite the alarming title, the authors noted that several investigations independently reported that coadministration of "ginseng" had no significant impact on the pharmacokinetics and pharmacodynamics of warfarin regarding its anticoagulation and INR (Lee SH *et al.*, 2008; Lee YH *et al.*, 2010; Zhu M *et al.*, 1999). However, the authors noted that more properly designed study to take into consideration of warfarin's effect on the synthesis of vitamin K dependent clotting factors (i.e. need time) is needed and cautioned against the concomitant administration of warfarin and "ginseng" in stroke patients. It may reduce the effects of alcohol by lowering blood alcohol concentration (Kiefer D and Pantuso T, 2003). It may reduce the absorption and increase the elimination of midazolam (a benzodiazepine) from the body, possibly through CYP3A induction (Malati CY *et al.*, 2012).

The British Herbal Compendium contraindicates the use of *P. ginseng* with stimulants, including excessive use of caffeine (Blumenthal M *et al.*, 2000). It may interact with caffeine to cause hypertension (Kiefer D and Pantuso T, 2003). Concomitant use of the herb with the monoamine oxidase inhibitor phenelzine (a type of antidepressant drug) may result in manic-like symptoms (Chen XW *et al.*, 2011). Two such cases have been reported in the WHO monographs (Joshi KG and Faubion MD, 2005). A case report of interaction with raltegravir (an antiretroviral drug) resulted in an acute elevation of liver enzymes, marked jaundice, and significant weight loss (Mateo-Carrasco H *et al.*, 2012). Another case report of interaction with imatinib in a patient with chronic myelogenous leukemia resulted in imatinib-induced hepatotoxicity (Bilgi N *et al.*, 2010).

Authors' notes: *P. ginseng* products appear to reduce the Prothrombin Time (PT) and INR of some patients on warfarin therapy to subtherapeutic levels in case reports, and the effect is reversible on withdrawal of the products. However, a study in ischemic stroke patients showed coadministration of *P. ginseng* and warfarin did not influence PT and INR (Lee SH *et al.*, 2008), while another study on patients with cardiac valve replacement showed slight decrease in INR with coadministration of Korean red ginseng, but there was no statistically significant differences (Lee YH *et al.*, 2010). The interactions of warfarin with medicinal herbs including ginseng have also been reviewed by Milić *et al.* (2014).

2.2 Red Ginseng

2.2.1 *Introduction*

Latin Name/Botanical Name: *Panax ginseng* C.A. Mey. (Araliaceae family)
Pharmaceutical Name: Radix et Rhizoma Ginseng Rubra
Other Names: 红参 (Hong Shen).
Origin: Eastern Siberia, Japan, North Korea, Northeast China
Method of preparation: *P. ginseng* collected, washed, steamed and dried.

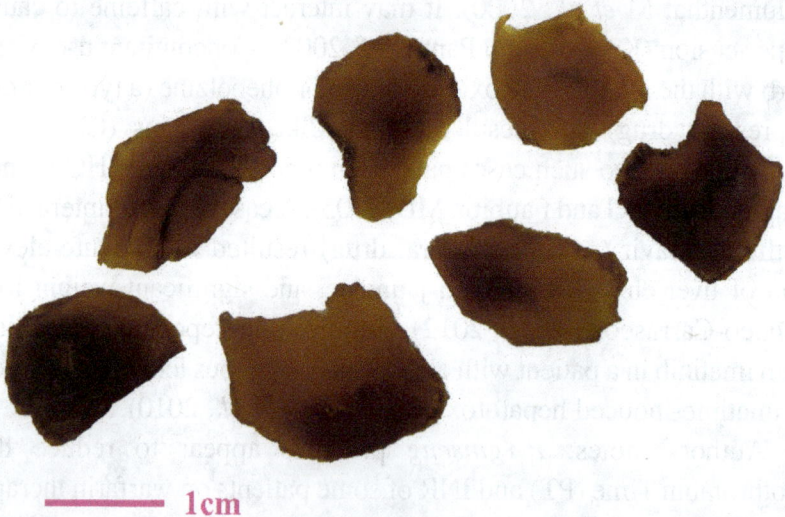

Figure 2.3   Photograph of sliced red ginseng.

2.2.2 *Phytoconstituents*

Red ginseng is *P. ginseng* that has been processed by steaming. The high-temperature conditions associated with steaming can induce certain ginsenosides to undergo structural conversion, producing new ginsenosides not present in raw *P. ginseng*. These new ginsenosides include Rg3 (Kim WY *et al.*, 2000), Rg5 (Kim WY *et al.*, 2000), F4 (Kim WY *et al.*, 2000), Rk1 (Park IH *et al.*, 2002b), Rk2 (Park IH *et al.*, 2002b), Rk3 (Park IH *et al.*, 2002b), Rs4 (Park IH *et al.*, 2002a), Rs5 (Park IH *et al.*, 2002a), Rs6 (Park IH *et al.*, 2002a) and Rs7 (Park IH *et al.*, 2002a).

2.2.3 *Pharmacological activities*

General reviews (Jia L *et al.*, 2009; Lü JM *et al.*, 2009; Zhao Z and Xiao P, 2009); Anti-allergy (Jung JH *et al.*, 2013; Jung JW *et al.*, 2011; Sumiyoshi M *et al.*, 2010); Anti-Alzheimer's (Heo JH *et al.*, 2011; Kim J *et al.*, 2013); Anti-arthritic (Jhun J *et al.*, 2014); Anti-bacterial (Bae M *et al.*, 2014); Anti-depressant (Lee KJ and Ji GE, 2014); Anti-diabetic (Jung HL and Kang HY, 2013; Kang KS *et al.*, 2013; Kim S *et al.*, 2011; Lee SH *et al.*, 2012; Quan HY *et al.*, 2013; Shishtar E *et al.*, 2014; Yuan HD *et al.*, 2012); Anti-hyperlipidemic (Kwak YS *et al.*, 2010); Anti-hypertensive (Jovanovski E *et al.*, 2014; Jeon BH *et al.*, 2000; Han KH *et al.*, 1998); Anti-inflammatory (Yang Y *et al.*, 2014); Anti-neoplastic (Choi YJ *et al.*, 2011; Seo EY and Kim WK, 2011, Ho YL *et al.*, 2012); Anti-obesity (Cho HM *et al.*, 2014; Lee H *et al.*, 2014); Anti-osteoporotic (Lee JH *et al.*, 2013); Anti-oxidative (Dong GZ *et al.*, 2013); Anti-platelet (Lee JG *et al.*, 2009; Lee JG *et al.*, 2010); Anti-ulcer (Oyagi A *et al.*, 2010); Anti-viral (Lee MH *et al.*, 2011; Yoo DG *et al.*, 2012); Fertility-enhancing (Jang M *et al.*, 2011); Hepatoprotective (Ki SH *et al.*, 2013; Park HM *et al.*, 2012; Park SJ *et al.*, 2013; Sohn SH *et al.*, 2013); Hypoglycemic (De Souza LR *et al.*, 2011); Immunomodulatory (Xu ML *et al.*, 2012); Memory-enhancing (Lee CH *et al.*, 2013); Cardioprotective (Ahn CM *et al.*, 2011; Ko HM *et al.*, 2013; Lee JS *et al.*, 2011; Lim KH *et al.*, 2013a; Lim KH *et al.*, 2013b; Lim KH *et al.*, 2014); Radioprotective (Hwang E *et al.*, 2013); Renoprotective (Choi HJ *et al.*, 2012); Skin-whitening (Oh CT *et al.*, 2013).

In addition, red *P. ginseng* exhibits potential therapeutic effects for the following conditions: Attention Deficit Hyperactivity Disorder (ADHD) (Lee SH *et al.*, 2011); Atopic Dermatitis (Kim HS *et al.*, 2011; Sohn EH *et al.*, 2011); Benign Prostate Hyperplasia (BPH) (Bae JS *et al.*, 2012); Cold hypersensitivity (Park KS *et al.*, 2014); Drug-induced hearing loss (Choung YH *et al.*, 2011); Erectile Dysfunction (ED) (Choi HK *et al.*, 1995; Jang DJ *et al.*, 2008; Kim SD *et al.*, 2013); Menopausal symptoms (Oh KJ *et al.*, 2010); Cyclosporine-induced Pancreatic injury (Lim SW *et al.*, 2013); Polycystic Ovarian Syndrome (PCOS) (Jung JH *et al.*, 2011). Furthermore, it may have beneficial effects on the visual process (Wahid F *et al.*, 2010) and protective effects against certain toxic compounds found in cigarette smoke (Lee SE and Park YS, 2014).

2.2.4 *Actions*

To greatly tonify the original qi, regain pulse and secure collapse, tonify qi and control the "blood" (please see Appendix 2) (The State Pharmacopoeia Commission of P.R. China, 2010b).

2.2.5 *Indications*

The State Pharmacopoeia Commission of P.R. China (2010b) states that the indications in TCM include "tending to collapse caused by body deficiency, coldness of limbs and faint pulse, qi failing to control the blood, flooding and spotting".

2.2.6 *Administration and dosage*

Three to 9 g a day, decocted alone and added into a compound decoction to be taken orally (The State Pharmacopoeia Commission of P.R. China, 2010b).

2.2.7 *Safety considerations*

Similar to ginseng root.

2.3 American Ginseng

2.3.1 *Introduction*

Latin Name/Botanical Name: *Panax quinquefolius* L. (Araliaceae family)
Pharmaceutical Name: Radix Panacis Quinquefolii
Other Names: 西洋参 (**Xi Yang Shen**), 花旗参 (**Hua Qi Shen**), 泡参 (**Pao Shen**) (For local names, please refer to Table 4.2)
Origin: North America, cultivated in North China

(a)

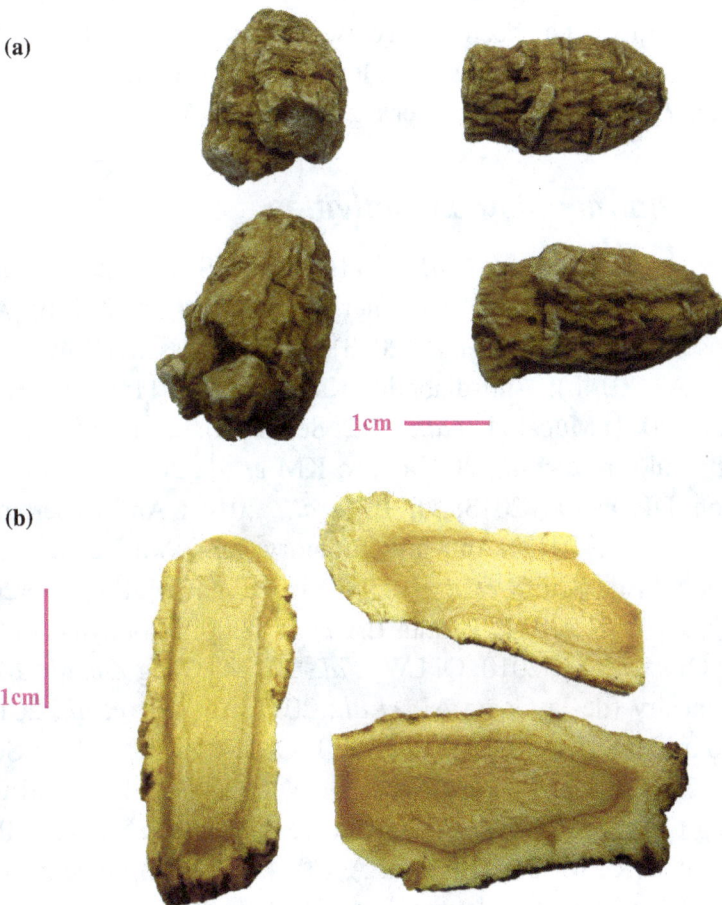

1cm

(b)

1cm

Figure 2.4   Photographs of *Panax quinquefolius* (**a**) main root, and (**b**) slices.

2.3.2 *Phytoconstituents*

P. quinquefolius contains saponins, polysaccharides, polyynes and flavonoids. Similar to *Panax ginseng*, the main active principles of *P. quinquefolius* are ginsenosides (Chen JH *et al.*, 2007; Court WA *et al.*, 1996; Dong L *et al.*, 2011; Wang AB *et al.*, 2005; Zhang CY *et al.*, 2011; Zhang K *et al.*, 2008). However, there are still differences between them. An important parameter used for differentiation is the presence of the ginsenoside Rf in *P. ginseng*, (which is not found in *P. quinquefolius*) and the presence of pseudoginsenoside F11 in *P. quinquefolius* (which is not found in *P. ginseng*). In addition, the ratio of Rg_1/Rb_1 has been widely used to distinguish between these two herbs. *P. quinquefolius* has a low Rg_1/Rb_1 ratio of less than 0.4, whereas *P. ginseng* has a higher Rg_1/Rb_1 ratio (Kim DH, 2012).

2.3.3 *Pharmacological activities*

General reviews (Qi LW *et al.*, 2011b; Yuan CS *et al.*, 2010; Zhao Z and Xiao P, 2010); Anti-Alzheimer's (Qi LW *et al.*, 2011b); Anti-atherosclerotic (Wang Z *et al.*, 2013); Anti-depressant (Rinwa P and Kumar A, 2014b); Anti-diabetic (Kasuli EG, 2011; Lee NH and Son CG, 2011; Mucalo I *et al.*, 2012; Sen S *et al.*, 2013a; Sen S *et al.* 2013b; Vuksan V *et al.*, 2000a; Yoo KM *et al.*, 2012); Anti-fatigue (Barton DL *et al.*, 2013; Qi B *et al.*, 2014); Anti-hypertensive (Mucalo I *et al.*, 2013); Anti-inflammatory (Ichikawa T *et al.*, 2009); Anti-neoplastic (Cui X *et al.*, 2010; King ML and Murphy LL, 2010; Miller SC *et al.*, 2011; Peralta EA *et al.*, 2009; Poudyal D *et al.*, 2013; Qi LW *et al.*, 2010; Qi LW *et al.*, 2011b; Wang Z *et al.*, 2013); Anti-obesity (de la Garza AL *et al.*, 2011; Yeo CR *et al.*, 2011a); Anti-oxidative (Kitts DD *et al.*, 2000; Qi LW *et al.*, 2011b; Sen S *et al.*, 2011); Anti-Parkinson's (Qi LW *et al.*, 2011b); Anti-ulcer (Huang CC *et al.*, 2013); Anti-ulcerative collitis (Jin Y *et al.*, 2010); Anxiolytic (Rinwa P and Kumar A, 2014a); Cardioprotective (Li J *et al.*, 2010); Cardioregulatory (Jiang M *et al.*, 2014); Hypoglycemic

(Vuksan V *et al.*, 2000b); Immunomodulatory (High KP *et al.*, 2012; Miller SC *et al.*, 2012; Yan J *et al.*, 2013); Memory-enhancing (Scholey A *et al.*, 2010); Neuroprotective (Xu H *et al.*, 2014); Radioprotective (Lee TK *et al.*, 2010).

In addition, *P. quinquefolius* exhibits potential therapeutic effects for the following conditions: Multiple Sclerosis (MS) (Bowie LE *et al.*, 2012); Common cold (Seida JK *et al.*, 2011); Menopausal symptoms (Shou C *et al.*, 2011); Premature ovarian failure (Ge P *et al.*, 2014).

2.3.4 *Actions*

To tonify qi and nourish yin, clear heat and engender fluid (The State Pharmacopoeia Commission of P.R. China, 2010c).

In TCM, *P. quinquefolius* is mainly used for cough, hemoptysis, thirst, irritability and debility (Zhao Z, 2004). As it is "cool" in nature, it is suitable for internal hotness and dryness as well as fatigue, wasting thirst (which may refer to diabetes mellitus), and dry mouth and throat (Bensky D *et al.*, 2004). Its neurologic indication is vexation (which may refer to mild anxiety) (The State Pharmacopoeia Commission of P.R. China 2010c).

2.3.5 *Indications*

Indications in TCM include "deficiency of qi and yin, deficiency heat with vexation and fatigue, panting and coughing with blood in phlegm, interior heat wasting thirst, dry mouth and throat" (The State Pharmacopoeia Commission of P.R. China, 2010d).

2.3.6 *Administration and dosage*

3 to 6 g a day, decocted alone and mixed with other decoction before taking orally (The State Pharmacopoeia Commission of P.R. China, 2010d).

2.3.7 Safety considerations

2.3.7.1 Side effects and interactions with other herbs

In TCM, *P. quinquefolius* is considered incompatible with *Veratri Nigri Radix et Rhizoma* and *Trogopterori* faeces (The State Pharmacopoeia Commission of P.R. China, 2010d) and they should not be taken together.

2.3.7.2 Interactions with drugs

Vitamin C enhances the anti-oxidative property of *P. quinquefolius*. (Li JP *et al.*, 2000). It has been shown to reduce the anti-coagulant effect of warfarin in a randomised, controlled trial (Yuan CS *et al.*, 2004). *P. quinquefolius* did not alter the pharmacokinetics of zido-vudine (Lee LS *et al.*, 2008) and indinavir (Andrade AS *et al.*, 2008).

2.4 San Qi or Tian Qi

2.4.1 *Introduction*

Latin Name/Botanical Name: *Panax notoginseng* (Burk.) F. H. Chen
(Araliaceae family)
Pharmaceutical Name: Radix et Rhizoma Notoginseng
Other Names: 三七 **(San Qi),** 田七 **(Tian Qi) (For local names,
please refer to Table 4.2)**
Origin: China (Guangxi & Yunnan)

(a)

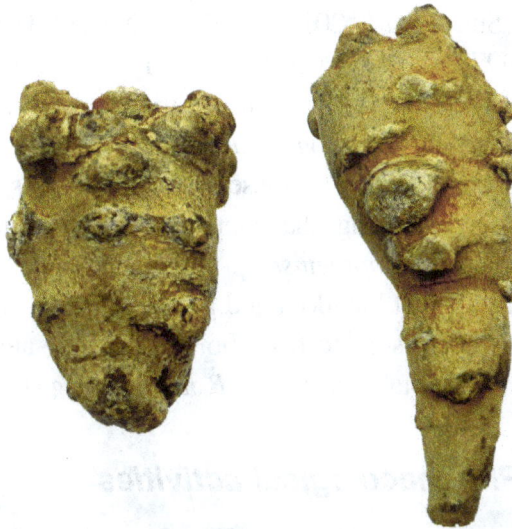

1cm

(b)

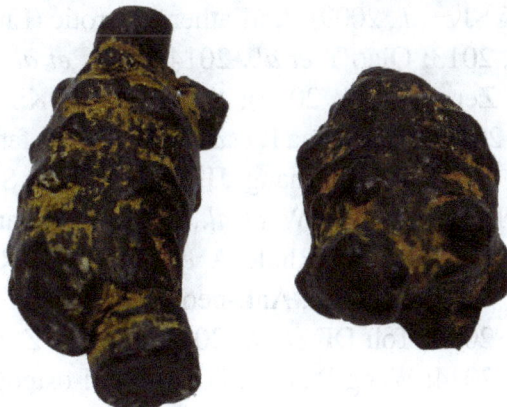

1cm

Figure 2.5 Photographs of *Panax notoginseng* which are (**a**) raw, and (**b**) semi-processed.

2.4.2 *Phytoconstituents*

P. notoginseng contains saponins (Fu HZ *et al.*, 2013; Zhang Y *et al.*, 2013), dencichine, flavonoids and polysaccharides (Dong TT *et al.*, 2003), as well as triacylgycerols such as trilinolein (Ng TB, 2006). Dencichine is an amino acid which has haemostatic activity. *P. notoginseng* root contains more saponins than *P. ginseng* and *P. quinquefolius* and some of the most abundant ginsenosides are Rb1 and Rg1 (Yang X *et al.*, 2014). In addition, unlike the other two herbs, *P. notoginseng* also contains an abundance of notoginsenosides, such as notoginsenoside R1 (Sun S *et al.*, 2010), A, B, C, D, E, G, H, I, J (Yoshikawa M *et al.*, 1997), L, M, N (Yoshikawa M *et al.*, 2001), Rw1 and Rw2 (Cui XM *et al.*, 2008). In contrast, the roots of *P. ginseng* only contain trace amounts of notoginsenoside R1 and R4 while *P. quinquefolius* does not contain any of these notoginsenosides (Choi KT, 2008). Another distinguishing characteristic is the absence of an oleanolic acid saponin in *P. notoginseng*. Oleanolic acid saponins occur commonly in the plant kingdom and ginsenoside Ro is one such example which has been isolated from both *P. ginseng* and *P. quinquefolius*. However, it is notably absent in *P. notoginseng* (Kim DH, 2012).

2.4.3 *Pharmacological activities*

General reviews (Ng TB, 2006; Zhao Y and Xiao P, 2009); Angiogenic (Hong SJ *et al.*, 2009); Anti-atherosclerotic (Liu G *et al.*, 2009; Liu Y *et al.*, 2013; Qiao Y *et al.*, 2014; Xu L *et al.*, 2011; Yuan Z *et al.*, 2011; Zeng Y *et al.*, 2012); Anti-diabetic (Kim JJ *et al.*, 2009; Tu Q *et al.*, 2011; Uzayisenga R *et al.*, 2014); Anti-fatigue (Liang MT *et al.*, 2005; Xu YX and Zhang JJ, 2013; Zhou S *et al.*, 2012); Anti-hyperlipidemic (Xia W *et al.*, 2011; Ji W and Gong BQ, 2007); Anti-inflammatory (Rhule A *et al.*, 2008; Rhule A *et al.*, 2006; Wang Y *et al.*, 2006); Anti-neoplastic (He F *et al.*, 2014; Park SC *et al.*, 2009; Toh DF *et al.*, 2011; Wang CZ *et al.*, 2009; Wang JR *et al.*, 2014; Wang P *et al.*, 2014); Anti-osteoporotic (Li XD *et al.*,

2010); Anti-oxidative (Qiang H *et al.*, 2010); Anti-platelet (Lau AJ *et al.*, 2009; Wang J *et al.*, 2008); Anti-ulcer (Huang CC *et al.*, 2013); Cardioprotective (Chen S *et al.*, 2011; Liu L *et al.*, 2008; Liu J *et al.*, 2014; Shang Q *et al.*, 2013; Yang X *et al.*, 2014; Yang XC *et al.*, 2014); Hypoglycemic (Liang MT *et al.*, 2012); Immunomodulatory (Spelman K *et al.*, 2011; Sun HX *et al.*, 2004); Neuroprotective (Jia D *et al.*, 2014; Si YC *et al.*, 2011, Zeng XS *et al.*, 2014; Zhou N *et al.*, 2014).

In addition, *P. notoginseng* exhibits potential therapeutic effects for the following conditions: Acute Lung Injury (ALI) (Chen YQ *et al.*, 2014; Rong L *et al.*, 2009); Erectile Dysfunction (ED) (Li H *et al.*, 2014; Lin F and Gou X, 2013); Haemorrhagic shock (Liu HZ *et al.*, 2014); Pulmonary fibrosis (Tsai KD *et al.*, 2011); Stroke (Chen X *et al.*, 2008; Liu L *et al.*, 2014). Furthermore, it appears to be able to increase the strength of repairing ligament (Ng GY and Wong RY, 2008).

In TCM, *P. notoginseng* is mainly used to improve blood circulation and remove blood clots, disperse swelling and relieve pain. It is indicated for different bleeding related disorders and pain related conditions (please see "Indications") (The State Pharmacopoeia Commission of P.R. China, 2010). In addition, this plant may be used for different kinds of heart disease and chest pain (Zhao Z, 2004).

2.4.4 *Actions*

To dissipate stasis and stanch bleeding, disperse swelling and relieve pain (The State Pharmacopoeia Commission of P.R. China, 2010e).

2.4.5 *Indications*

Include "hemoptysis, hematemesis, epistaxis, hematochezia, flooding and spotting, traumatic bleeding, stabbing pain in chest and abdomen, swelling and pain caused by injuries from falls" (The State Pharmacopoeia Commission of P.R. China, 2010e).

2.4.6 *Administration and dosage*

a) 3 to 9 g; b) Ground into powder and 1 to 3 g taken orally with water each time; and c) "appropriate quantity for external use" but the quantity has not been specified (The State Pharmacopoeia Commission of P.R. China, 2010e).

2.4.7 *Safety considerations*

2.4.7.1 *Use during pregnancy and lactation*

"Used with caution in pregnancy" (The State Pharmacopoeia Commission of P.R. China, 2010e) — as *P. notoginseng* can improve blood circulation and remove blood clots, it may lead to miscarriages and should be avoided in pregnancy.

2.4.7.2 *Interactions with drugs*

P. notoginseng is reported to enhance the anti-cancer effects of cisplatin (an alkylating agent) (Yu ML *et al.,* 2012) and 5-fluorouracil (an anti-metabolite) (Wang CZ *et al.,* 2007). *P. notoginseng* has been shown to interact with caffeine, increasing its elimination from the body possibly via the induction of CYP1A2 (Liu R *et al.,* 2012).

Authors' notes: Traditionally, it is also boiled in soup and taken by young boys apparently to help them grow taller and bigger. The raw form has therapeutic effects and should only be taken under the advice and supervision of a qualified TCM practitioner. The steamed form is considered as a tonic for the blood. When steamed, additional saponins are formed, including a known anti-cancer compound 20(S)-Rg3.

References

Ahn CM, Hong SJ, Choi SC, Park JH, Kim JS, Lim DS (2011). Red ginseng extract improves coronary flow reserve and increases absolute numbers of various circulating angiogenic cells in patients with first ST-segment elevation acute myocardial infarction. *Phytother Res* **25**(2): 239–249.

An X, Zhang AL, Yang AW, Lin L, Wu D, Guo X, Shergis JL, Thien FC, Worsnop CJ, Xue CC (2011). Oral ginseng formulae for stable chronic obstructive pulmonary disease: a systematic review. *Respir Med* **105**(2): 165–176.

Andrade AS, Hendrix C, Parsons TL, Caballero B, Yuan CS, Flexner CW, Dobs AS, Brown TT (2008). Pharmacokinetic and metabolic effects of American ginseng (*Panax quinquefolius*) in healthy volunteers receiving the HIV protease inhibitor indinavir. *BMC Complement Altern Med* **8**: 50.

Aryal B, Maskey D, Kim MJ, Yang JW, Kim HG (2011). Effect (HN) of ginseng on calretinin expression in mouse hippocampus following exposure to 835 MHz radiofrequency. *J Ginseng Res* **35**(2): 138–148.

Avsar U, Karakus E, Halici Z, Bayir Y, Bilen H, Aydin A, Avsar UZ, Ayan A, Aydin S, Karadeniz A (2013). Prevention of bone loss by *Panax ginseng* in a rat model of inflammation-induced bone loss. *Cell Mol Biol* **59** (Suppl.): OL1835–OL1841.

Bae JS, Park HS, Park JW, Li SH, Chun YS (2012). Red ginseng and 20(S)-Rg3 control testosterone-induced prostate hyperplasia by deregulating androgen receptor signaling. *J Nat Med* **66**(3): 476–485.

Bae M, Jang S, Lim JW, Kang J, Bak EJ, Cha JH, Kim H (2014). Protective effect of Korean Red Ginseng extract against *Helicobacter pylori*-induced gastric inflammation in Mongolian gerbils. *J Ginseng Res* **38**(1): 8–15.

Bahrke MS, Morgan WR (2000). Evaluation of the ergogenic properties of ginseng: an update. *Sports Med* **29**(2): 113–133.

Barton DL, Liu H, Dakhil SR, Linquist B, Sloan JA, Nichols CR, McGinn TW, Stella PJ, Seeger GR, Sood A, Loprinzi CL (2013). Wisconsin Ginseng (*Panax quinquefolius*) to improve cancer-related fatigue: a randomized, double-blind trial, N07C2. *J Natl Cancer Inst* **105**(16): 1230–1238.

Bensky D, Clavey S, Stöger E (2004). *Chinese Herbal Medicine: Materia Medica*. 3rd ed. Seattle, WA: Eastland Press.

Bilgi N, Bell K, Ananthakrishnan AN, Atallah E (2010). Imatinib and *Panax ginseng*: a potential interaction resulting in liver toxicity. *Ann Pharmacother* **44**(5): 926–928.

Blumenthal M, Goldberg A, Brinckmann J (2000). *Herbal Medicine Expanded Commission E Monographs*. 1st Boston: Integrative Medicine Communications.

Bowie LE, Roscoe WA, Lui EM, Smith R, Karlik SJ (2012). Effects of an aqueous extract of North American ginseng on MOG(35-55)-induced EAE in mice. *Can J Physiol Pharmacol* **90**(7): 933–939.

Calderón MM, Chairez CL, Gordon LA, Alfaro RM, Kovacs JA, Penzak SR (2014). Influence of *Panax ginseng* on the steady state pharmacokinetic profile of lopinavir-ritonavir in healthy volunteers. *Pharmacotherapy* **34**(11): 1151–1158.

Chan LY, Chiu PY, Lau TK (2003). An *in-vitro* study of ginsenoside Rb1-induced teratogenicity using a whole rat embryo culture model. *Hum Reprod* **18**(10): 2166–2168.

Chen JH, Xie MY, Fu ZH, Lee FSC, Wang XR (2007). Development of a quality evaluation system for *Panax quinquefolium* L. based on HPLC chromatographic fingerprinting of seven major ginsenosides. *Microchem J* **85**: 201–208.

Chen S, Liu J, Liu X, Fu Y, Zhang M, Lin Q, Zhu J, Mai L, Shan Z, Yu X, Yang M, Lin S (2011). *Panax notoginseng* saponins inhibit ischemia-induced apoptosis by activating PI3K/Akt pathway in cardiomyocytes. *J Ethnopharmacol* **137**(1): 263–270.

Chen S, Wang Z, Huang Y, O'Barr SA, Wong RA, Yeung S, Chow MS (2014). Ginseng and anticancer drug combination to improve cancer chemotherapy: a critical review. *Evid Based Complement Alternat Med* 168940.

Chen X, Zhou M, Li Q, Yang J, Zhang Y, Zhang D, Kong S, Zhou D, He L (2008). Sanchi for acute ischaemic stroke. *Cochrane Database Syst Rev* (4):CD006305.

Chen XW, Serag ES, Sneed KB, Liang J, Chew H, Pan SY, Zhou SF (2011). Clinical herbal interactions with conventional drugs: from molecules to maladies. *Curr Med Chem* **18**(31): 4836–4850.

Chen YQ, Rong L, Qiao JO (2014). Anti inflammatory effects of *Panax notoginseng* saponins ameliorate acute lung injury induced by oleic acid and lipopolysaccharide in rats. *Mol Med Rep* **10**(3): 1400–1408.

Cheng H, Li S, Fan Y, Gao X, Hao M, Wang J, Zhang X, Tai G, Zhou Y (2011). Comparative studies of the antiproliferative effects of ginseng polysaccharides on HT-29 human colon cancer cells. *Med Oncol* **28**(1): 175–181.

Cho HM, Kang YH, Yoo H, Yoon SY, Kang SW, Chang EJ, Song Y (2014). *Panax* red ginseng extract regulates energy expenditures by modulating PKA-dependent lipid mobilization in adipose tissue. *Biochem Biophys Res Commun* **447**(4): 644–648.

Cho IH (2012). Effects of *Panax ginseng* in neurodegenerative diseases. *J Ginseng Res* **36**(4): 342–353.

Choi HJ, Kim EJ, Shin YW, Park JH, Kim DH, Kim NJ (2012). Protective effect of heat-processed ginseng (sun ginseng) in the adenine-induced renal failure rats. *J Ginseng Res* **36**(3): 270–276.

Choi HK, Seong DH, Rha KH (1995). Clinical efficacy of Korean red ginseng for erectile dysfunction. *Int J Impot Res* **7**(3): 181–186.

Choi IY, Kim SJ, Kim MC, Kim HL, Shin HJ, Kang TH, Jeong HJ, Shim JS, Kim JH, Yang DC, Hong SH, Kim HM, Um JY (2010). Inhibitory effects of the transgenic *Panax ginsengs* on phorbol ester plus A23187-induced IL-6 production and cyclooxygenase-2 via suppression of NF-κB and MAPKs in HMC-1. *Immunopharmacol Immunotoxicol* **33**(1): 205–210.

Choi KT (2008). Botanical characteristics, pharmacological effects and medicinal components of Korean Panax ginseng C A Meyer. *Acta Pharmacol Sin* **29**: 1109–1118.

Choi YJ, Choi H, Cho CH, Park JW (2011). Red ginseng deregulates hypoxia-induced genes by dissociating the HIF-1 dimer. *J Nat Med* **65**(2): 344–352.

Choung YH, Kim SW, Tian C, Min JY, Lee HK, Park SN, Lee JB, Park K (2011). Korean red ginseng prevents gentamicin-induced hearing loss in rats. *Laryngoscope* **121**(6): 1294–1302.

Chung SH, Choi CG, Park SH (2001). Comparisons between white ginseng radix and rootlet for antidiabetic activity and mechanism in KKAy mice. *Arch Pharm Res* **24**(3): 214–218.

Court WA, Hendel JG, Elmi J (1996). Reversed-phase high-performance liquid chromatographic determination of ginsenosides of *Panax quinquefolium*. *J Chromatogr A* **755**: 11–17.

Cui X, Jin Y, Poudyal D, Chumanevich AA, Davis T, Windust A, Hofseth A, Wu W, Habiger J, Pena E, Wood P, Nagarkatti M, Nagarkatti PS, Hofseth L (2010). Mechanistic insight into the ability of American ginseng to suppress colon cancer associated with colitis. *Carcinogenesis* **31**(10): 1734–1741.

Cui XM, Jiang ZY, Zeng J, Zhou JM, Chen JJ, Zhang XM, Xu LS, Wang Q (2008). Two new dammarane triterpene glycosides from the rhizomes of Panax notoginseng. *J Asian Nat Prod Res* **10**(9–10): 845–849.

Dallard BE, Baravalle C, Andreotti C, Ortega HH, Neder V, Calvinho LF (2011). Intramammary inoculation of *Panax ginseng* extract in cows at drying off enhances early mammary involution. *J Dairy Res* **78**(1): 63–71.

Dang H, Chen Y, Liu X, Wang Q, Wang L, Jia W, Wang Y (2009). Antidepressant effects of ginseng total saponins in the forced swimming test and chronic mild stress models of depression. *Prog Neuropsychopharmacol Biol Psychiatry* **33**(8): 1417–1424.

De la Garza AL, Milagro FI, Boque N, Campión J, Martínez JA (2011). Natural inhibitors of pancreatic lipase as new players in obesity treatment. *Planta Med* **77**(8): 773–785.

De Souza LR, Jenkins AL, Sievenpiper JL, Jovanovski E, Rahelić D, Vuksan V (2011). Korean red ginseng (*Panax ginseng* C.A. Meyer) root fractions: differential effects on postprandial glycemia in healthy individuals. *J Ethnopharmacol* **137**(1): 245–250.

Dong L, Zhang CY, Chen SL (2011). HPLC-UV-ELSD characteristic figure and chemical pattern recognition of *Panacis Quinquefolii Radix*. *Yao Xue Xue Bao* **46**(2): 198–202.

Dong TT, Cui XM, Song ZH, Zhao KJ, Ji ZN, Lo CK, Tsim KW (2003). Chemical assessment of roots of *Panax notoginseng* in China: regional and seasonal variations in its active constituents. *J Agric Food Chem* 2003 **51**(16): 4617–4623.

Dong GZ, Jang EJ, Kang SH, Cho IJ, Park SD, Kim SC, Kim YW (2013). Red ginseng abrogates oxidative stress via mitochondria protection mediated by LKB1-AMPK pathway. *BMC Complement Altern Med* **13**: 64.

Doo JP, Chang HL (2015). Review of cases of patient risk associated with ginseng abuse and misuse. *J Ginseng Res* **39**(2): 89–93.

Fu HZ, Zhong RJ, Zhang DM, Wang D (2013) A new protopanaxadiol-type ginsenoside from the roots of *Panax notoginseng*. *J Asian Nat Prod Res* [Epub ahead of print].

Fu YQ, Hua C, Zhou J, Cheng BR, Zhang J (2013). Protective effects of ginseng total saponins against hepatic ischemia/reperfusion injury in experimental obstructive jaundice rats. *Pharm Biol* **51**(12): 1545–1551.

Ge P, Xing N, Ren Y, Zhu L, Han D, Kuang H, Li J (2014). Preventive effect of american ginseng against premature ovarian failure in a rat model. *Drug Dev Res* [Epub ahead of print].

Geng J, Dong J, Ni H, Lee MS, Wu T, Jiang K, Wang G, Zhou AL, Malouf R (2010). Ginseng for cognition. *Cochrane Database Syst Rev* (12): CD007769.

Guo J, Gan XT, Haist JV, Rajapurohitam V, Zeidan A, Faruq NS, Karmazyn M (2011). Ginseng inhibits cardiomyocyte hypertrophy and heart failure via NHE-1 inhibition and attenuation of calcineurin activation. *Circ Heart Fail* **4**(1): 79–88.

Guo N, Ablajan K, Fan B, Yan H, Yu Y, Dou D (2013). Simultaneous determination of seven ginsenosides in Du Shen Tang decoction by rapid resolution liquid chromatography (RRLC) coupled with tandem mass spectrometry. *Food Chem* **141**(4): 4046–4050.

Han H, Chen Y, Bi H, Yu L, Sun C, Li S, Oumar SA, Zhou Y (2011). *In vivo* antimalarial activity of ginseng extracts. *Pharm Biol* **49**(3): 283–289.

Han KH, Choe SC, Kim HS, Sohn DW, Nam KY, Oh BH, Lee MM, Park YB, Choi YS, Seo JD, Lee YW (1998). Effect of red ginseng on blood pressure in patients with essential hypertension and white coat hypertension. *Am J Chin Med* **26**(2): 199–209.

Hankins A (2009). Producing and marketing wild simulated ginseng in forest and agroforestry system. Virginia Cooperative Extension, Publication 354–312. Available at http://pubs.ext.vt.edu/354/354-312/354-312.html, accessed 1 Feb 2015.

Hassan AM, Abdel-Aziem SH, El-Nekeety AA, Abdel-Wahhab MA (2014). *Panax ginseng* extract modulates oxidative stress, DNA fragmentation and up-regulate gene expression in rats sub chronically treated with aflatoxin B1 and fumonisin B1. *Cytotechnology* [Epub ahead of print].

He F, Ding Y, Liang C, Song SB, Dou DQ, Song GY, Kim YH (2014). Antitumor effects of dammarane-type saponins from steamed Notoginseng. *Pharmacog Mag* **10**(39): 314–317.

Heo JH, Lee ST, Oh MJ, Park HJ, Shim JY, Chu K, Kim M (2011). Improvement of cognitive deficit in Alzheimer's disease patients by long term treatment with korean red ginseng. *J Ginseng Res* **35**(4): 457–461.

Herrmann F, Sporer F, Tahrani A, Wink M (2013). Antitrypanosomal properties of *Panax ginseng* C. A. Meyer: new possibilities for a remarkable traditional drug. *Phytother Res* **27**(1): 86–98.

High KP, Case D, Hurd D, Powell B, Lesser G, Falsey AR, Siegel R, Metzner-Sadurski J, Krauss JC, Chinnasami B, Sanders G, Rousey S, Shaw EG (2012). A randomized, controlled trial of *Panax quinquefolius* extract (CVT-E002) to reduce respiratory infection in patients with chronic lymphocytic leukemia. *J Support Oncol* **10**(5): 195–201.

Ho CC, Tan HM (2011). Rise of herbal and traditional medicine in erectile dysfunction management. *Curr Urol Rep* **12**(6): 470–478.

Ho YL, Li KC, Chao W, Chang YS, Huang GJ (2012). Korean red ginseng suppresses metastasis of human hepatoma SK-Hep1 cells by inhibiting matrix metalloproteinase-2/-9 and urokinase plasminogen activator. *Evid Based Complement Alternat Med* 965846.

Hong SJ, Wan JB, Zhang Y, Hu G, Lin HC, Seto SW, Kwan YW, Lin ZX, Wang YT, Lee SM (2009). Angiogenic effect of saponin extract from *Panax notoginseng* on HUVECs *in vitro* and zebrafish *in vivo*. *Phytother Res* **23**(5): 677–686.

Huang CC, Chen YM, Wang DC, Chiu CC, Lin WT, Huang CY, Hsu MC (2013). Cytoprotective effect of American ginseng in a rat ethanol gastric ulcer model. *Molecules* **19**(1): 316–326.

Hwang E, Lee TH, Park SY, Yi TH, Kim SY (2014). Enzyme-modified *Panax ginseng* inhibits UVB-induced skin aging through the regulation of procollagen type I and MMP-1 expression. *Food Funct* **5**(2): 265–274.

Hwang E, Sun ZW, Lee TH, Shin HS, Park SY, Lee DG, Cho BG, Sohn H, Kwon OW, Kim SY, Yi TH (2013). Enzyme-processed Korean red ginseng extracts protects against skin damage induced by UVB irradiation in hairless mice. *J Ginseng Res* **37**(4): 425–434.

Hwang I, Ahn G, Park E, Ha D, Song JY, Jee Y (2011). An acidic polysaccharide of *Panax ginseng* ameliorates experimental autoimmune encephalomyelitis and induces regulatory T cells. *Immunol Lett* **138**(2): 169–178.

Ichikawa T, Li J, Nagarkatti P, Nagarkatti M, Hofseth LJ, Windust A, Cui T (2009). American ginseng preferentially suppresses STAT/iNOS signaling in activated macrophages. *J Ethnopharmacol* **125**(1): 145–150.

Janetzky K, Morreale AP (1997). Probable interaction between warfarin and ginseng. *Am J Health Syst Pharm* **54**(6): 692–693.

Jang DJ, Lee MS, Shin BC, Lee YC, Ernst E (2008). Red ginseng for treating erectile dysfunction: a systematic review. *Br J Clin Pharmacol* **66**(4): 444–450.

Jang HA, Cho S, Kang SG, Ko YH, Kang SH, Bae JH, Cheon J, Kim JJ, Lee JG (2012). The relaxant effect of ginseng saponin on the bladder and prostatic urethra: an *in vitro* and *in vivo* study. *Urol Int* **88**(4): 463–469.

Jang HI, Shin HM (2010). Wild *Panax ginseng* (*Panax ginseng* C.A. Meyer) protects against methotrexate-induced cell regression by enhancing the immune response in RAW 264.7 macrophages. *Am J Chin Med* **38**(5): 949–960.

Jang M, Min JW, In JG, Yang DC (2011). Effects of red ginseng extract on the epididymal sperm motility of mice exposed to ethanol. *Int J Toxicol* **30**(4): 435–442.

Jeon BH, Kim CS, Kim HS, Park JB, Nam KY, Chang SJ (2000). Effect of Korean red ginseng on blood pressure and nitric oxide production. *Acta Pharmacol Sin* **21**(12): 1095–1100.

Jeong CS (2002). Effect of butanol fraction of Panax ginseng head on gastric lesion and ulcer. *Arch Pharm Res* **25**(1): 61–66.

Jhun J, Lee J, Byun JK, Kim EK, Woo JW, Lee JH, Kwok SK, Ju JH, Park KS, Kim HY, Park SH, Cho ML (2014). Red ginseng extract ameliorates autoimmune arthritis via regulation of STAT3 pathway, Th17/Treg balance, and osteoclastogenesis in mice and human. *Mediators Inflamm* 351856.

Ji W, Gong BQ (2007). Hypolipidemic effects and mechanisms of *Panax notoginseng* on lipid profile in hyperlipidemic rats. *J Ethnopharmacol* **113**(2): 318–324.

Jia D, Deng Y, Gao J, Liu X, Chu J, Shu Y (2014). Neuroprotective effect of *Panax notoginseng* plysaccharides against focal cerebral ischemia reperfusion injury in rats. *Int J Biol Macromol* **63**: 177–180.

Jia L, Zhao Y (2009). Current evaluation of the millennium phytomedicine — ginseng (I): etymology, pharmacognosy, phytochemistry, market and regulations. *Curr Med Chem* **16**(19): 2475–2484.

Jia L, Zhao Y, Liang XJ (2009). Current evaluation of the millennium phytomedicin — ginseng (II): collected chemical entities, modern pharmacology, and clinical applications emanated from traditional Chinese medicine. *Curr Med Chem* **16**(22): 2924–2942.

Jiang M, Murias JM, Chrones T, Sims SM, Lui E, Noble EG (2014). American ginseng acutely regulates contractile function of rat heart. *Front Pharmacol* **5**: 43.

Jiang X, Blair EY, McLachlan AJ (2006). Investigation of the effects of herbal medicines on warfarin response in healthy subjects: a population pharmacokinetic-pharmacodynamic modeling approach. *J Clin Pharmacol* **46**(11): 1370–1378.

Jin Y, Hofseth AB, Cui X, Windust AJ, Poudyal D, Chumanevich AA, Matesic LE, Singh NP, Nagarkatti M, Nagarkatti PS, Hofseth LJ (2010). American ginseng suppresses colitis through p53-mediated apoptosis of inflammatory cells. *Cancer Prev Res (Phila)* **3**(3): 339–347.

Joshi KG, Faubion MD (2005). Mania and psychosis associated with St. John's Wort and ginseng. *Psychiatry (Edgmont)* **2**(9): 56–61.

Jovanovski E, Bateman EA, Bhardwaj J, Fairgrieve C, Mucalo I, Jenkins AL, Vuksan V (2014). Effect of Rg3-enriched Korean red ginseng (*Panax ginseng*) on arterial stiffness and blood pressure in healthy individuals: a randomized controlled trial. *J Am Soc Hypertens* **8**(8): 537–541.

Jung HL, Kang HY (2013). Effects of Korean red ginseng supplementation on muscle glucose uptake in high-fat fed rats. *Chin J Nat Med* **11**(5): 494–499.

Jung JH, Kang IG, Kim DY, Hwang YJ, Kim ST (2013). The effect of Korean red ginseng on allergic inflammation in a murine model of allergic rhinitis. *J Ginseng Res* **37**(2): 167–175.

Jung JH, Park HT, Kim T, Jeong MJ, Lim SC, Nah SY, Cho IH, Park SH, Kang SS, Moon CJ, Kim JC, Kim SH, Bae CS (2011). Therapeutic effect of Korean red ginseng extract on infertility caused by polycystic ovaries. *J Ginseng Res* **35**(2): 250–255.

Jung JW, Kang HR, Ji GE, Park MS, Song WJ, Kim MH, Kwon JW, Kim TW, Park HW, Cho SH, Min KU (2011). Therapeutic effects of fermented red ginseng in allergic rhinitis: a randomized, double-blind, placebo-controlled study. *Allergy Asthma Immunol Res* **3**(2): 103–110.

Kalkan Y, Kapakin KA, Kara A, Atabay T, Karadeniz A, Simsek N, Karakus E, Can I, Yildirim S, Ozkanlar S, Sengul E (2012). Protective effect of *Panax ginseng* against serum biochemical changes and apoptosis in kidney of rats treated with gentamicin sulphate. *J Mol Histol* **43**(5): 603–613.

Kang KS, Ham J, Kim YJ, Park JH, Cho EJ, Yamabe N (2013). Heat-processed *Panax ginseng* and diabetic renal damage: active components and action mechanism. *J Ginseng Res.* **37**(4): 379–388.

Kang S, Min H (2012). Ginseng, the "immunity boost": the effects of *Panax ginseng* on immune system. *J Ginseng Res* **36**(4): 354–368.

Karakus E, Karadeniz A, Simsek N, Can I, Kara A, Yildirim S, Kalkan Y, Kisa F (2011). Protective effect of *Panax ginseng* against serum biochemical changes and apoptosis in liver of rats treated with carbon tetrachloride (CCl4). *J Hazard Mater* **195**: 208–213.

Karmazyn M, Moey M, Gan XT (2011). Therapeutic potential of ginseng in the management of cardiovascular disorders. *Drugs* **71**(15): 1989–2008.

Kasuli EG (2011). Are alternative supplements effective treatment for diabetes mellitus? *Nutr Clin Pract* **26**(3): 352–355.

Ki SH, Yang JH, Ku SK, Kim SC, Kim YW, Cho IJ (2013). Red ginseng extract protects against carbon tetrachloride-induced liver fibrosis. *J Ginseng Res* **37**(1): 45–53.

Kiefer D, Pantuso T (2003). *Panax ginseng. Am Fam Physician* **68**(8): 1539–1542.

Kim DH (2012). Chemical diversity of Panax ginseng, Panax quinquifolium, and Panax notoginseng. *J Ginseng Res* **36**(1): 1–15.

Kim DY, Yang WM (2011). *Panax ginseng* ameliorates airway inflammation in an ovalbumin-sensitized mouse allergic asthma model. *J Ethnopharmacol* **136**(1): 230–235.

Kim H, Lee HJ, Kim DJ, Kim TM, Moon HS, Choi H (2013). *Panax ginseng* exerts antiproliferative effects on rat hepatocarcinogenesis. *Nutr Res* **33**(9): 753–760.

Kim HG, Cho JH, Yoo SR, Lee JS, Han JM, Lee NH, Ahn YC, Son CG (2013). Antifatigue effects of Panax ginseng C.A. Meyer: a randomised, double-blind, placebo-controlled trial. *PLoS One* **8**(4): e61271.

Kim HG, Yoo SR, Park HJ, Lee NH, Shin JW, Sathyanath R, Cho JH, Son CG (2011). Antioxidant effects of Panax ginseng C.A. Meyer in healthy subjects: a randomized, placebo-controlled clinical trial. *Food Chem Toxicol* **49**(9): 2229–2235.

Kim HJ, Kang HJ, Seo JY, Lee CH, Kim YS, Kim JS (2011). Antiobesity effect of oil extract of ginseng. *J Med Food* **14**(6): 573–583.

Kim HJ, Kim P, Shin CY (2013). A comprehensive review of the therapeutic and pharmacological effects of ginseng and ginsenosides in central nervous system. *J Ginseng Res* **37**(1): 8–29.

Kim HK (2013). Pharmacokinetics of ginsenoside Rb1 and its metabolite compound K after oral administration of Korean Red Ginseng extract. *J Ginseng Res* **37**(4): 451–456.

Kim HS, Kim DH, Kim BK, Yoon SK, Kim MH, Lee JY, Kim HO, Park YM (2011). Effects of topically applied Korean red ginseng and its genuine constituents on atopic dermatitis-like skin lesions in NC/Nga mice. *Int Immunopharmacol* **11**(2): 280–285.

Kim J, Kim SH, Lee DS, Lee DJ, Kim SH, Chung S, Yang HO (2013). Effects of fermented ginseng on memory impairment and β-amyloid reduction in Alzheimer's disease experimental models. *J Ginseng Res* **37**(1): 100–107.

Kim JH (2012). Cardiovascular diseases and *Panax ginseng*: a review on molecular mechanisms and medical applications. *J Ginseng Res* **36**(1): 16–26.

Kim JH, Kang JW, Kim M, Lee DH, Kim H, Choi HS, Kim EJ, Chung IM, Chung IY, Yoon DY (2011). The liquid *Panax ginseng* inhibits epidermal growth factor-induced metalloproteinase 9 and cyclooxygenase 2 expressions via inhibition of inhibitor factor kappa-B-alpha and extracellular signal-regulated kinase in NCI-H292 human airway epithelial cells. *Am J Rhinol Allergy* **25**(2): e55–e59.

Kim JJ, Xiao H, Tan Y, Wang ZZ, Paul Seale J, Qu X (2009). The effects and mechanism of saponins of *Panax notoginseng* on glucose metabolism in 3T3-L1 cells. *Am J Chin Med* **37**(6): 1179–1189.

Kim S, Shin BC, Lee MS, Lee H, Ernst E (2011). Red ginseng for type 2 diabetes mellitus: a systematic review of randomized controlled trials. *Chin J Integr Med* **17**(12): 937–944.

Kim SD, Kim YJ, Huh JS, Kim SW, Sohn DW (2013). Improvement of erectile function by Korean red ginseng (*Panax ginseng*) in a male rat model of metabolic syndrome. *Asian J Androl* **15**(3): 395–399.

Kim TH, Jeon SH, Hahn EJ, Paek KY, Park JK, Youn NY, Lee HL (2009). Effects of tissue-cultured mountain ginseng (Panax ginseng CA Meyer) extract on male patients with erectile dysfunction. *Asian J Androl* **11**(3): 356–361.

Kim WY, Kim JM, Han SB, Lee SK, Kim ND, Park MK, Kim CK, Park JH (2000). Steaming of ginseng at high temperature enhances biological activity. *J Nat Prod* **63**(12): 1702–1704.

Kim YS, Cho IH, Jeong MJ, Jeong SJ, Nah SY, Cho YS, Kim SH, Go A, Kim SE, Kang SS, Moon CJ, Kim JC, Kim SH, Bae CS (2011). Therapeutic effect of total ginseng saponin on skin wound healing. *J Ginseng Res* **35**(3): 360–367.

King ML, Murphy LL (2010). Role of cyclin inhibitor protein p21 in the inhibition of HCT116 human colon cancer cell proliferation by American ginseng (*Panax quinquefolius*) and its constituents. *Phytomedicine* **17**(3–4): 261–268.

Kitts DD, Wijewickreme AN, Hu C (2000). Antioxidant properties of a North American ginseng extract. *Mol Cell Biochem* **203**(1–2): 1–10.

Ko HM, Joo SH, Kim P, Park JH, Kim HJ, Bahn GH, Kim HY, Lee J, Han SH, Shin CY, Park SH (2013). Effects of Korean red ginseng extract on tissue plasminogen activator and plasminogen activator inhibitor-1 expression in cultured rat primary astrocytes. *J Ginseng Res* **37**(4): 401–412.

Kuo SC, Teng CM, Lee JC, Ko FN, Chen SC, Wu TS (1990). Antiplatelet components in Panax ginseng. *Planta Med* **56**(2): 164–167.

Kurz A, Perneczky R (2011). Amyloid clearance as a treatment target against Alzheimer's disease. J *Alzheimers Dis* **24**(Suppl. 2): 61–73.

Kwak YS, Kyung JS, Kim JS, Cho JY, Rhee MH (2010). Anti-hyperlipidemic effects of red ginseng acidic polysaccharide from Korean red ginseng. *Biol Pharm Bull* **33**(3): 468–472.

Lau AJ, Toh DF, Chua TK, Pang YK, Woo SO, Koh HL (2009). Antiplatelet and anticoagulant effects of *Panax notoginseng*: comparison of raw and steamed *Panax notoginseng* with *Panax ginseng* and Panax quinquefolium. *J Ethnopharmacol* **125**(3): 380–386.

Lee B, Kim H, Shim I, Lee H, Hahm DH (2011a). Wild ginseng attenuates anxiety- and depression-like behaviors during morphine withdrawal. *J Microbiol Biotechnol* **21**(10): 1088–1096.

Lee B, Kwon S, Yeom M, Shim I, Lee H, Hahm DH (2011b). Wild ginseng attenuates repeated morphine-induced behavioral sensitization in rats. *J Microbiol Biotechnol* **21**(7): 757–765.

Lee B, Park J, Kwon S, Park MW, Oh SM, Yeom MJ, Shim I, Lee HJ, Hahm DH (2010). Effect of wild ginseng on scopolamine-induced acetylcholine depletion in the rat hippocampus. *J Pharm Pharmacol* **62**(2): 263–271.

Lee CH, Kim JM, Kim DH, Park SJ, Liu X, Cai M, Hong JG, Park JH, Ryu JH (2013). Effects of Sun ginseng on memory enhancement and hippocampal neurogenesis. *Phytother Res* **27**(9): 1293–1299.

Lee DC, Lau AS (2011). Effects of *Panax ginseng* on tumor necrosis factor-α-mediated inflammation: a mini-review. *Molecules* **16**(4): 2802–2816.

Lee H, Kim M, Shik Shin S, Yoon M (2014). Ginseng treatment reverses obesity and related disorders by inhibiting angiogenesis in female db/db mice. *J Ethnopharmacol* **155**(2): 1342–1352.

Lee JG, Lee YY, Kim SY, Pyo JS, Yun-Choi HS, Park JH (2009). Platelet antiaggregating activity of ginsenosides isolated from processed ginseng. *Pharmazie* **64**(9): 602–604.

Lee JG, Lee YY, Wu B, Kim SY, Lee YJ, Yun-Choi HS, Park JH (2010). Inhibitory activity of ginsenosides isolated from processed ginseng on platelet aggregation. *Pharmazie* **65**(7): 520–522.

Lee JH, Lee HJ, Yang M, Moon C, Kim JC, Bae CS, Jo SK, Jang JS, Kim SH (2013). Effect of Korean red ginseng on radiation-induced bone loss in C3H/HeN mice. *J Ginseng Res* **37**(4): 435–441.

Lee JS, Choi HS, Kang SW, Chung JH, Park HK, Ban JY, Kwon OY, Hong HP, Ko YG (2011). Therapeutic effect of Korean red ginseng on inflammatory cytokines in rats with focal cerebral ischemia/reperfusion injury. *Am J Chin Med* **39**(1): 83–94.

Lee JS, Ko EJ, Hwang HS, Lee YN, Kwon YM, Kim MC, Kang SM (2014). Antiviral activity of ginseng extract against respiratory syncytial virus infection. *Int J Mol Med* **34**(1): 183–190.

Lee KJ, Ji GE (2014). The effect of fermented red ginseng on depression is mediated by lipids. *Nutr Neurosci* **17**(1): 7–15.

Lee LS, Cho CW, Hong HD, Lee YC, Choi UK, Kim YC (2013). Hypolipidemic and antioxidant properties of phenolic compound-rich extracts from white ginseng (*Panax ginseng*) in cholesterol-fed rabbits. *Molecules* **18**(10): 12548–12560.

Lee LS, Wise SD, Chan C, Parsons TL, Flexner C, Lietman PS (2008). Possible differential induction of phase 2 enzyme and antioxidant pathways by American ginseng, *Panax quinquefolius*. *J Clin Pharmacol* **48**(5): 599–609.

Lee MH, Lee BH, Jung JY, Cheon DS, Kim KT, Choi C (2011). Antiviral effect of Korean red ginseng extract and ginsenosides on murine norovirus and feline calicivirus as surrogates for human norovirus. *J Ginseng Res* **35**(4): 429–435.

Lee NH, Son CG (2011). Systematic review of randomized controlled trials evaluating the efficacy and safety of ginseng. *J Acupunt Meridian Stud* **4**(2): 85–97.

Lee SE, Park YS (2014). Korean Red Ginseng water extract inhibits COX-2 expression by suppressing p38 in acrolein-treated human endothelial cells. *J Ginseng Res* **38**(1): 34–39.

Lee SH, Ahn YM, Ahn SY, Doo HK, Lee BC (2008). Interaction between warfarin and *Panax ginseng* in ischemic stroke patients. *J Altern Complement Med* **14**(6): 715–721.

Lee SH, Lee HJ, Lee YH, Lee BW, Cha BS, Kang ES, Ahn CW, Park JS, Kim HJ, Lee EY, Lee HC (2012). Korean red ginseng (*Panax ginseng*) improves insulin sensitivity in high-fat-fed Sprague-Dawley rats. *Phytother Res* **26**(1): 145–147.

Lee SH, Park WS, Lim MH (2011). Clinical effects of Korean red ginseng on attention deficit hyperactivity disorder in children: an observational study. *J Ginseng Res* **35**(2): 226–234.

Lee TK, O'Brien KF, Wang W, Johnke RM, Sheng C, Benhabib SM, Wang T, Allison RR (2010). Radioprotective effect of American ginseng on human lymphocytes at 90 minutes postirradiation: a study of 40 cases. *J Altern Complement Med* **16**(5): 561–567.

Lee NH, Son CG (2011). Systematic review of randomized controlled trials evaluating the efficacy and safety of ginseng. *J Acupunct Meridian Stud* **4**(2): 85–97.

Lee ST, Chu K, Sim JY, Heo JH, Kim M (2008). Panax ginseng enhances cognitive performance in Alzheimer disease. *Alzheimer Dis Assoc Disord* **22**(3): 222–226.

Lee YH, Lee BK, Choi YJ, Yoon IK, Chang BC, Gwak HS (2010). Interaction between warfarin and Korean red ginseng in patients with cardiac valve replacement. *Int J Cardiol* **145**(2): 275–276.

Li H, He WY, Lin F, Gou X (2014). *Panax notoginseng* saponins improve erectile function through attenuation of oxidative stress, restoration of Akt activity and protection of endothelial and smooth muscle cells in diabetic rats with erectile dysfunction. *Urol Int* **93**(1): 92–99.

Li J, Ichikawa T, Jin Y, Hofseth LJ, Nagarkatti P, Nagarkatti M, Windust A, Cui T (2010). An essential role of Nrf2 in American ginseng-mediated anti-oxidative actions in cardiomyocytes. *J Ethnopharmacol* **130**(2): 222–230.

Li JP, Huang M, Teoh H, Man RY (2000). Interactions between *Panax quinquefolium* saponins and vitamin C are observed *in vitro*. *Mol Cell Biochem* **204**(1–2): 77–82.

Li XD, Chang B, Chen B, Liu ZY, Liu DX, Wang JS, Hou GQ, Huang DY, Du SX (2010). *Panax notoginseng* saponins potentiate osteogenesis of bone marrow stromal cells by modulating gap junction intercellular communication activities. *Cell Physiol Biochem* **26**(6): 1081–1092.

Li YC (1999). "中药材真伪鉴别彩色图谱大全". 1st ed. Chengdu: Sichuan Science and Technology Press.

Liang MT, Lau WY, Sokmen B, Spalding TW, Chuang WJ (2012). Effects of *Panax notoginseng* (Chinese ginseng) and acute exercise on postprandial glycemia in non-diabetic adults. *J Complement Integr Med* **4**: 8.

Liang MT, Podolka TD, Chuang WJ (2005). *Panax notoginseng* supplementation enhances physical performance during endurance exercise. *J Strength Cond Res* **19**(1): 108–114.

Lim KH, Cho JY, Kim B, Bae BS, Kim JH (2014). Red ginseng (*Panax ginseng*) decreases isoproterenol-induced cardiac injury via antioxidant properties in porcine. *J Med Food* **17**(1): 111–118.

Lim KH, Kang CW, Choi JY, Kim JH (2013a). Korean red ginseng induced cardioprotection against myocardial ischemia in guinea pig. *Korean J Physiol Pharmacol* **17**(4): 283–289.

Lim KH, Ko D, Kim JH (2013b). Cardioprotective potential of Korean red ginseng extract on isoproterenol-induced cardiac injury in rats. *J Ginseng Res* **37**(3): 273–282.

Lim SW, Doh KC, Jin L, Piao SG, Heo SB, Zheng YF, Bae SK, Chung BH, Yang CW (2013). Oral administration of ginseng ameliorates cyclosporine-induced pancreatic injury in an experimental mouse model. *PLoS One* **8**(8): e72685.

Lin F, Gou X (2013). *Panax notoginseng* saponins improve the erectile dysfunction in diabetic rats by protecting the endothelial function of the penile corpus cavernosum. *Int J Impot Res* **25**(6): 206–211.

Liu G, Wang B, Zhang J, Jiang H, Liu F (2009). Total panax notoginsenosides prevent atherosclerosis in apolipoprotein E-knockout mice: Role of downregulation of CD40 and MMP-9 expression. *J Ethnopharmacol.* **126**(2): 350–354.

Liu HZ, Liu ZL, Zhao SP, Sun CZ, Yang MS (2014). Protective mechanism of *Panax notoginseng* saponins on rat hemorrhagic shock model in recovery stage. *Cell Biochem Biophys* [Epub ahead of print].

Liu J, Wang Y, Qiu L, Yu Y, Wang C (2014). Saponins of *Panax notoginseng*: chemistry, cellular targets and therapeutic opportunities in cardiovascular diseases. *Expert Opin Investig Drugs* **23**(4): 523–539.

Liu L, Shi R, Shi Q, Cheng Y, Huo Y (2008). Protective effect of saponins from *Panax notoginseng* against doxorubicin-induced cardiotoxicity in mice. *Planta Med* **74**(3): 203–209.

Liu L, Zhu L, Zou Y, Liu W, Zhang X, Wei X, Hu B, Chen J (2014). *Panax notoginseng* saponins promotes stroke recovery by influencing expression of Nogo-A, NgR and p75NGF, *in vitro* and *in vivo*. *Biol Pharm Bull* **37**(4): 560–568.

Liu R, Qin M, Hang P, Liu Y, Zhang Z, Liu G (2012). Effects of *Panax notoginseng* saponins on the activities of CYP1A2, CYP2C9, CYP2D6 and CYP3A4 in rats *in vivo*. *Phytother Res* **26**(8): 1113–1118.

Liu Y, Hao F, Zhang H, Cao D, Lu X, Li X (2013). *Panax notoginseng* saponins promote endothelial progenitor cell mobilization and attenuate atherosclerotic lesions in apolipoprotein E knockout mice. *Cell Physiol Biochem* **32**(4): 814–826.

Liu ZQ (2012). Chemical insights into ginseng as a resource for natural antioxidants. *Chem Rev* **112**(6): 3329–3355.

Lobina C, Carai MA, Loi B, Gessa GL, Riva A, Cabri W, Petrangolini G, Morazzoni P, Colombo G (2014). Protective effect of Panax ginseng in cisplatin-induced cachexia in rats. *Future Oncol* **10**(7): 1203–1214.

Lü JM, Yao Q, Chen C (2009). Ginseng compounds: an update on their molecular mechanisms and medical applications." *Curr Vasc Pharmacol* **7**(3): 293–302.

Malati CY, Robertson SM, Hunt JD, Chairez C, Alfaro RM, Kovacs JA, Penzak SR (2012). Influence of *Panax ginseng* on cytochrome P450 (CYP)3A and P-glycoprotein (P-gp) activity in healthy participants. *J Clin Pharmacol* **52**(6): 932–939.

Mateo-Carrasco H, Gálvez-Contreras MC, Fernández-Ginés FD, Nguyen TV (2012). Elevated liver enzymes resulting from an interaction between Raltegravir and *Panax ginseng*: a case report and brief review. *Drug Metabol Drug Interact* **27**(3): 171–175.

Milić N, Milosević N, Golocorbin Kon S, Bozić T, Abenavoli L, Borrelli F (2014). Warfarin interactions with medicinal herbs. *Nat Prod Commun* **9**(8): 1211–1216.

Miller SC, Delorme D, Shan JJ (2011). Extract of North American ginseng (*Panax quinquefolius*), administered to leukemic, juvenile mice extends their life span. *J Complement Integr Med* 8.

Miller SC, Ti L, Shan JJ (2012). The sustained influence of short term exposure to a proprietary extract of North American ginseng on the hemopoietic cells of the bone marrow, spleen and blood of adult and juvenile mice. *Phytother Res* **26**(5): 675–681.

Moey M, Gan XT, Huang CX, Rajapurohitam V, Martínez-Abundis E, Lui EM, Karmazyn M (2012). Ginseng reverses established cardiomyocyte hypertrophy and postmyocardial infarction-induced hypertrophy and heart failure. *Circ Heart Fail* **5**(4): 504–514.

Mucalo I, Jovanovski E, Rahelić D, Božikov V, Romić Z, Vuksan V (2013). Effect of American ginseng (*Panax quinquefolius* L.) on arterial stiffness in subjects with type-2 diabetes and concomitant hypertension. *J Ethnopharmacol* **150**(1): 148–153.

Mucalo I, Rahelić D, Jovanovski E, Bozikov V, Romić Z, Vuksan V (2012). Effect of American ginseng (*Panax quinquefolius* L.) on glycemic control in type 2 diabetes. *Coll Antropol* **36**(4): 1435–1440.

National Center for Complementary and Alternative Medicine (2012). *Ginseng*. Retrieved 1 Nov 2014. from http://NCCIH.nih.gov/health/asianginseng/ataglance.htm

Nah SY (2014). Ginseng ginsenoside pharmacology in the nervous system: involvement in the regulation of ion channels and receptors. *Front Physiol* **5**: 98.

Ng GY, Wong RY (2008). Ultrasound phonophoresis of *Panax notoginseng* improves the strength of repairing ligament: a rat model. *Ultrasound Med Biol* **34**(12): 1919–1923.

Ng TB (2006). Pharmacological activity of sanchi ginseng (*Panax notoginseng*). *J Pharm Pharmacol* **58**(8): 1007–1019.

Oh CT, Park JI, Jung YR, Joo YA, Shin DH, Cho HJ, Ahn SM, Lim YH, Park CK, Hwang JS (2013). Inhibitory effect of Korean red ginseng on melanocyte proliferation and its possible implication in GM-CSF-mediated signalling. *J Ginseng Res* **37**(4): 389–400.

Oh KJ, Chae MJ, Lee HS, Hong HD, Park K (2010). Effects of Korean red ginseng on sexual arousal in menopausal women: placebo-controlled, double-blind crossover clinical study. *J Sex Med* **7**(4 Pt. 1): 1469–1477.

Oliynyk S, Oh S (2013). Actoprotective effect of ginseng: improving mental and physical performance. *J Ginseng Res* **37**(2): 144–166.

Ong WY, Farooqui T, Koh HL, Farooqui AA, Ling EA (2015). Protective effects of ginseng on neurological disorders. *Front Aging Neurosci* **7**:129.

Oyagi A, Ogawa K, Kakino M, Hara H (2010). Protective effects of a gastrointestinal agent containing Korean red ginseng on gastric ulcer models in mice. *BMC Complement Altern Med* **10**: 45.

Park BG, Jung HJ, Cho YW, Lim HW, Lim CJ (2013). Potentiation of antioxidative and anti-inflammatory properties of cultured wild ginseng root extract through probiotic fermentation. *J Pharm Pharmacol* **65**(3): 457–464.

Park E, Hwang I, Song JY, Jee Y (2011). Acidic polysaccharide of *Panax ginseng* as a defense against small intestinal damage by whole-body gamma irradiation of mice. *Acta Histochem* **113**(1): 19–23.

Park EH, Kim DR, Kim HY, Park SK, Chang MS (2014). *Panax ginseng* induces the expression of CatSper genes and sperm hyperactivation. *Asian J Androl* [Epub ahead of print].

Park HJ, Han ES, Park DK (2010). The ethyl acetate extract of PGP (*Phellinus linteus* grown on *Panax ginseng*) suppresses B16F10 melanoma cell proliferation through inducing cellular differentiation and apoptosis. *J Ethnopharmacol* **132**(1): 115–121.

Park HM, Kim SJ, Mun AR, Go HK, Kim GB, Kim SZ, Jang SI, Lee SJ, Kim JS, Kang HS (2012). Korean red ginseng and its primary ginsenosides inhibit ethanol-induced oxidative injury by suppression of the MAPK pathway in TIB-73 cells. *J Ethnopharmacol* **141**(3): 1071–1076.

Park IH, Han SB, Kim JM, Piao L, Kwon SW, Kim NY, Kang TL, Park MK, Park JH (2002a). Four new acetylated ginsenosides from processed ginseng (sun ginseng). *Arch Pharm Res* **25**(6): 837–841.

Park IH, Kim NY, Han SB, Kim JM, Kwon SW, Kim HJ, Park MK, Park JH (2002b). Three new dammarane glycosides from heat-processed ginseng. *Arch Pharm Res* **25**(4): 428–432.

Park KS, Park KI, Kim JW, Yun YJ, Kim SH, Lee CH, Park JW, Lee JM (2014). Efficacy and safety of Korean red ginseng for cold hypersensitivity in the hands and feet: a randomized, double-blind, placebo-controlled trial. *J Ethnopharmacol* [Epub ahead of print].

Park SC, Yoo HS, Park C, Cho CK, Kim GY, Kim WJ, Lee YW, Choi YH (2009). Induction of apoptosis in human lung carcinoma cells by the water extract of *Panax notoginseng* is associated with the activation of caspase-3 through downregulation of Akt. *Int J Oncol* **35**(1): 121–127.

Park SJ, Lee JR, Jo MJ, Park SM, Ku SK, Kim SC (2013). Protective effects of Korean red ginseng extract on cadmium-induced hepatic toxicity in rats. *J Ginseng Res* **37**(1): 37–44.

Pei L, Shaozhen H, Gengting D, Tingbo C, Liang L, Hua Z (2013). Effectiveness of *Panax ginseng* on acute myocardial ischemia reperfusion injury was abolished by flutamide via endogenous testosterone-mediated Akt pathway. *Evid Based Complement Alternat Med* doi: 10.1155/2013/817826

Peralta EA, Murphy LL, Minnis J, Louis S, Dunnington GL (2009). American ginseng inhibits induced COX-2 and NFKB activation in breast cancer cells. *J Surg Res* **157**(2): 261–267.

Poudyal D, Cui X, Le PM, Hofseth AB, Windust A, Nagarkatti M, Nagarkatti PS, Schetter AJ, Harris CC, Hofseth LJ (2013). A key role of microRNA-29b for the suppression of colon cancer cell migration by American ginseng. *PLoS One* **8**(10): e75034.

Qadir MI, Tahir M, Lone KP, Munir B, Sami W (2011). Protective role of ginseng against gentamicin-induced changes in kidney of albino mice. J *Ayub Med Coll Abbottabad* **23**(4): 53–57.

Qi B, Liu L, Zhang H, Zhou GX, Wang S, Duan XZ, Bai XY, Wang SM, Zhao DQ (2014). Anti-fatigue effects of proteins isolated from *Panax quinquefolium*. *J Ethnopharmacol* **153**(2): 430–434.

Qi LW, Wang CZ, Yuan CS (2010). American ginseng: potential structure-function relationship in cancer chemoprevention. *Biochem Pharmacol* **80**(7): 947–954.

Qi LW, Wang CZ, Du GJ, Zhang ZY, Calway T, Yuan CS (2011a). Metabolism of ginseng and its interactions with drugs. *Curr Drug Metab* **12**(9): 818–822.

Qi LW, Wang CZ, Yuan CS (2011b). Ginsenosides from American ginseng: chemical and pharmacological diversity. *Phytochemistry* **72**(8): 689–699.

Qiang H, Zhang C, Shi ZB, Yang HQ, Wang KZ (2010). Protective effects and mechanism of *Panax notoginseng* saponins on oxidative stress-induced damage and apoptosis of rabbit bone marrow stromal cells. *Chin J Integr Med* **16**(6): 525–530.

Qiao Y, Zhang PJ, Lu XT, Sun WW, Liu GL, Ren M, Yan L, Zhang JD (2014). *Panax notoginseng* saponins inhibits atherosclerotic plaque angiogenesis by down-regulating vascular endothelial growth factor and nicotinamide adenine dinucleotide phosphate oxidase subunit 4 expression. *Chin J Integr Med* [Epub ahead of print].

Quan HY, Kim do Y, Chung SH (2013). Korean red ginseng extract alleviates advanced glycation end product-mediated renal injury. *J Ginseng Res* **37**(2): 187–193.

Raghavendran HR, Rekha S, Shin JW, Kim HG, Wang JH, Park HJ, Choi MK, Cho JH, Son CG (2011). Effects of Korean ginseng root extract on cisplatin-induced emesis in a rat-pica model. *Food Chem Toxicol* **49**(1): 215–221.

Raghavendran HR, Sathyanath R, Shin J, Kim HK, Han JM, Cho J, Son CG (2012). *Panax ginseng* modulates cytokines in bone marrow toxicity and myelopoiesis: ginsenoside Rg1 partially supports myelopoiesis. *PLoS One* **7**(4): e33733.

Ramesh T, Kim SW, Hwang SY, Sohn SH, Yoo SK, Kim SK (2012). *Panax ginseng* reduces oxidative stress and restores antioxidant capacity in aged rats. *Nutr Res* **32**(9): 718–726.

Rastogi V, Santiago-Moreno J, Doré S (2015). Ginseng: a promising neuroprotective strategy in stroke. *Front Cell Neurosci* **8**: 457.

Rhule A, Navarro S, Smith JR, Shepherd DM (2006). *Panax notoginseng* attenuates LPS-induced pro-inflammatory mediators in RAW264.7 cells. *J Ethnopharmacol* **106**(1): 121–128.

Rhule A, Rase B, Smith JR, Shepherd DM (2008). Toll-like receptor ligand-induced activation of murine DC2.4 cells is attenuated by *Panax notoginseng*. *J Ethnopharmacol* **116**(1): 179–186.

Rinwa P, Kumar A (2014a). Modulation of nitrergic signalling pathway by American ginseng attenuates chronic unpredictable stress-induced cognitive impairment, neuroinflammation, and biochemical alterations. *Naunyn Schmiedebergs Arch Pharmacol* **387**(2): 129–141.

Rinwa P, Kumar A (2014b). *Panax quinquefolium* involves nitric oxide pathway in olfactory bulbectomy rat model. *Physiol Behav* **129**: 142–151.

Rong L, Chen Y, He M, Zhou X (2009). *Panax notoginseng* saponins attenuate acute lung injury induced by intestinal ischaemia/reperfusion in rats. *Respirology* **14**(6): 890–898.

Rosado MF (2003). Thrombosis of a prosthetic aortic valve disclosing a hazardous interaction between warfarin and a commercial ginseng product. *Cardiology* **99**: 111.

Scholey A, Ossoukhova A, Owen L, Ibarra A, Pipingas A, He K, Roller M, Stough C (2010). Effects of American ginseng (*Panax quinquefolius*) on neurocognitive function: an acute, randomised, double-blind, placebo-controlled, crossover study. *Psychopharmacology (Berl)* **212**(3): 345–356.

Seida JK, Durec T, Kuhle S (2011). North American (*Panax quinquefolius*) and Asian ginseng (*Panax ginseng*) preparations for prevention of the common cold in healthy adults: a systematic Review. *Evid Based Complement Alternat Med* 282151.

Sen S, Chen S, Feng B, Wu Y, Lui E, Chakrabarti S (2011). American ginseng (*Panax quinquefolius*) prevents glucose-induced oxidative stress and associated endothelial abnormalities. *Phytomedicine* **18**(13): 1110–1117.

Sen S, Chen S, Wu Y, Feng B, Lui EK, Chakrabarti S (2013a). Preventive effects of North American ginseng (*Panax quinquefolius*) on diabetic retinopathy and cardiomyopathy. *Phytother Res* **27**(2): 290–298.

Sen S, Querques MA, Chakrabarti S (2013b). North American Ginseng (*Panax quinquefolius*) prevents hyperglycemia and associated pancreatic abnormalities in diabetes. *J Med Food* **16**(7): 587–592.

Seo EY, Kim WK (2011). Red ginseng extract reduced metastasis of colon cancer cells *in vitro* and *in vivo*. *J Ginseng Res* **35**(3): 315–324.

Shang Q, Xu H, Liu Z, Chen K, Liu J (2013). Oral *Panax notoginseng* preparation for coronary heart disease: a systematic review of randomized controlled trials. *Evid Based Complement Alternat Med* 940125.

Shao J, Jia L (2013). Potential serious interactions between nutraceutical ginseng and warfarin in patients with ischemic stroke. *Trends Pharmacol Sci* **34**(2): 85–86.

Shishtar E, Sievenpiper JL, Djedovic V, Cozma AI, Ha V, Jayalath VH, Jenkins DJ, Meija SB, de Souza RJ, Jovanovski E, Vuksan V (2014). The effect of ginseng (the genus *Panax*) on glycemic control: a systematic review and meta-analysis of randomized controlled clinical trials. *PLoS One* **9**(9): e107391.

Shou C, Li J, Liu Z (2011). Complementary and alternative medicine in the treatment of menopausal symptoms. *Chin J Integr Med* **17**(12): 883–888.

Si YC, Zhang JP, Xie CE, Zhang LJ, Jiang XN (2011). Effects of *Panax notoginseng* saponins on proliferation and differentiation of rat hippocampal neural stem cells. *Am J Chin Med* **39**(5): 999–1013.

Sohn EH, Jang SA, Lee CH, Jang KH, Kang SC, Park HJ, Pyo S (2011). Effects of Korean red ginseng extract for the treatment of atopic dermatitis-like skin lesions in mice. *J Ginseng Res* **35**(4): 479–486.

Sohn SH, Kim SK, Kim YO, Kim HD, Shin YS, Yang SO, Kim SY, Lee SW (2013). A comparison of antioxidant activity of Korean white and red ginsengs on H_2O_2-induced oxidative stress in HepG2 hepatoma cells. *J Ginseng Res* **37**(4): 442–450.

Song XG (2009). "中药调剂与鉴别彩色图谱". 1st ed. Beijing: China Medical Science Press.

Spelman K, Aldag R, Hamman A, Kwasnik EM, Mahendra MA, Obasi TM, Morse J, Williams EJ (2011). Traditional herbal remedies that influence cell adhesion molecule activity. *Phytother Res* **25**(4): 473–483.

Spolarich AE, Andrews L (2007). An examination of the bleeding complications associated with herbal supplements, antiplatelet and anticoagulant medications. *J Dent Hyg* **81**(3): 67.

Suleymanova E, Gulyaev M, Chepurnova N (2014). Ginseng extract attenuates early MRI changes after status epilepticus and decreases subsequent reduction of hippocampal volume in the rat brain. *Epilepsy Res* **108**(2): 223–231.

Sumiyoshi M, Sakanaka M, Kimura Y (2010). Effects of Red Ginseng extract on allergic reactions to food in Balb/c mice. *J Ethnopharmacol* **132**(1): 206–212.

Sun HX, Ye YP, Pan HJ, Pan YJ (2004). Adjuvant effect of *Panax notoginseng* saponins on the immune responses to ovalbumin in mice. *Vaccine* **22**(29–30): 3882–3889.

Sun S, Wang CZ, Tone R, Li XL, Fishbein A, Wang Q, He TC, Du W, Yuan CS (2010). Effects of steaming the root of Panax notoginseng on chemical composition and anticancer activities. *Food Chem* **118**: 307–314.

Teng CM, Kuo SC, Ko FN, Lee JC, Lee LG, Chen SC, Huang TF (1989). Antiplatelet actions of panaxynol and ginsenosides isolated from ginseng. *Biochim Biophys Acta* **990**(3): 315–320.

The State Pharmacopoeia Commission of P.R. China (2010a: p210; 2010b: p211; 2010c: p310; 2010d: p311; 2010e: p299; 2010f: p6). *Pharmacopoeia of the People's Republic of China*. Volume 1. Beijing: China Medical Science Press [English version].

The State Pharmacopoeia Commission of P.R. China (2000). *Pharmacopoeia of the People's Republic of China*. Volume 1. Beijing: Beijing Chemical Industry Press, p. 184 [Chinese version].

Toh DF, Patel DN, Chan EC, Teo A, Neo SY, Koh HL (2011). Antiproliferative effects of raw and steamed extracts of *Panax notoginseng* and its ginsenoside constituents on human liver cancer cells. *Chin Med* **6**: 4.

Tsai KD, Yang SM, Lee JC, Wong HY, Shih CM, Lin TH, Tseng MJ, Chen W (2011). *Panax notoginseng* attenuates bleomycin-induced pulmonary fibrosis in mice. *Evid Based Complement Alternat Med* 404761.

Tu Q, Qin J, Dong H, Lu F, Guan W (2011). Effects of *Panax notoginoside* on the expression of TGF-β1 and Smad-7 in renal tissues of diabetic rats. *J Huazhong Univ Sci Technolog Med Sci* **31**(2): 190–193.

Uzayisenga R, Ayeka PA, Wang Y (2014). Anti-diabetic potential of *Panax notoginseng* saponins (PNS): a review. *Phytother Res* **28**(4): 510–516.

Van Kampen JM, Baranowski DB, Shaw CA, Kay DG (2014). *Panax ginseng* is neuroprotective in a novel progressive model of Parkinson's disease. *Exp Gerontol* **50**: 95–105.

Verma P, Sharma P, Parmar J, Sharma P, Agrawal A, Goyal PK (2011). Amelioration of radiation-induced hematological and biochemical alterations in Swiss albino mice by *Panax ginseng* extract. *Integr Cancer Ther* **10**(1): 77–84.

Viana VM, Ervin J, Donovan RZ, Elliot C, Gholz H (eds.) (1996). Certification of forest products. Issues and Perspectives. Washington: Island Press.

Vuksan V, Sievenpiper JL, Koo VY, Francis T, Beljan-Zdravkovic U, Xu Z, Vidgen E (2000a). American ginseng (*Panax quinquefolius* L) reduces postprandial glycemia in nondiabetic subjects and subjects with type 2 diabetes mellitus. *Arch Intern Med* **160**(7): 1009–1013.

Vuksan V, Stavro MP, Sievenpiper JL, Koo VY, Wong E, Beljan-Zdravkovic U, Francis T, Jenkins AL, Leiter LA, Josse RG, Xu Z (2000b). American ginseng improves glycemia in individuals with normal glucose tolerance: effect of dose and time escalation. *J Am Coll Nutr* **19**(6): 738–744.

Wahid F, Jung H, Khan T, Hwang KH, Kim YY (2010). Effects of red ginseng extract on visual sensitivity and ERG b-wave of bullfrog's eye. *Planta Med* **76**(5): 426–432.

Wang AB, Wang CZ, Wu JA, Osinski J, Yuan CS (2005). Determination of major ginsenosides in *Panax quinquefolius* (American ginseng) using high-performance liquid chromatography. *Phytochem Anal* **16**: 272–277.

Wang CZ, Calway T, Yuan CS (2012). Herbal medicines as adjuvants for cancer therapeutics. *Am J Chin Med* **40**(4): 657–669.

Wang CZ, Luo X, Zhang B, Song WX, Ni M, Mehendale S, Xie JT, Aung HH, He TC, Yuan CS (2007). Notoginseng enhances anti-cancer effect of 5-fluorouracil on human colorectal cancer cells. *Cancer Chemother Pharmacol* **60**(1): 69–79.

Wang CZ, Xie JT, Fishbein A, Aung HH, He H, Mehendale SR, He TC, Du W, Yuan CS (2009). Antiproliferative effects of different plant parts of *Panax notoginseng* on SW480 human colorectal cancer cells. *Phytother Res* **23**(1): 6–13.

Wang J, Huang ZG, Cao H, Wang YT, Hui P, Hoo C, Li SP (2008). Screening of anti-platelet aggregation agents from Panax notoginseng using human platelet extraction and HPLC-DAD-ESI-MS/MS. *J Sep Sci* **31**(6–7): 1173–1180.

Wang JR, Yau LF, Zhang R, Xia Y, Ma J, Ho HM, Hu P, Hu M, Liu L, Jiang ZH (2014). Transformation of ginsenosides from notoginseng by artificial gastric juice can increase cytotoxicity toward cancer cells. *J Agric Food Chem* **62**(12): 2558–2573.

Wang LE, Lee TF (1998). Effect of ginseng saponins on exercise performance in non-trained rats. *Planta Med* **64**(2): 130–133.

Wang P, Cui J, Du X, Yang Q, Jia C, Xiong M, Yu X, Li L, Wang W, Chen Y, Zhang T (2014). *Panax notoginseng* saponins (PNS) inhibits breast cancer metastasis. *J Ethnopharmacol* **154**(3): 663–671.

Wang XJ (2009). "中药鉴定学." 1st ed. Beijing: Higher Education Press.

Wang Y, Peng D, Huang W, Zhou X, Liu J, Fang Y (2006). Mechanism of altered TNF-alpha expression by macrophage and the modulatory effect of *Panax notoginseng* saponins in scald mice. *Burns* **32**(7): 846–852.

Wang Z, Wang Y, Zhao X (2013). Panax quinquefolium diolsaponins dose-dependently inhibits the proliferation of vascular smooth muscle cells by downregulating proto-oncogene expression. *Indian J Pharmacol* **45**(5): 483–489.

Wong VK, Cheung SS, Li T, Jiang ZH, Wang JR, Dong H, Yi XQ, Zhou H, Liu L (2010). Asian ginseng extract inhibits *in vitro* and *in vivo* growth of mouse lewis lung carcinoma via modulation of ERK-p53 and NF-κB signaling. *J Cell Biochem* **111**(4): 899–910.

World Health Organization (2002). *WHO Monographs on Selected Medicinal Plants.* World Health Organization, Retrieved from http://apps.who.int/medicinedocs/en/d/Js2200e/

Wu H, Høiby N, Yang L, Givskov M, Song Z (2014). Effects of *radix ginseng* on microbial infections: a narrative review. *J Tradit Chin Med* **34**(2): 227–233.

Wu H, Lee B, Yang L, Wang H, Givskov M, Molin S, Høiby N, Song Z, (2011)."Effects of ginseng on *Pseudomonas aeruginosa* motility and biofilm formation." FEMS Immunol Med Microbiol. 62(1):49–56.

Xia W, Sun C, Zhao Y, Wu L (2011). Hypolipidemic and antioxidant activities of sanchi (radix notoginseng) in rats fed with a high fat diet. *Phytomedicine* **18**(6): 516–520.

Xu H, Yu X, Qu S, Chen Y, Wang Z, Sui D (2014). Protective effect of *Panax quinquefolium* 20(S)-protopanaxadiol saponins, isolated from

Pana quinquefolium, on permanent focal cerebral ischemic injury in rats. *Exp Ther Med* **7**(1): 165–170.

Xu L, Liu JT, Liu N, Lu PP, Pang X (2011). Effects of *Panax notoginseng* saponins on proliferation and apoptosis of vascular smooth muscle cells. *J Ethnopharmacol* **137**(1): 226–230.

Xu ML, Kim HJ, Choi YR, Kim HJ (2012). Intake of Korean red ginseng extract and saponin enhances the protection conferred by vaccination with inactivated influenza a virus. *J Ginseng Res* **36**(4): 396–402.

Xu Y, Ding J, Ma XP, Ma YH, Liu ZQ, Lin N (2014). Treatment with *Panax ginseng* antagonizes the estrogen decline in ovariectomized mice. *Int J Mol Sci* **15**(5): 7827–7840.

Xu YX, Zhang JJ (2013). Evaluation of anti-fatigue activity of total saponins of Radix notoginseng. *Indian J Med Res* **137**(1): 151–155.

Yamada N, Araki H, Yoshimura H (2011). Identification of antidepressant-like ingredients in ginseng root (*Panax ginseng* C.A. Meyer) using a menopausal depressive-like state in female mice: participation of 5-HT2A receptors. *Psychopharmacology (Berl)* **216**(4): 589–599.

Yan J, Ma Y, Zhao F, Gu W, Jiao Y (2013). Identification of immunomodulatory signatures induced by American ginseng in murine immune cells. *Evid Based Complement Alternat Med* 972814.

Yang WM, Park SY, Kim HM, Park EH, Park SK, Chang MS (2011). Effects of *Panax ginseng* on glial cell-derived neurotrophic factor (GDNF) expression and spermatogenesis in rats. *Phytother Res* **25**(2): 308–311.

Yang WZ, Hu Y, Wu WY, Ye M, Guo DA (2014). Saponins in the genus Panax L. (Araliaceae): a systematic review of their chemical diversity. *Phytochemistry* **106**: 7–24.

Yang X, Xiong X, Wang J (2014). Sanqi *Panax notoginseng* injection for angina pectoris. *Evid Based Complement Alternat Med* 963208.

Yang XC, Xiong XJ, Wang HR, Wang J (2014). Protective effects of *Panax notoginseng* saponins on cardiovascular diseases: a comprehensive overview of experimental studies. *Evid Based Complement Alternat Med* 204840.

Yang Y, Yang WS, Yu T, Sung GH, Park KW, Yoon K, Son YJ, Hwang H, Kwak YS, Lee CM, Rhee MH, Kim JH, Cho JY (2014). ATF-2/

CREB/IRF-3-targeted anti-inflammatory activity of Korean red ginseng water extract. *J Ethnopharmacol* **154**(1): 218–228.

Yeo CR, Lee SM, Popovich DG (2011a). Ginseng (*Panax quinquefolius*) reduces cell growth, lipid acquisition and increases adiponectin expression in 3T3-L1 cells. *Evid Based Complement Alternat Med* 610625.

Yeo CR, Yang C, Wong TY, Popovich DG (2011b). A quantified ginseng (*Panax ginseng* C.A. Meyer) extract influences lipid acquisition and increases adiponectin expression in 3T3-L1 cells. *Molecules* **16**(1): 477–492.

Yoo DG, Kim MC, Park MK, Song JM, Quan FS, Park KM, Cho YK, Kang SM (2012). Protective effect of Korean red ginseng extract on the infections by H1N1 and H3N2 influenza viruses in mice. *J Med Food* **15**(10): 855–862.

Yoo KM, Lee C, Lo YM, Moon B (2012). The hypoglycemic effects of American red ginseng (*Panax quinquefolius* L.) on a diabetic mouse model. *J Food Sci* **77**(7): H147–H152.

Yoshikawa M, Morikawa T, Yashiro K, Murakami T, Matsuda H (2001). Bioactive saponins and glycosides. XIX. Notoginseng (3): immunological adjuvant activity of notoginsenosides and related saponins: structures of notoginsenosides-L, -M, and -N from the roots of Panax notoginseng (Burk.) F. H. Chen. *Chem Pharm Bull (Tokyo)* **49**(11): 1452–1456.

Yoshikawa M, Murakami T, Ueno T, Yashiro K, Hirokawa N, Murakami N, Yamahara J, Matsuda H, Saijoh R, Tanaka O (1997). Bioactive saponins and glycosides. VIII. Notoginseng (1): new dammarane-type triterpene oligoglycosides, notoginsenosides-A, -B, -C, and -D, from the dried root of Panax notoginseng (Burk.) F.H. Chen. *Chem Pharm Bull (Tokyo)* **45**(6): 1039–1045.

Yu ML, Zhang CL, Yuan DD, Tong XH, Tao L (2012). *Panax notoginseng* saponins enhance the cytotoxicity of cisplatin via increasing gap junction intercellular communication. *Biol Pharm Bull* **35**(8): 1230–1237.

Yuan CS, Wang CZ, Wicks SM, Qi LW (2010). Chemical and pharmacological studies of saponins with a focus on American ginseng. *J Ginseng Res* **34**(3): 160–167.

Yuan CS, Wei G, Dey L, Karrison T, Nahlik L, Maleckar S, Kasza K, Ang-Lee M, Moss J (2004). Brief communication: American ginseng reduces warfarin's effect in healthy patients: a randomized, controlled trial. *Ann Intern Med* **141**(1): 23–27.

Yuan HD, Kim JT, Kim SH, Chung SH (2012). Ginseng and diabetes: the evidences from *in vitro*, animal and human studies. *J Ginseng Res* **36**(1): 27–39.

Yuan Z, Liao Y, Tian G, Li H, Jia Y, Zhang H, Tan Z, Li X, Deng W, Liu K, Zhang Y (2011). *Panax notoginseng* saponins inhibit Zymosan A induced atherosclerosis by suppressing integrin expression, FAK activation and NF-κB translocation. *J Ethnopharmacol* **138**(1): 150–155.

Zeng XS, Zhou XS, Luo FC, Jia JJ, Qi L, Yang ZX, Zhang W, Bai J (2014). Comparative analysis of the neuroprotective effects of ginsenosides Rg1 and Rb1 extracted from *Panax notoginseng* against cerebral ischemia. *Can J Physiol Pharmacol* **92**(2): 102–108.

Zeng Y, Song JX, Shen XZ (2012). Herbal remedies supply a novel prospect for the treatment of atherosclerosis: a review of current mechanism studies. *Phytother Res* **26**(2): 159–167.

Zhang CY, Dong L, Wang J, Chen SL (2011). Simultaneous determination of ten ginsenosides in panacis quinquefolii radix by ultra performance liquid chromatography and quality evaluation based on chemometric methods. *Pharmazie* **66**(8): 553–559.

Zhang GJ (2004). "现代实用中药鉴别技术". Beijing: People's Medical Publishing House.

Zhang K, Wang X, Ding L, Li J, Qu CL, Chen LG, Jin HY, Zhang HQ (2008). Determination of seven major ginsenosides in different parts of *Panax quinquefolius* L. (American Ginseng) with different ages. *Chem Res Chinese Univ* **24**: 707–711.

Zhang Y, Han LF, Sakah KJ, Wu ZZ, Liu LL, Agyemang K, Gao XM, Wang T (2013). Bioactive protopanaxatriol type saponins isolated from the roots of *Panax notoginseng* (burk.) f. H. Chen. *Molecules* **18**(9): 10352–10366.

Zhao Z, Hong Kong Baptist University. School of Chinese Medicine (2004). *An Illustrated Chinese Materia Medica in Hong Kong*

[Xianggang Zhong Yao Cai Tu Jian]. 1st ed. Hong Kong: School of Chinese Medicine, Hong Kong Baptist University.

Zhao Z, Xiao P (2009). *Encyclopedia of Medicinal Plants*. Volume 2. Shanghai: Shanghai World Publishing Corporation.

Zhao Z, Xiao P, (2010). *Encyclopedia of Medicinal Plants*. Volume 3. Shanghai: Shanghai World Publishing Corporation.

Zheng SD, Wu HJ, Wu DL (2012). Roles and mechanisms of ginseng in protecting heart. *Chin J Integr Med* **18**(7): 548–555.

Zhou H, Hou SZ, Luo P, Zeng B, Wang JR, Wong YF, Jiang ZH, Liu L (2011). Ginseng protects rodent hearts from acute myocardial ischemia-reperfusion injury through GR/ER-activated RISK pathway in an endothelial NOS-dependent mechanism. *J Ethnopharmacol* **135**(2): 287–298.

Zhou N, Tang Y, Keep RF, Ma X, Xiang J (2014). Antioxidative effects of *Panax notoginseng* saponins in brain cells. *Phytomedicine*. **21**(10): 1189–1195.

Zhou S, Wang Y, Tian H, Huang Q, Gao Y, Zhang G (2012). Anti-fatigue effects of *Panax notoginseng* in simulation plateau-condition mice. *Pharmacogn Mag* **8**(31): 197–201.

Zhu M, Chan KW, Ng LS, Chang Q, Chang S, Li RC (1999). Possible influences of ginseng on the pharmacokinetics and pharmacodynamics of warfarin in rats. *J Pharm Pharmacol* **51**(2): 175–180.

Other Plants That are Termed "Ginseng"

CHAPTER **3**

This chapter discusses two plants, namely the Siberian ginseng or Ci Wu Jia (*Eleutherococcus senticosus,* also known as *Acanthopanax senticosus*) and the five-leaf ginseng or Jiao Gu Lan (*Gynostemma pentaphyllum*). Unlike the herbs introduced in Chapter 2, these two herbs are not from the genus Panax.

3.1 Siberian Ginseng

3.1.1 *Introduction*

Latin Name/ Botanical Name: *Eleutherococcus senticosus Rupr. et Maxim*

Synonym *Acanthopanax senticosus* (Rupr. et Maxim.) Harms (Araliaceae family)

Pharmaceutical Name: Radix et Rhizoma seu Caulis Acanthopanacis Senticosi

Origin: Southeast Asia, Northern China, Democratic People's Republic of Korea, Japan and Southeastern part of the Russian Federation

Other Names: 刺五加 (Ci Wu Jia), Ussurian thorny, pepperbush, Taiga root

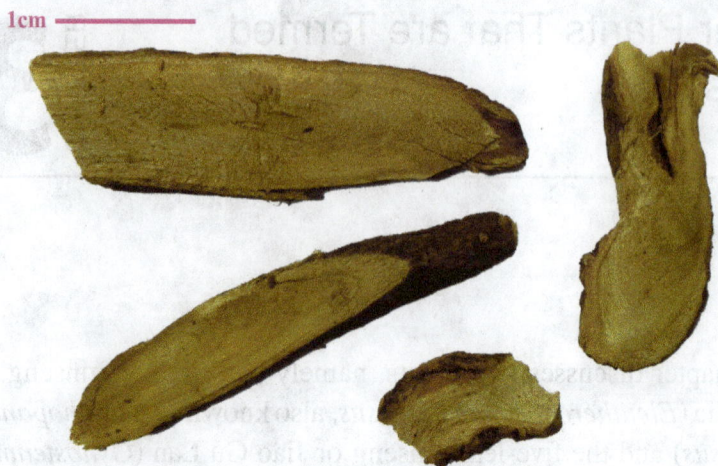

Figure 3.1 Photograph of *Eleutherococcus senticocus* slices.

3.1.2 *Phytoconstituents*

E. senticosus contains triterpenoid saponins, polysaccharides, lignans, coumarins and flavones (Huang L *et al.*, 2011, Zhao Z and Xiao P, 2009), syringin (eleutheroside B), eleutheroside E, isofraxidin (Bai Y *et al.*, 2011) and glycans such as eleutherans A, B, C, D, E, F and G (Hikino H *et al.*, 1986). Among these, phenolic compounds such as syringin (eleutheroside B) (Niu HS *et al.*, 2008) and eleutheroside E are considered to be the most active components. Unlike herbs from the genus Panax, *E. senticosus* does not contain ginsenosides.

3.1.3 *Pharmacological activities*

General reviews (Bleakney TL, 2008; Deyama T *et al.*, 2011; Huang L *et al.*, 2011; Zhao Z and Xiao P, 2009); Anti-Alzheimer's (Bai Y *et al.*, 2011; Tohda C *et al.*, 2008); Anti-arthritic (He C *et al.*, 2014; Takahashi Y *et al.*, 2014); Anti-depressant (Jin L *et al.*, 2013; Wu F *et al.*, 2013); Anti-diabetic (Ahn J *et al.*, 2013; Liu TP *et al.*,

2005; Niu HS *et al.*, 2008; Park SH *et al.*, 2006); Anti-fatigue (Huang LZ *et al.*, 2011a; Huang LZ *et al.*, 2011b; Kuo J *et al.*, 2010; Rhim YT *et al.*, 2007); Anti-inflammatory (Huang L *et al.*, 2011; Kim HJ *et al.*, 2014; Lin QY *et al.*, 2008b; Kim HS *et al.*, 2012; Zhang N *et al.*, 2012); Anti-neoplastic (Hacker B and Medon PJ, 1984; Hibasami H *et al.*, 2000; Huang L *et al.*, 2011; Yoon TJ *et al.*, 2004); Anti-obesity (Cha YS *et al.*, 2004); Anti-osteoporotic (Hwang YC *et al.*, 2009; Lim DW *et al.*, 2013); Anti-oxidative (Kim KJ *et al.*, 2010; Liang Q *et al.*, 2010; Wang X *et al.*, 2010); Anti-Parkinson's (Li XZ *et al.*, 2013; Li XZ *et al.*, 2014; Liu SM *et al.*, 2012); Anti-ulcer (Fujikawa T *et al.*, 1996); Anti-viral (Glatthaar-Saalmuller B *et al.*, 2001); Anxiolytic (Huang L *et al.*, 2011; Soya H *et al.*, 2008); Hepatoprotective (Huang L *et al.*, 2011, Smalinskiene A *et al.*, 2009); Immunomodulatory (Han J *et al.*, 2014; Li W *et al.*, 2013; Shen ML *et al.*, 1991); Neuroprotective (Bu Y *et al.*, 2005; Lee D *et al.*, 2012).

In addition, *E. senticosus* exhibits potential protective effects against the following conditions: Cadmium poisoning (Smalinskiene A *et al.*, 2014); Endotoxic shock (Lin QY *et al.*, 2008a).

3.1.4 *Actions*

To reinforce qi, to invigorate the function of the spleen and the kidney, and to calm the mind (The State Pharmacopoeia Commission of P.R. China 2010f).

3.1.5 *Indications*

The Expanded Commission E approved *E. senticosus* as a "tonic in times of fatigue and debility, declining capacity for work or concentration, and during convalescences". Other uses for *E. senticosus* are for "chronic inflammatory conditions and traditionally for functional asthenia" (Blumenthal M *et al.*, 2000). In TCM context, indications for *E. senticosus* include "Spleen–Lung qi deficiency, weak constitution and lack of strength, anepithymia (loss of appetite), dual deficiency of lung and kidney, chronic cough and dyspnea of deficiency type, limp aching in lower back and knees caused by kidney deficiency, insomnia and dream-disturbed sleep" (The State Pharmacopoeia Commission of P.R. China, 2010f).

3.1.6 *Dosage and administration*

a) 9 to 27 g (The State Pharmacopoeia Commission of P.R. China, 2010f).
b) Unless otherwise prescribed, 2 to 3 g per day of powdered or cut root for teas for up to three months, as well as aqueous alcoholic extracts for internal use. A repeated course is feasible.
c) Infusion: 2 to 3 g in 150 ml of water (b and c: Blumenthal M *et al.*, 2000).

3.1.7 *Safety considerations*

3.1.7.1 *Side effects and interactions with other herbs*

E. senticosus is generally considered to be milder in activity than the more stimulating *Panax ginseng* (Blumenthal M *et al.*, 2000). The Expanded Commission E reported its side effects as "None known", although it noted that the herb is contraindicated in people with hypertension (Blumenthal M *et al.*, 2000; Farnsworth NR, 1985). However, the glycosides contained in *E. senticosus* have been shown to lower blood pressure (McGuffin M *et al.*, 1997).

3.1.7.2 *Use during pregnancy and lactation*

No restrictions known (Blumenthal M *et al.*, 2000).

3.1.7.3 *Interaction with drugs*

While no herb–drug interaction has been reported in the Expanded Commission E Monographs (Blumenthal M *et al.*, 2000), *E. senticosus* has been shown to increase the transport of digoxin (a cardiac glycoside) and decrease the transport of cephalexin (an antibiotic) across human intestinal cell line (Takahashi T *et al.*, 2010), which leads to a increase and decrease in efficacy of the two drugs, respectively.

3.2 Five-Leaf Ginseng or Jiao Gu Lan

3.2.1 *Introduction*

Latin Name/Botanical Name: *Gynostemma pentaphyllum* **(Thunb.) Makino (Cucurbitaceae family)**

Pharmaceutical Name: Herba Gynostemmae Pentaphylli

Origin: Widely distributed throughout China, India, Myanmar, Korea, and Japan

Other Names: 绞股蓝 **(Jiao Gu Lan)**

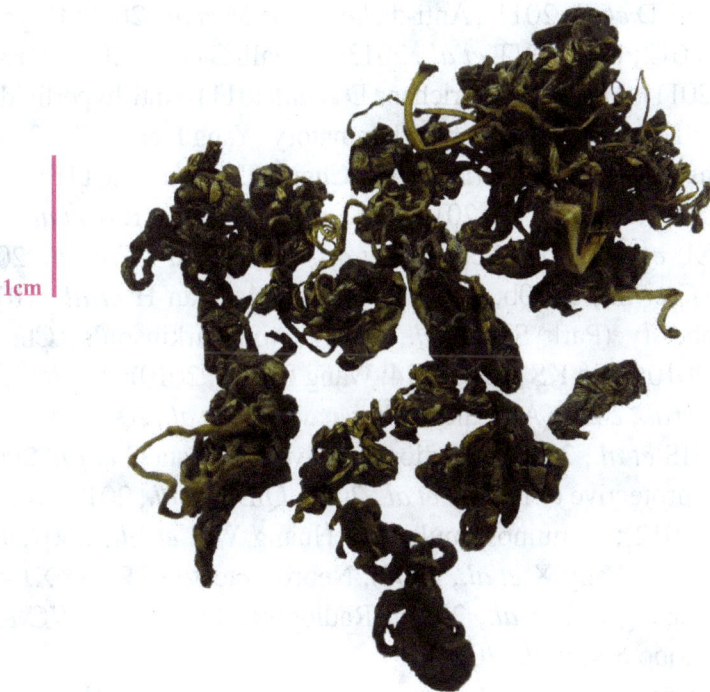

1cm

Figure 3.2   Photograph of dried *Gynostemma pentaphyllum*.

3.2.2 *Phytoconstituents*

G. pentaphyllum contains saponins (Kao TH *et al.*, 2008), flavo-noids (Kao TH *et al.*, 2008), chlorophyll (Tsai YC *et al.*, 2010b), carotenoids (Tsai YC *et al.*, 2010b) and polysaccharides (Chi A *et al.*, 2012). Its major active principles are gypenosides, a type of saponin and examples include gypenosides III, VII (Circosta C *et al.*, 2005a), XVII (Meng X *et al.*, 2014), XLIX (Huang TH *et al.*, 2006) and LXXIV (Joh EH *et al.*, 2010). Similar to *P. ginseng, G. pentaphyllum* contains ginsenosides Rb1, Rb3, Rd and F2 (Lu JG *et al.*, 2013).

3.2.3 *Pharmacological activities*

General review (Zhao Z and Xiao P, 2010); Anti-Alzheimer's (Zhang G *et al.*, 2011); Anti-asthmatic (Circosta C *et al.*, 2005b; Huang WC *et al.*, 2008; Liou CJ *et al.*, 2010); Anti-bacterial (Srichana D *et al.*, 2011); Anti-diabetic (Ge M *et al.*, 2009; Huyen VT *et al.*, 2012; Huyen VT *et al.*, 2013; Megalli S *et al.*, 2007; Yassin K *et al.*, 2011); Anti-fungal (Srichana D *et al.*, 2011); Anti-hyperlipidemic (Yang YH *et al.*, 2013); Anti-inflammatory (Yang F *et al.*, 2013); Anti-neoplastic (Chen DJ *et al.*, 2014; Cheng TC *et al.*, 2011; Hsu HY *et al.*, 2011; Lin JJ *et al.*, 2011; Liu J *et al.*, 2014; Lu KW *et al.*, 2010; Piao XL *et al.*, 2013; Schild L *et al.*, 2010; Tsai YC *et al.*, 2010a; Tsai YC *et al.*, 2010b; Yan H *et al.*, 2014a; Yan H *et al.*, 2014b); Anti-obesity (Park SH *et al.*, 2014); Anti-Parkinson's (Choi HS *et al.*, 2010; Shin KS *et al.*, 2014; Wang P *et al.*, 2010); Anti-oxidative (Chi A *et al.*, 2012); Anti-ulcer (Rujjanawate C *et al.*, 2004); Anxiolytic (Choi HS *et al.*, 2013); Cardioprotective (Circosta C *et al.*, 2005a); Hepatoprotective (Chen JC *et al.*, 2008; Qin R *et al.*, 2012; Müller C *et al.*, 2012); Immunostimulatory (Huang WC *et al.*, 2007; Liu J *et al.*, 2014; Yang X *et al.*, 2008); Neuroprotective (Wang XJ *et al.*, 2014; Zhang GL *et al.*, 2011); Radioprotective (Chen WC *et al.*, 1996; Lobo SN *et al.*, 2014).

Although *G. pentaphyllum* is consumed as an herbal tea, its use in TCM is limited and it is not included in the Chinese Pharmacopoeia.

3.2.4 *Safety considerations*

3.2.4.1 *Interactions with drugs*

Gypenosides showed strong interaction with dextromethorphan (antitussive) via CYP2D6 inhibition, weak interaction with paclitaxel (chemotherapy drug) via CYP2C8 inhibition, weak interaction with midazolam (benzodiazepine) and testosterone (steroid hormone) via CYP3A4 inhibition and weak interaction with tolbutamide (oral hypoglycemic agent) via CYP2C9 inhibition (He M *et al.*, 2013).

References

Ahn J, Um MY, Lee H, Jung CH, Heo SH, Ha TY (2013). Eleutheroside E, an active component of *Eleutherococcus senticosus*, ameliorates insulin resistance in type 2 diabetic db/db mice. *Evid Based Complement Alternat Med* 934183.

Bai Y, Tohda C, Zhu S, Hattori M, Komatsu K (2011). Active components from Siberian ginseng (*Eleutherococcus senticosus*) for protection of amyloid β(25-35)-induced neuritic atrophy in cultured rat cortical neurons. *J Nat Med* **65**(3–4): 417–423.

Bleakney TL (2008). Deconstructing an adaptogen: *Eleutherococcus senticosus*. *Holist Nurs Pract* **22**(4): 220–224.

Blumenthal M, Goldberg A, Brinckmann J (2000). *Herbal Medicine Expanded Commission E Monographs*. 1st ed. Boston: Integrative Medicine Communications.

Bu Y, Jin ZH, Park SY, Baek S, Rho S, Ha N, Park SK, Kim H, Kim SY (2005). Siberian ginseng reduces infarct volume in transient focal cerebral ischaemia in Sprague-Dawley rats. *Phytother Res* **19**(2): 167–169.

Cha YS, Rhee SJ, Heo YR (2004). *Acanthopanax senticosus* extract prepared from cultured cells decreases adiposity and obesity indices in C57BL/6J mice fed a high fat diet. *J Med Food* **7**(4): 422–429.

Chen DJ, Liu HM, Xing SF, Piao XL (2014). Cytotoxic activity of gypenosides and gynogenin against non-small cell lung carcinoma A549 cells. *Bioorg Med Chem Lett* **24**(1): 186–191.

Chen JC, Tsai CC, Chen LD, Chen HH, Wang WC (2008). Therapeutic effect of gypenoside on chronic liver injury and fibrosis induced by CCl4 in rats. *Am J Chin Med* **28**(2): 175–185.

Chen WC, Hau DM, Chen KT, Wang MI, Lin IH (1996). Protective effects of *Gynostemma pentaphyllum* in gamma-irradiated mice. *Am J Chin Med* **24**(1): 83–92.

Cheng TC, Lu JF, Wang JS, Lin LJ, Kuo HI, Chen BH (2011). Antiproliferation effect and apoptosis mechanism of prostate cancer cell PC-3 by flavonoids and saponins prepared from *Gynostemma pentaphyllum*. *J Agric Food Chem* **59**(20): 11319–11329.

Chi A, Tang L, Zhang J, Zhang K (2012). Chemical composition of three polysaccharides from *Gynostemma pentaphyllum* and their antioxidant activity in skeletal muscle of exercised mice. *Int J Sport Nutr Exerc Metab* **22**(6): 479–485.

Choi HS, Park MS, Kim SH, Hwang BY, Lee CK, Lee MK (2010). Neuroprotective effects of herbal ethanol extracts from *Gynostemma pentaphyllum* in the 6-hydroxydopamine-lesioned rat model of Parkinson's disease. *Molecules* **15**(4): 2814–2824.

Choi HS, Zhao TT, Shin KS, Kim SH, Hwang BY, Lee CK, Lee MK, (2013). Anxiolytic effects of herbal ethanol extract from *Gynostemma pentaphyllum* in mice after exposure to chronic stress. *Molecules* **18**(4): 4342–4356.

Circosta C, De Pasquale R, Occhiuto F (2005a). Cardiovascular effects of the aqueous extract of *Gynostemma pentaphyllum* Makino. *Phytomedicine* **12**(9): 638–643.

Circosta C, De Pasquale R, Palumbo DR, Occhiuto F (2005b). Bronchodilatory effects of the aqueous extract of *Gynostemma pentaphyllum* and gypenosides III and VIII in anaesthetized guinea-pigs. *J Pharm Pharmacol* **57**(8): 1053–1058.

Deyama T, Nishibe S, Nakazawa Y (2001). Constituents and pharmacological effects of Eucommia and Siberian ginseng. *Acta Pharmacol Sin* **22**(12): 1057–1070.

Farnsworth NR (1985). Siberian ginseng (*Eleutherococus senticosus*): current status as an adaptogen. In Wagner H, Hikino H, Farnsworth NR (eds). *Economic and Medicinal Plant Research*. Volume 1. London: Academic Press.

Fujikawa T, Yamaguchi A, Morita I, Takeda H, Nishibe S (1996). Protective effects of *Acanthopanax senticosus* Harms from Hokkaido and its components on gastric ulcer in restrained cold water stressed rats. *Biol Pharm Bull* **19**(9): 1227–1230.

Ge M, Ma S, Tao L, Guan S (2009). The effect of gypenosides on cardiac function and expression of cytoskeletal genes of myocardium in diabetic cardiomyopathy rats. *Am J Chin Med* **37**(6): 1059–1068.

Glatthaar-Saalmüller B, Sacher F, Esperester A (2001). Antiviral activity of an extract derived from roots of *Eleutherococcus senticosus*. *Antiviral Res* **50**(3): 223–228.

Hacker B, Medon PJ (1984). Cytotoxic effects of *Eleutherococcus senticosus* aqueous extracts in combination with N6-(delta 2-isopentenyl)-adenosine and 1-beta-D-arabinofuranosylcytosine against L1210 leukemia cells. *J Pharm Sci* **73**(2): 270–272.

Han J, Bian L, Liu X, Zhang F, Zhang Y, Yu N (2014). Effects of *Acanthopanax senticosus* polysaccharide supplementation on growth performance, immunity, blood parameters and expression of pro-inflammatory cytokines genes in challenged weaned piglets. *Asian-Australas J Anim Sci* **27**(7): 1035–1043.

He C, Chen X, Zhao C, Qie Y, Yan Z, Zhu X (2014). Eleutheroside E ameliorates arthritis severity in collagen-induced arthritis mice model by suppressing inflammatory cytokine release. *Inflammation* **37**(5): 1533–1543.

He M, Jiang J, Qiu F, Liu S, Peng P, Gao C, Miao P (2013). Inhibitory effects of gypenosides on seven human cytochrome P450 enzymes *in vitro*. *Food Chem Toxicol* **57**: 262–265.

Hibasami H, Fujikawa T, Takeda H, Nishibe S, Satoh T, Fujisawa T, Nakashima K (2000). Induction of apoptosis by *Acanthopanax senticosus* HARMS and its component, sesamin in human stomach cancer KATO III cells. *Oncol Rep* **7**(6): 1213–1216.

Hikino H, Takahashi M, Otake K, Konno C (1986). Isolation and hypoglycemic activity of eleutherans A, B, C, D, E, F, and G: glycans of *Eleutherococcus senticosus* roots. *J Nat Prod* **49**(2): 293–297.

Hsu HY, Yang JS, Lu KW, Yu CS, Chou ST, Lin JJ, Chen YY, Lin ML, Chueh FS, Chen SS, Chung JG (2011). An experimental study on the antileukemia effects of gypenosides *in vitro* and *in vivo*. *Integr Cancer Ther* **10**(1): 101–112.

Huang L, Zhao H, Huang B, Zheng C, Peng W, Qin L (2011). *Acanthopanax senticosus*: review of botany, chemistry and pharmacology. *Pharmazie* **66**(2): 83–97.

Huang LZ, Huang BK, Ye Q, Qin LP (2011a). Bioactivity-guided fractionation for anti-fatigue property of *Acanthopanax senticosus*. *J Ethnopharmacol* **133**(1): 213–219.

Huang LZ, Wei L, Zhao HF, Huang BK, Rahman K, Qin LP (2011b). The effect of Eleutheroside E on behavioral alterations in murine sleep deprivation stress model. *Eur J Pharmacol* **658**(2–3): 150–155.

Huang TH, Li Y, Razmovski-Naumovski V, Tran VH, Li GQ, Duke CC, Roufogalis BD (2006). Gypenoside XLIX isolated from *Gynostemma pentaphyllum* inhibits nuclear factor-kappaB activation via a PPAR-alpha-dependent pathway. *J Biomed Sci* **13**(4): 535–548.

Huang WC, Kuo ML, Li ML, Yang RC, Liou CJ, Shen JJ (2007). Extract of *Gynostemma pentaphyllum* enhanced the production of antibodies and cytokines in mice. *Yakugaku Zasshi* **127**(5): 889–896.

Huang WC, Kuo ML, Li ML, Yang RC, Liou CJ, Shen JJ (2008). *Gynostemma pentaphyllum* decreases allergic reactions in a murine asthmatic model. *Am J Chin Med* **36**(3): 579–592.

Huyen VT, Phan DV, Thang P, Hoa NK, Ostenson CG (2013). *Gynostemma pentaphyllum* tea improves insulin sensitivity in type 2 diabetic patients. *J Nutr Metab* 765383.

Huyen VT, Phan DV, Thang P, Ky PT, Hoa NK, Ostenson CG (2012). Antidiabetic effects of add-on *Gynostemma pentaphyllum* extract therapy with sulfonylureas in type 2 diabetic patients. *Evid Based Complement Altern Med* 452313.

Hwang YC, Jeong IK, Ahn KJ, Chung HY (2009). The effects of *Acanthopanax senticosus* extract on bone turnover and bone mineral density in Korean postmenopausal women. *J Bone Miner Metab* **27**(5): 584–590.

Jin L, Wu F, Li X, Li H, Du C, Jiang Q, You J, Li S, Xu Y (2013). Antidepressant effects of aqueous extract from *Acanthopanax senticosus* in mice. *Phytother Res* **27**(12): 1829–1833.

Joh EH, Yang JW, Kim DH (2010). Gypenoside LXXIV ameliorates scopolamine-induced learning deficit in mice. *Planta Med* **76**(8): 793–795.

Kao TH, Huang SC, Inbaraj BS, Chen BH (2008). Determination of flavonoids and saponins in *Gynostemma pentaphyllum* (Thunb.) Makino by liquid chromatography-mass spectrometry. *Anal Chim Acta* **626**(2): 200–211.

Kim HJ, McLean D, Pyee J, Kim J, Park H (2014). Extract from *Acanthopanax senticosus* prevents LPS-induced monocytic cell adhesion via suppression of LFA-1 and Mac-1. *Can J Physiol Pharmacol* **92**(4): 278–284.

Kim HS, Park SY, Kim EK, Ryu EY, Kim YH, Park G, Lee SJ (2012). *Acanthopanax senticosus* has a heme oxygenase-1 signaling-dependent effect on *Porphyromonas gingivalis* lipopolysaccharide-stimulated macrophages. *J Ethnopharmacol* **142**(3): 819–828.

Kim KJ, Hong HD, Lee OH, Lee BY (2010). The effects of *Acanthopanax senticosus* on global hepatic gene expression in rats subjected to heat environmental stress. *Toxicology* **278**(2): 217–223.

Kuo J, Chen KW, Cheng IS, Tsai PH, Lu YJ, Lee NY (2010). The effect of eight weeks of supplementation with *Eleutherococcus senticosus* on endurance capacity and metabolism in human. *Chin J Physiol* **53**(2): 105–111.

Lee D, Park J, Yoon J, Kim MY, Choi HY, Kim H (2012). Neuroprotective effects of *Eleutherococcus senticosus* bark on transient global cerebral ischemia in rats. *J Ethnopharmacol* **139**(1): 6–11.

Li W, Luo Q, Jin LH (2013). *Acanthopanax senticosus* extracts have a protective effect on *Drosophila* gut immunity. *J Ethnopharmacol* **146**(1): 257–263.

Li XZ, Zhang SN, Lu F, Liu CF, Wang Y, Bai Y, Wang N, Liu SM (2013). Cerebral metabonomics study on Parkinson's disease mice treated with extract of *Acanthopanax senticosus* harms. *Phytomedicine* **20**(13): 1219–1229.

Li XZ, Zhang SN, Wang KX, Liu SM, Lu F (2014). iTRAQ-based quantitative proteomics study on the neuroprotective effects of extract of *Acanthopanax senticosus* harm on SH-SY5Y cells overexpressing A53T mutant α-synuclein. *Neurochem Int* **72**: 37–47.

Liang Q, Yu X, Qu S, Xu H, Sui D (2010). *Acanthopanax senticosides* B ameliorates oxidative damage induced by hydrogen peroxide in cultured neonatal rat cardiomyocytes. *Eur J Pharmacol* **627**(1–3): 209–215.

Lim DW, Kim JG, Lee Y, Cha SH, Kim YT (2013). Preventive effects of *Eleutherococcus senticosus* bark extract in OVX-induced osteoporosis in rats. *Molecules* **18**(7): 7998–8008.

Lin JJ, Hsu HY, Yang JS, Lu KW, Wu RS, Wu KC, Lai TY, Chen PY, Ma CY, Wood WG, Chung JG (2011). Molecular evidence of anti-leukemia activity of gypenosides on human myeloid leukemia HL-60 cells *in vitro* and *in vivo* using a HL-60 cells murine xenograft model. *Phytomedicine* **18**(12): 1075–1085.

Lin QY, Jin LJ, Cao ZH, Li HQ, Xu YP (2008a). Protective effect of *Acanthopanax senticosus* extract against endotoxic shock in mice. *J Ethnopharmacol* **118**(3): 495–502.

Lin QY, Jin LJ, Cao ZH, Lu YN, Xue HY, Xu YP (2008b). *Acanthopanax senticosus* suppresses reactive oxygen species production by mouse peritoneal macrophages *in vitro* and *in vivo*. *Phytother Res* **22**(6): 740–745.

Liou CJ, Huang WC, Kuo ML, Yang RC, Shen JJ (2010). Long-term oral administration of *Gynostemma pentaphyllum* extract attenuates airway inflammation and Th2 cell activities in ovalbumin-sensitized mice. *Food Chem Toxicol* **48**(10): 2592–2598.

Liu J, Zhang L, Ren Y, Gao Y, Kang L, Qiao Q (2014). Anticancer and immunoregulatory activity of *Gynostemma pentaphyllum* polysaccharides in H22 tumor-bearing mice. *Int J Biol Macromol* **69**: 1–4.

Liu SM, Li XZ, Huo Y, Lu F (2012). Protective effect of extract of *Acanthopanax senticosus* Harms on dopaminergic neurons in Parkinson's disease mice. *Phytomedicine* **19**(7): 631–638.

Liu TP, Lee CS, Liou SS, Liu IM, Cheng JT (2005). Improvement of insulin resistance by *Acanthopanax senticosus* root in fructose-rich chow-fed rats. *Clin Exp Pharmacol Physiol* **32**(8): 649–654.

Lobo SN, Qi YQ, Liu QZ (2014). The effect of *Gynostemma pentaphyllum* extract on mouse dermal fibroblasts. *ISRN Dermatol* 202876.

Lu JG, Zhu L, Lo KY, Leung AK, Ho AH, Zhang HY, Zhao ZZ, Fong DW, Jiang ZH (2013). Chemical differentiation of two taste variants of *Gynostemma pentaphyllum* by using UPLC-Q-TOF-MS and HPLC-ELSD. *J Agric Food Chem* **61**(1): 90–97.

Lu KW, Chen JC, Lai TY, Yang JS, Weng SW, Ma YS, Tang NY, Lu PJ, Weng JR, Chung JG (2010). Gypenosides causes DNA damage and inhibits expression of DNA repair genes of human oral cancer SAS cells. *In Vivo* **24**(3): 287–291.

McGuffin M, Hobbs C, Upton R, Goldberg A (1997). *American Herbal Product Association's Botanical Safety Handbook*. Boca Raton: CRC Press.

Megalli S, Davies NM, Roufogalis BD (2007). Anti-hyperlipidemic and hypoglycemic effects of *Gynostemma pentaphyllum* in the Zucker fatty rat. *J Pharm Pharm Sci* **9**(3): 281–291.

Meng X, Wang M, Sun G, Ye J, Zhou Y, Dong X, Wang T, Lu S, Sun X (2014). Attenuation of Aβ25-35-induced parallel autophagic and apoptotic cell death by gypenoside XVII through the estrogen receptor-dependent activation of Nrf2/ARE pathways. *Toxicol Appl Pharmacol* **279**(1): 63–75.

Müller C, Gardemann A, Keilhoff G, Peter D, Wiswedel I, Schild L (2012). Prevention of free fatty acid-induced lipid accumulation, oxidative stress, and cell death in primary hepatocyte cultures by a *Gynostemma pentaphyllum* extract. *Phytomedicine* **19**(5): 395–401.

Niu HS, Liu IM, Cheng JT, Lin CL, Hsu FL (2008). Hypoglycemic effect of syringin from *Eleutherococcus senticosus* in streptozotocin-induced diabetic rats. *Planta Med* **74**(2): 109–113.

Park SH, Huh TL, Kim SY, Oh MR, Tirupathi Pichiah PB, Chae SW, Cha YS (2014). Antiobesity effect of *Gynostemma pentaphyllum* extract (actiponin): a randomized, double-blind, placebo-controlled trial. *Obesity (Silver Spring)* **22**(1): 63–71.

Park SH, Lee SG, Kang SK, Chung SH (2006). *Acanthopanax senticosus* reverses fatty liver disease and hyperglycemia in ob/ob mice. *Arch Pharm Res* **29**(9): 768–776.

Piao XL, Wu Q, Yang J, Park SY, Chen DJ, Liu HM (2013). Dammarane-type saponins from heat-processed *Gynostemma pentaphyllum* show fortified activity against A549 cells. *Arch Pharm Res* **36**(7): 874–879.

Qin R, Zhang J, Li C, Zhang X, Xiong A, Huang F, Yin Z, Li K, Qin W, Chen M, Zhang S, Liang L, Zhang H, Nie H, Ye W (2012). Protective effects of gypenosides against fatty liver disease induced by high fat and cholesterol diet and alcohol in rats. *Arch Pharm Res* **35**(7): 1241–1250.

Rhim YT, Kim H, Yoon SJ, Kim SS, Chang HK, Lee TH, Lee HH, Shin MC, Shin MS, Kim CJ (2007). Effect of *Acanthopanax senticosus* on 5-hydroxytryptamine synthesis and tryptophan hydroxylase expression in the dorsal raphe of exercised rats. *J Ethnopharmacol* **114**(1): 38–43.

Rujjanawate C, Kanjanapothi D, Amornlerdpison D (2004). The anti-gastric ulcer effect of *Gynostemma pentaphyllum* Makino. *Phytomedicine* **11**(5): 431–435.

Schild L, Chen BH, Makarov P, Kattengell K, Heinitz K, Keilhoff G (2010). Selective induction of apoptosis in glioma tumour cells by a *Gynostemma pentaphyllum* extract. *Phytomedicine* **17**(8–9): 589–597.

Shen ML, Zhai SK, Chen HL, Luo YD, Tu GR, Ou DW (1991). Immunomopharmacological effects of polysaccharides from *Acanthopanax senticosus* on experimental animals. *Int J Immunopharmacol* **13**(5): 549–554.

Shin KS, Zhao TT, Choi HS, Hwang BY, Lee CK, Lee MK (2014). Effects of gypenosides on anxiety disorders in MPTP-lesioned mouse model of Parkinson's disease. *Brain Res* **1567**: 57–65.

Smalinskiene A, Lesauskaite V, Zitkevicius V, Savickiene N, Savickas A, Ryselis S, Sadauskiene I, Ivanov L (2009). Estimation of the combined effect of *Eleutherococcus senticosus* extract and cadmium on liver cells. *Ann N Y Acad Sci* **1171**: 314–320.

Smalinskiene A, Savickiene N, Zitkevicius V, Pangonyte D, Sadauskiene I, Kasauskas A, Ivanov L, Lesauskaite V, Savickas A, Rodovičius H (2014). Effect of *Acanthopanax senticosus* on the accumulation of cadmium and on the immune response of spleen cells. *J Toxicol Environ Health A* **77**(21): 1311–1318.

Soya H, Deocaris CC, Yamaguchi K, Ohiwa N, Saito T, Nishijima T, Kato M, Tateoka M, Matsui T, Okamoto M, Fujikawa T (2008). Extract from *Acanthopanax senticosus* harms (Siberian ginseng) activates NTS and SON/PVN in the rat brain. *Biosci Biotechnol Biochem* **72**(9): 2476–2480.

Srichana D, Taengtip R, Kondo S (2011). Antimicrobial activity of *Gynostemma pentaphyllum* extracts against fungi producing aflatoxin and fumonisin and bacteria causing diarrheal disease. *Southeast Asian J Trop Med Public Health* **42**(3): 704–710.

Takahashi T, Kaku T, Sato T, Watanabe K, Sato J (2010). Effects of *Acanthopanax senticosus* HARMS extract on drug transport in human intestinal cell line Caco-2. *J Nat Med* **64**(1): 55–62.

Takahashi Y, Tanaka M, Murai R, Kuribayashi K, Kobayashi D, Yanagihara N, Watanabe N (2014). Prophylactic and therapeutic effects of *Acanthopanax senticosus* harms extract on murine collagen-induced arthritis. *Phytother Res* **28**(10): 1513–1519.

The State Pharmacopoeia Commission of P.R. China (2010a: p210; 2010b: p211; 2010c: p310; 2010d: p311; 2010e: p299; 2010f: p6). *Pharmacopoeia of the People's Republic of China*. Volume 1. Beijing: China Medical Science Press [English version].

The State Pharmacopoeia Commission of P.R. China (2000). *Pharmacopoeia of the People's Republic of China*. Volume 1. Beijing: Beijing Chemical Industry Press, p. 184 [Chinese version].

Tohda C, Ichimura M, Bai Y, Tanaka K, Zhu S, Komatsu K (2008). Inhibitory effects of *Eleutherococcus senticosus* extracts on amyloid beta(25-35)-induced neuritic atrophy and synaptic loss. *J Pharmacol Sci* **107**(3): 329–339.

Tsai YC, Lin CL, Chen BH (2010a). Preparative chromatography of flavonoids and saponins in *Gynostemma pentaphyllum* and their antiproliferation effect on hepatoma cell. *Phytomedicine* **18**(1): 2–10.

Tsai YC, Wu WB, Chen BH (2010b). Preparation of carotenoids and chlorophylls from *Gynostemma pentaphyllum* (Thunb.) Makino and their antiproliferation effect on hepatoma cell. *J Med Food* **13**(6): 1431–1442.

Wang P, Niu L, Gao L, Li WX, Jia D, Wang XL, Gao GD (2010). Neuroprotective effect of gypenosides against oxidative injury in the substantia nigra of a mouse model of Parkinson's disease. *J Int Med Res* **38**(3): 1084–1092.

Wang X, Hai CX, Liang X, Yu SX, Zhang W, Li YL (2010). The protective effects of *Acanthopanax senticosus* Harms aqueous extracts against oxidative stress: role of Nrf2 and antioxidant enzymes. *J Ethnopharmacol* **127**(2): 424–432.

Wang XJ, Sun T, Kong L, Shang ZH, Yang KQ, Zhang QY, Jing FM, Dong L, Xu XF, Liu JX, Xin H, Chen ZY (2014). Gypenosides pretreatment protects the brain against cerebral ischemia and increases neural stem cells/progenitors in the subventricular zone. *Int J Dev Neurosci* **33**: 49–56.

Wu F, Li H, Zhao L, Li X, You J, Jiang Q, Li S, Jin L, Xu Y (2013). Protective effects of aqueous extract from *Acanthopanax senticosus* against corticosterone-induced neurotoxicity in PC12 cells. *J Ethnopharmacol* **148**(3): 861–868.

Yan H, Wang X, Niu J, Wang Y, Wang P, Liu Q (2014a). Anti-cancer effect and the underlying mechanisms of gypenosides on human colorectal cancer SW-480 cells. *PLoS One* **9**(4): e95609.

Yan H, Wang X, Wang Y, Wang P, Xiao Y (2014b). Antiproliferation and anti-migration induced by gypenosides in human colon cancer SW620 and esophageal cancer Eca-109 cells. *Hum Exp Toxicol* **33**(5): 522–533.

Yang F, Shi H, Zhang X, Yang H, Zhou Q, Yu LL (2013). Two new saponins from tetraploid jiaogulan (*Gynostemma pentaphyllum*), and their anti-inflammatory and alpha-glucosidase inhibitory activities. *Food Chem* **141**(4): 3606–3613.

Yang X, Zhao Y, Yang Y, Ruan Y (2008). Isolation and characterization of immunostimulatory polysaccharide from an herb tea, *Gynostemma pentaphyllum* Makino. *J Agric Food Chem* **56**(16): 6905–6909.

Yang YH, Yang J, Jiang QH (2013). Hypolipidemic effect of gypenosides in experimentally induced hypercholesterolemic rats. *Lipids Health Dis* **12**: 154.

Yassin K, Huyen VT, Hoa KN, Ostenson CG (2011). Herbal extract of *Gynostemma pentaphyllum* decreases hepatic glucose output in type 2 diabetic goto-kakizaki rats. *Int J Biomed Sci* **7**(2): 131–136.

Yoon TJ, Yoo YC, Lee SW, Shin KS, Choi WH, Hwang SH, Ha ES, Jo SK, Kim SH, Park WM (2004). Anti-metastatic activity of *Acanthopanax senticosus* extract and its possible immunological mechanism of action. *J Ethnopharmacol* **93**(2–3): 247–253.

Zhang G, Zhao Z, Gao L, Deng J, Wang B, Xu D, Liu B, Qu Y, Yu J, Li J, Gao G (2011). Gypenoside attenuates white matter lesions induced by chronic cerebral hypoperfusion in rats. *Pharmacol Biochem Behav* **99**(1): 42–51.

Zhang, GL, Deng JP, Wang BH, Zhao ZW, Li J, Gao L, Liu BL, Xong JR, Guo XD, Yan ZQ, Gao GD (2011). Gypenosides improve cognitive impairment induced by chronic cerebral hypoperfusion in rats by suppressing oxidative stress and astrocytic activation. *Behav Pharmacol* **22**(7): 633–644.

Zhang N, Van Crombruggen K, Holtappels G, Bachert C (2012). A herbal composition of *Scutellaria baicalensis* and *Eleutherococcus senticosus* shows potent anti-inflammatory effects in an *ex vivo* human mucosal tissue model. *Evid Based Complement Altern Med* 673145.

Zhao Z, Xiao P (2009). *Encyclopedia of Medicinal Plants*. Volume 1. Shanghai: Shanghai World Publishing Corporation.

Zhao Z, Xiao P (2010). *Encyclopedia of Medicinal Plants*. Volume 4. Shanghai: Shanghai World Publishing Corporation.

Ginseng Products in Singapore

4.1 Introduction

Most papers on Chinese Proprietary Medicine (CPM) focus on adulterations, heavy metals or poisonous ingredients in these products (Koh HL and Woo S, 2000; Yee SK *et al.*, 2005).

Many commercially available health products (e.g. CPM) and food products contain "ginseng". The word "ginseng" has been used to refer to herbs of different species in the genus Panax as well as other plants. Health products containing Panax species are commonly used (Kang E *et al.*, 2012; Smith L *et al.*, 2004; Froiland K *et al.*, 2004; Ayranci U *et al.*, 2005). Since such products are readily available from supermarkets, herbal stores, health supplements stores and pharmacies, the consumers may rely on the information on the packaging or labels to help them make a decision before they purchase. In Chapters 2 and 3, detailed information on *Panax ginseng* (ginseng root), *Panax notoginseng* (San Qi or Tian Qi), *Panax quinquefolius* (American ginseng), *Eleutherococcus senticosus* (Siberian ginseng) and *Gynostemma pentaphyllum* (five-leaf ginseng) were presented. Different Panax species have different active ingredients and different uses. It is important that the correct herb is used. Furthermore, it is important for the information on these products to be comprehensive and clear and that they comply with the labeling and other regulations of Singapore. There may be errors in the labeling or incomplete labeling.

Table 4.1 List of plants which have been referred to as "ginseng" but which do not belong to the genus Panax.

No.	Latin name	Common name(s)
1	*Angelica sinensis*	Female ginseng, also commonly known as Dong Quai
2	*Eleutherococcus senticosus* (syn. *Acanthopanax senticosus*)	Siberian ginseng, also commonly known as 刺五加 (Ci Wu Jia)
3	*Eurycoma longifolia*	Malaysian ginseng, Tongkat Ali
4	*Gynostemma pentaphyllum*	Southern ginseng, also commonly known as Jiao Gu Lan, five-leaf ginseng
5	*Lepidium meyenii*	Peruvian ginseng, also commonly known as Maca
6	*Oplopanax horridus*	Alaskan ginseng
7	*Pfaffia paniculata*	Brazillian ginseng
8	*Pseudostellaria heterophylla*	Prince ginseng, also commonly known as 太子参 (Tai Zi Shen)
9	*Withania somnifera*	Indian ginseng, Ashwagandha

Table 4.1 shows a list of plants which have been referred to as "ginseng" but which do not belong to the genus Panax. They include *E. senticosus* and *G. pentaphyllum*, both of which are subjects of Chapter 3, as well as *Angelica sinensis* (Dong Quai or female ginseng) and *Eurycoma longifolia* (Tongkat ali or Malaysian ginseng), and *Withania somnifera* (Ashwaganda or Indian ginseng).

Table 4.2 shows a list of different plant species in the genus Panax and their geographical locations. (The *New York Times*, 2015).

4.2 Survey of Products

In Singapore, health products include drugs (pharmaceuticals), medical devices and complementary health products. Complementary

Table 4.2 List of plants in the genus Panax and their geographical locations.

No.	Scientific name / Pharmaceutical name	Local/Other name(s)	Geographical distribution
1	*Panax ginseng*	Bang chui	Eastern Siberia
	Radix ginseng	Chosen ninjin	Japan
		Di Jing	North Korea
		Gao Li Shen	
		Ginseng	Northeast China
		Ginsengwurzel	
		Goryo insam	
		Hakusan	
		Higeninjin	
		Hong Shen	
		Jen seng	
		Jenshen	
		Jin pi	
		Kao Li Shen	
		Korean ginseng	
		Li Shen	
		Min jin	
		Nhan sam	
		Nin jin	
		Nin zin	
		Niu huan	
		Oriental ginseng	
		Otane ninjin	
		Panax schinseng Nees	
		Ren Shen	
		Ren Xian	
		San-pi	
		Shan shen	
		Shen Cao	
		Sheng-sai-seng	
		T'ang-seng	
		Tyosenninzin	

(Continued)

Table 4.2 (*Continued*)

No.	Scientific name / Pharmaceutical name	Local/Other name(s)	Geographical distribution
		Yakuyo ninjin	
		Yehshan-seng	
		Yuan Shen	
2	*Panax notoginseng*	Jin Bu Huan	China (Guangxi and Yunnan)
	Panax pseudoginseng var. notoginseng	Pan long Qi	
	Radix notoginseng	Sam chil	
		San chi	
		San Qi	
		Tian chi	
		Tian Qi	
3	*Panax quinquefolius*	American ginseng	North America, cultivated in North China
	Radix Panacis quinquefolii	Hua Qi Shen	
		Mei Guo Ren Shen	
		Pao Shen	
		Sei yo jin	
		Seoyangsam	
		Xi Yang Ren Shen	
		Xi Yang Shen	
		Yang Shen	
4	*Panax japonicus*	Japanese ginseng or Zhu Jie Shen	A big territory from North India to Japan
5	*Panax japonicus var. angustifolius*	Xia Ye Zhu Jie Shen	Bhutan China (Guizhuo, Sichuan and Yunnan) India, Northeast India Nepal Northeast Thailand

(*Continued*)

Table 4.2   (*Continued*)

No.	Scientific name / Pharmaceutical name	Local/Other name(s)	Geographical distribution
6	*Panax japonicus var. bipinnatifidus*	Ge Da Qi	China (Gansu, Hubei Shaanxi, Sichuan, Xizang and Yunnan)
7	*Panax japonicus var. japonicus*	Yuan Bian Zhong or Zhu Jie Shen	East China Japan Korea Vietnam
8	*Panax japonicus var. major*	Zu Tzi Seng, Zhu Zi Shen	Myanmar Nepal South China Vietnam
9	*Panax stipuleanatus, Panax vietnamensis*	Ping Bian San Qi	China (Yunnan) Vietnam
10	*Panax zingiberensis*	Jiang Zhuang San Qi	China (Yunnan)
11	*Panax pseudoginseng*	Jia Ren Shen	Eastern Himalayas and Nepal

health products include CPM (finished products in the final dosage form produced according to a TCM method), other Traditional Medicine and homeopathic medicine, health supplements (those with vitamins and/or minerals) and traditional medicinal materials. Traditional medicinal materials include medicinal materials from plants, animals or minerals in their natural states, or in processed forms that have undergone simple processing, such as cutting or drying. Examples of such materials are those used in TCM, traditional Indian medicine, traditional Malay medicine (Jamu) and also herbal medicines from other countries. With regards to legislations, the following acts and regulations are available: the Medicines Act, the Health Products Act, the Poisons Act, the Sale of Drugs Act, the Medicines (Advertisement and Sale) Act etc. The control of health products is under the purview of the Health Sciences Authority (HSA). Products that are presently subjected to licensing requirements under HSA include drugs and CPM but not health supplements. On the other hand, food and supplements of food nature come under the purview of the Agri-Food and Veterinary Authority (AVA). The import and sale of these products in Singapore are governed by the Sale of Food Act and the Food Regulations. Importers are required to ensure that the food products they intend to import comply with the requirements of the Food Regulations, including the labelling requirements. Interested readers can find out more from the Health Sciences Authority website (http://www.hsa.gov.sg/content/hsa/en/ Health_Products_Regulation/Complementary_Health_Products/ Overview.html) or from the Statutes of Singapore (http://statutes.agc. gov.sg/aol/home.w3p).

To help educate the general public about ginseng and ginseng products, we decided to find out the products available in the local market that consist of the word "ginseng". We first collated information of commercially available health and food products in local medical and health shops in Singapore that are labelled to contain "ginseng" or "Panax" on their packaging. Next, we checked if the product labels provide all recommended information required by the Ministry of Health (MOH) such as name, brand, expiry date, manufacturer, batch number, ingredients, dosage, indication, and side effects.

Information on CPM, health supplements and food supplements were collated if the word "ginseng" or "Panax" is present on their packaging. The information collated includes name of product in English, brand, ingredients, actions and indications, dosage, side effects, contraindications, cautions, manufacturer, batch number, expiry date and price. The information is collated from three stores selling herbal/health products and two pharmacies, namely, FairPrice 24 hours at HDB Clementi Branch, GNC Lot 1 Shopper's Mall Branch (GNC), Guardian Health and Beauty Lot 1 Shopper's Mall Branch (Guardian), Sinchong Meheco and Unity Pharmacy, NTUC Healthcare Hougang Mall Branch with a total of 342 relevant products.

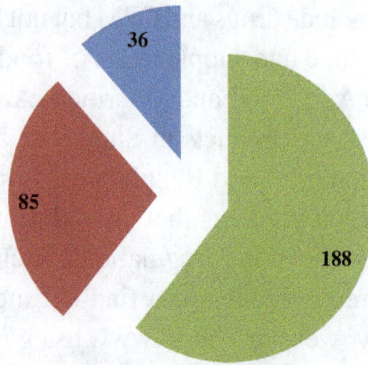

Figure 4.1   The number of products containing the word "Panax" or "ginseng" on the packaging surveyed.

A total of 342 product labels were recorded in our database. Products of the same brand and name were counted separately only if the ingredients, dosage forms, and/or information on the packaging were not similar. Products with different packaging sizes were considered as repeats and only one is used in the study as long as the dosage strength, ingredients and labeling were similar. After excluding 32 products which were repeated in our database and one product without information in English, the remaining 309 products were categorized into three groups (CPM, health supplements and food products). Figure 4.1 shows the breakdown of 309 products.

4.2.1   *Information on product label: name, brand and manufacturer*

All collated products had names on their packages and 96.5% (298) had mentioned their brand. Although it is a requirement for all the labeling information to be in English, it is found that the labels of 12 products were mostly in Korean. Therefore, the information on these packages was not comprehensible by the majority of consumers in Singapore.

Figure 4.2 shows the number of different products that included the following information on the packaging: name, brand, batch number, manufacturer, expiry date, name of ingredients, recommended daily dosage, indications, contraindications, cautions, interactions and side effects. Figure 4.3 shows the corresponding data as percentages.

Manufacturer's information was reported in 96.1% of all of products. Approximately 10% of the products had not reported their batch numbers in their labels. Batch number is important for tracking the batch of products produced at the same time, particularly important should there be any manufacturing or quality control issues.

Information on expiry date was found to be absent in five (2.6%) of CPMs, 12 (14%) of health supplements and four (11.1%) of food products. Expiry date is very important for all products and the failure to state the expiry date on the packaging may pose a risk to the consumers because expired products may no longer be effective, be of good quality or safe.

4.2.2 *Products composition*

4.2.2.1 *Four Panax species, E. senticosus and G. pentaphyllum*

Figure 4.4 shows the number of collated products, listing each plant specie in their ingredient list. Four species from the genus Panax, namely, *P. ginseng, P. quinquefolius, P. notoginseng* and *P. pseudoginseng*, and two species from other genera, namely *E. senticosus and G. pentaphyllum*, were listed on products as ingredients. The majority were labelled to contain *P. ginseng*, followed by *P. notoginseng* and *P. quinquefolius*. Interestingly, we were not able to find information on the specific Panax species of 31 of these products based on the information provided on the packaging. As can be seen, there were 19 products listed as "others". These are the products with combinations of two or more of the six plant species. The

Information

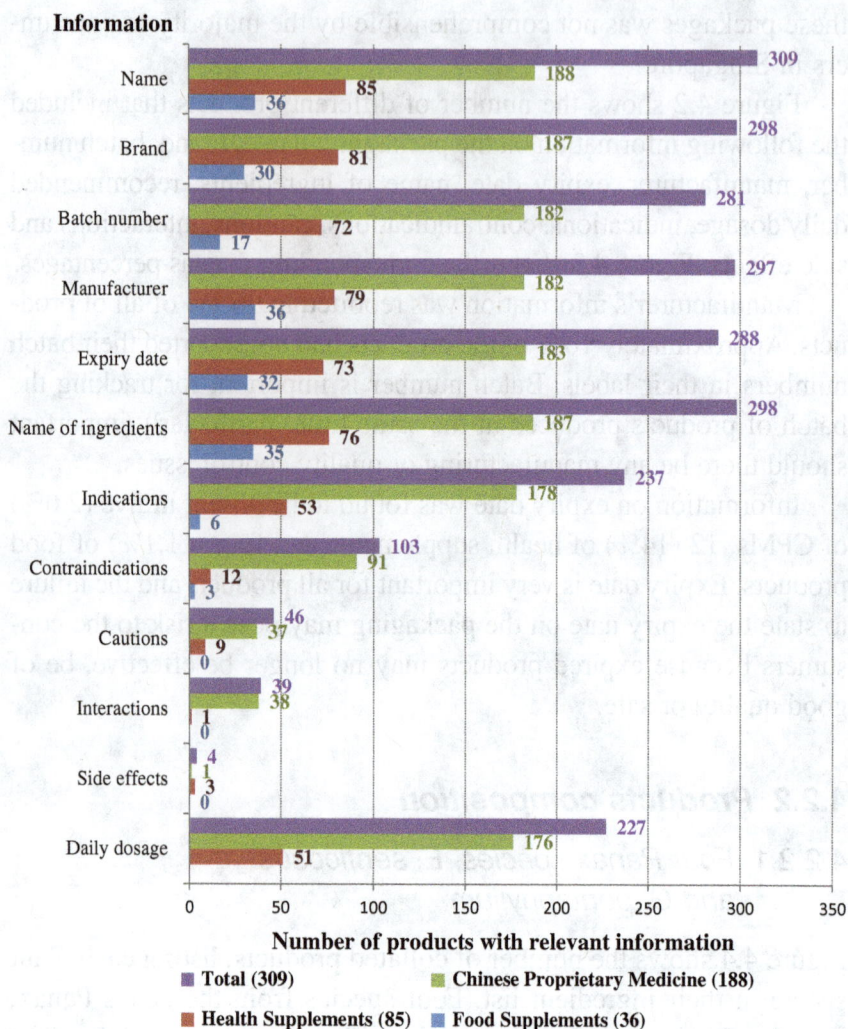

Figure 4.2   The <u>number</u> of different products that included the following information on the packaging: name, brand, batch number, manufacturer, expiry date, name of ingredients, recommended daily dosage, indications, contraindications, cautions, interactions and side effects. Recommended daily dosage is not applicable for Food Supplements (FS).

Information

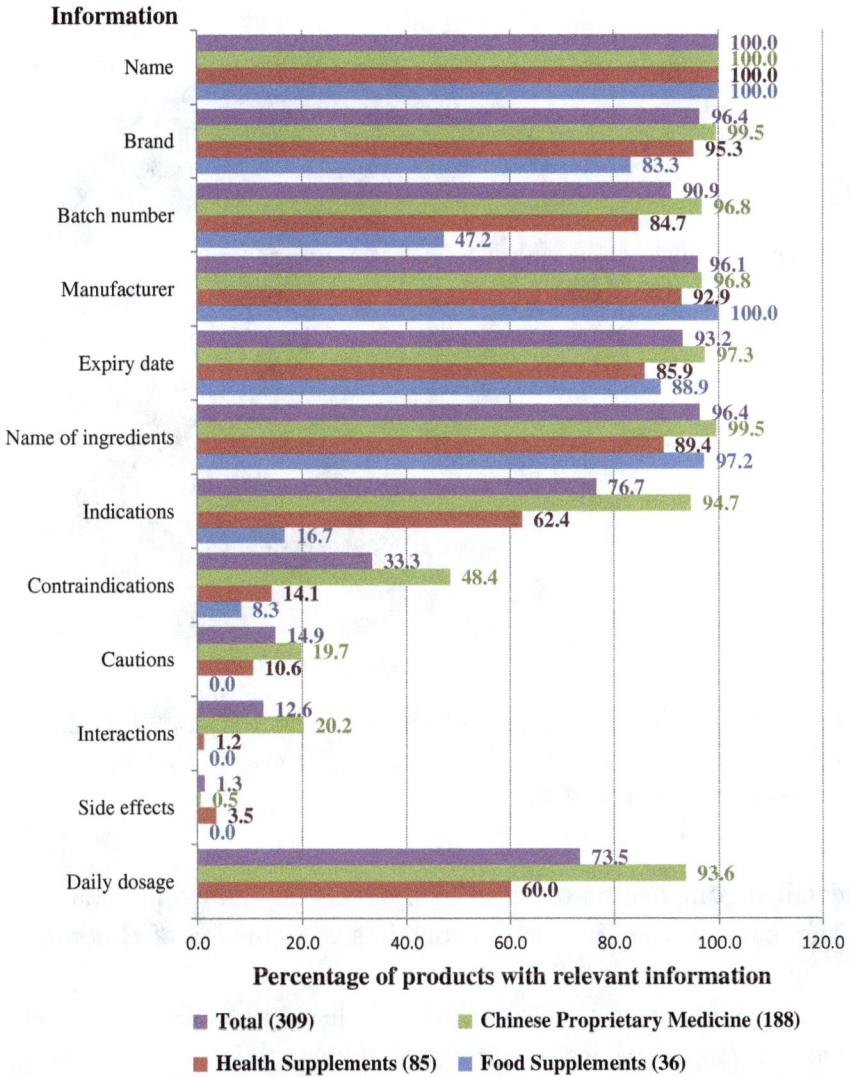

Figure 4.3 The percentage of different products that included the following information on the packaging: name, brand, batch number, manufacturer, expiry date, name of ingredients, recommended daily dosage, indications, contraindications, cautions, interactions and side effects. Recommended daily dosage is not applicable for Food Supplements (FS).

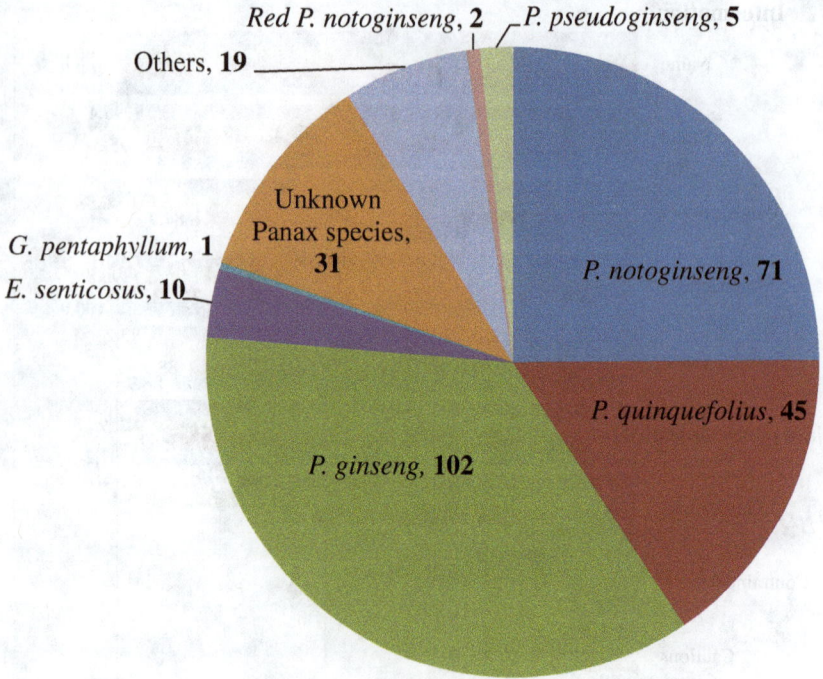

Figure 4.4   Presence of 4 Panax species (*P. ginseng*, *P. quinquefolius*, *P. notoginseng*, and *P. pseudoginseng*), *E. senticosus* and *G. pentaphyllum* found in label claims of products in the study.

detailed composition of these 19 products are shown in Table 4.3. The majority were labelled to contain a combination of *P. notoginseng* and *P. quinquefolius*.

The number of products with single listed ingredients indicating the four *Panax* species (*P. ginseng*, *P. quinquefolius*, *P. notoginseng*, *P. pseudoginseng*), *E. senticosus* and *G. pentaphyllum* are shown in Table 4.4 based on the label claims. The majority of these products were labelled to contain *P. notoginseng*.

The four different *Panax* species, *E. senticosus* and *G. pentaphyllum* are all said to have different properties and actions according to the TCM concept. Therefore, it is essential to use the right species for the

Table 4.3 Combination of two or more "ginseng" types in 19 products listed as "Others" in Figure 4.4.

Red P. ginseng	P. ginseng	P. notoginseng	P. quinquefolius	P. pseudoginseng	Korean ginseng	American ginseng	Siberian ginseng	No. of products
	X	X	X					9
	X	X						4
				X				1
						X		1
						X		1
					X	X		2
X					X	X	X	1

Table 4.4   Number of products with the four Panax species (*P. ginseng*, *P. quinquefolius*, *P. notoginseng*, and *P. pseudoginseng*), *E. senticosus* and *G. pentaphyllum* found in products with single listed ingredients.

Herb	Number of Products
P. ginseng	3
Red *P. ginseng*	1
P. notoginseng	18
Steamed *P. notoginseng*	2
E. senticosus	2
G. pentaphyllum	1
Korean ginseng	5
Red Korean ginseng	4
American ginseng	5

right indication. Misidentification or use of incorrect Panax species might have opposite effects and lead to complications.

4.2.2.2 *Listed ingredients*

Among 309 collated products, 298 ones had listed their ingredients. Besides the six plant species in Section 4.2.2.1, many products had listed other ingredients. These ingredients could be excipients, herbal ingredients, animal originated ingredients, minerals or vitamins. Figure 4.5 shows the number of listed ingredients in the products. The ingredients may be of herbal and animal origins. The majority of products had 5 to 10 ingredients listed in their labels. The maximum number was 64 (Health Maintenance Capsules from Nature's Green®).

For herbal ingredients, different plant parts can be used. For Panax species and *E. senticosus*, the roots are used. For *G. pentaphyllum*, the leaves and vine are used. In taxonomy, fungi are not considered to be in the plant kingdom. However, at this juncture, it is important to note that in TCM, fungi are usually considered as plants (Chang HM *et al.*, 2000). Hence, in this book, all ingredients with fungal origin (e.g.,

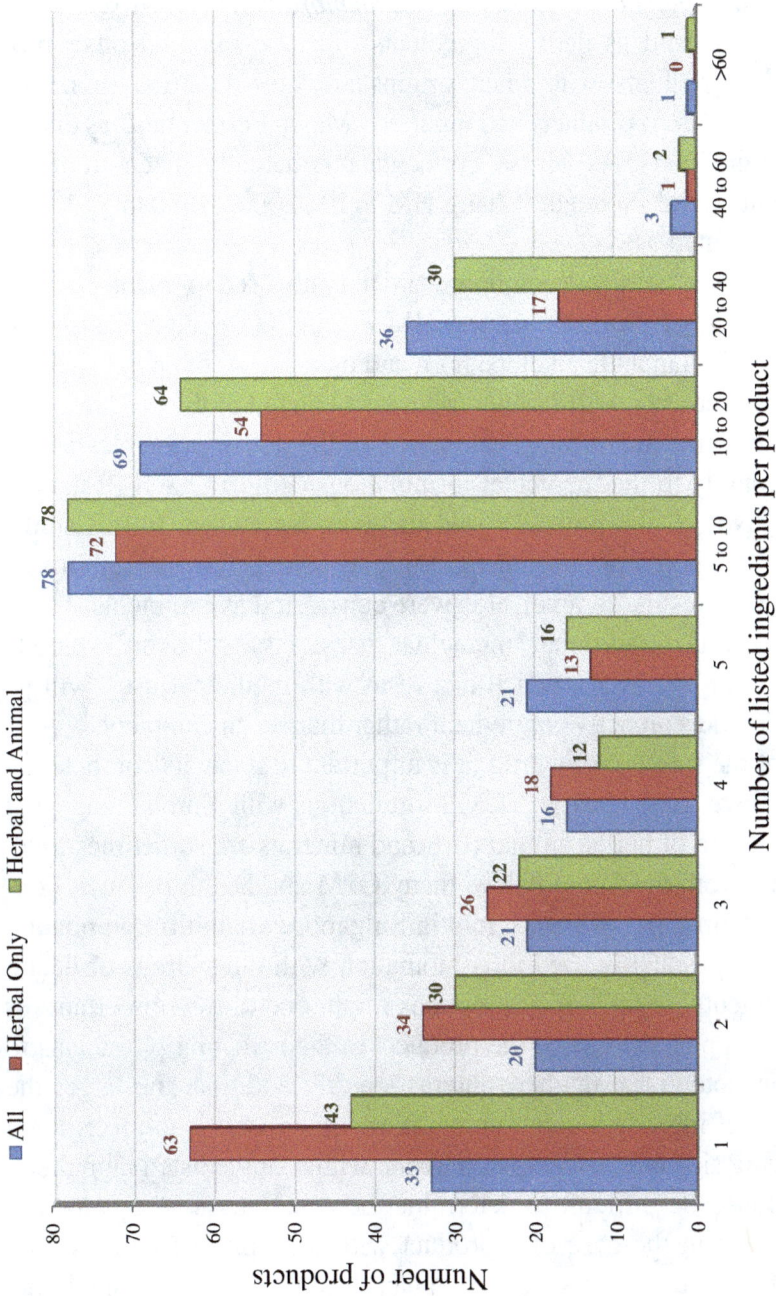

Figure 4.5   The number of listed ingredients.

Poria, Glossy ganoderma, Astragalus membranaceus, Cordyceps) are also categorized as herbal ingredients. Specific oils and other processed ingredients with plant origins are not classified as herbal ingredients. Two products had reported "Massa Fermentata" as one of their ingredients. As Massa Fermentata is actually made from six different herbal products (Chang HM *et al.*, 2000; Hijikata Y, 2006), it was counted as six.

In TCM, "herb" is a common word not only used for plants but also include animal products (Chang HM *et al.*, 2000). Ingredients with animal origin include antelope horn and tiger penis. Table 4.3 shows a list of ingredients with animal origin encountered in the products.

Excipients are substances other than the active principles added intentionally to the medicinal formulations (Pifferi G and Restani P, 2003). Not all the product listed the excipients used. In this study, substances such as sweeteners, artificial colors, flavors, stabilizers, water, oils, resins, caramel, etc., were considered as excipients. Those with specific traditional medicinal uses, e.g., "dragon's blood" (Zhao Z *et al.*, 2004), which is a resin with medicinal uses, will be considered as an active ingredient rather than as an excipient.

For the safe use of a drug, it is important to know its composition and dosage to be used. In TCM formulations with a broad range and composition of herbs, animal parts and minerals are sometimes used. As seen from the figure below, many CPM and health products containing "ginseng" or Panax sold in Singapore are multi-component. If such a product is used in combination with other drugs or health supplements, drug–herb interactions might occur. It is important for users to report the use of the products to their treating physicians to prevent potential drug–herb interactions. In addition, the larger the number of ingredients in a preparation, the greater is the likelihood of having side effects compared to one with a single listed ingredient. It will also be difficult to determine the exact cause of a particular side effect in the case of a product with multiple ingredients. The use of more than one specie of Panax or multiple ingredients in the

Table 4.5 The list of ingredients with animal origins listed on the products.

Ingredient	Remarks
Agkistrodan japonicae	Snake
Arisaema cum bile	Arisaematis (herbal) + bile of oxen
Beeswax	Natural wax produced in beehive
Bombryx batryticatus	Stiff silk worm
Bombryx masculus	Male silk worm
Calculus bovis	The gall stones of oxen
Carapax et Plastrum Testudinis	The shell of *Chinemys reevesii* (turtle)
Carapax trionycis	Water turtle shell
Cauda cervi	The tail of deer
Colla Corii asini	The skin of donkey (donkey-hide gelatin)
Colla Cornus cervi	The skin of horn of deer (antler glue)
Concha Haliotidis	Abalone shell
Concha Ostreae	Oyster shell
Cornu Bubali	Water Buffalo horn
Cornu Cervi degelatinatum	Deer horn (deglelatin)
Cornu Cervi pantotrichum	Deer horn (pilose antler)
Cornu Cervi parvum	Proximal parts horn of deer (deer velvet)
Cornu Saigae taaricae	The horn of Saiga (antelope)
Dens draconis	Fossilized teeth (Long chi- Dens Draconis Preparata)
Eupolyphaga seu steleophaga	Dried female ground beetle
Foetus Cervi	Deer fetus
Formica fusca	Ant
Gecko	Lizard
Hirudo	Leech, a blood sucking worm
Honey	Honey
Ligamentium Cervi	Deer ligaments
Lumbricus	Earthworm
Mel (feng mi)	Honey
Moschus	Deer musk secretions

(*Continued*)

Table 4.5   (*Continued*)

Ingredient	Remarks
Ootheca mantidis	Egg case of praying mantis
Os draconis	Skeleton fossil of prehistoric mammals like hipparion (ancient horse), rhinoceros, deer, oxen, etc
Os Sepia	Cuttlefish skeleton (Cuttlebone)
Penis Canitis	Reproductive organ of male dogs
Penis Cervi	Reproductive organ of male deer
Penis Otariae	Reproductive organ of male seal
Periostracum Serpentis	The skin of snake
Pheretima	Earthworm
Propolis	Part of beehive
Pullus Cum Osse Nigro	Dark boned/ dark skinned chicken (乌鸡)
Royal Jelly	The oral section of worker bees used as the diet of queen bees
Scolopendra	Centipede
Scorpio	Scorpion
Sheng yu	Fish
Snake gall	Bile of snake
Testis et Penis Bovis	Reproductive organ of ox
Testis et Penis Cans	Reproductive organ of male dogs
Young deer	An immature deer
Zaocys	Snake

formulation may seem to provide additional benefits to the consumers. However, it may pose problem in identifying the causative herb should there be an adverse event.

4.2.3 *Dosage forms*

Among the 309 products, 36 were in powder or small granular forms and their dosages were within the range of 1.5–6 grams per dose. Such dosages may be difficult to measure. The risks of over-dosage or insufficient treatment are high. Patient may also not adhere to the correct dosage. Convenient dosage forms such as capsules and tablets improve compliance.

Table 4.6 shows the distribution of different dosage forms in the different types of products. While it is assumed that all the ingredients including the excipients are stated on the packaging, it might be possible that in some products, only the herbal ingredients were labeled. The majority of the health products are in solid oral dosage forms (200, 73 %), most commonly as capsules followed by tablets. Topical forms are generally used for rheumatic conditions or to treat injuries. Interestingly, one product could be used both orally and topically (Yunnan Baiyao Tincture). Thus, it was counted twice, both as liniment and as oral liquid. Health products have specific pharmaceutical dosage forms while food products do not exist in pharmaceutical dosage forms. Since the dosage form is one of the

Table 4.6 Distribution of dosage forms in CPM and HS surveyed.

State	Dosage forms	Chinese Proprietary Medicine (n)	Health Supplements (n)	Health products with single listed ingredients (n)
Oral Solid	Capsule	85	16	13
	Caplet/ Pill/ Tablet	40	19	8
	Granules	4	0	0
	Powder	31	1	9
	Slice	0	2	0
	Softgel	0	2	0
Oral Liquid	Oral Liquid	18	24	4
	Sachet	2	0	2
	Tea	3	9	5
Topical	Liniment	6	6	0
	Plaster	0	6	0
Total		189*	85	41

*One CPM product can be used both orally or topically.

criteria differentiating health products from food products, food products are excluded in Table 4.6.

As can be seen from Figure 4.3, more than 96 % of oral CPMs had information on recommended daily dosages while about 70 % of health supplements had similar information. Under the Health Products Act in Singapore, information on recommended daily dosage is required for CPMs and Health Supplements but is not applicable to food products and topical health products.

4.2.4 *Indications*

As shown in Figure 4.3, 95 % of CPM products had reported the indications clearly — 50% for health supplements and less than 14% for food products reported their indications for usage. Eleven health supplements and one food product had mentioned their indications indirectly. It means that after explaining the traditional usage of some herbs, they had mentioned that the product contains those specific herbs.

A total of 636 indications was reported in all products. Most of the products had claimed to be effective for some traditional uses such as improving yin–yang balance, nourishing different Zang–Fu organ systems, enhancing Qi, etc. It is beyond the scope of this book to subcategorise such indications. Improvement in circulatory system followed by analgesic effects were the most commonly reported conventional indications. In addition, effects on mental problems and nervous system were also commonly encountered with a total of 59 products claiming to have such effects.

Conventional medicine and TCM are two different medical systems. TCM concepts are different from conventional medicine. The body–organ system (Zang–Fu) in TCM is different from what is known in anatomy and conventional medicine (Yuen JWM *et al.*, 2012). In other words, although they use similar words to describe the conditions, the anatomical and physiological meanings of "spleen", "kidney", "heart", "lung", etc., in TCM may not have the similar meaning in modern medicine (Chen P, 2004). In addition, some common words like "blood" are used differently in TCM and conventional medicine (Chai K, 2007). The regulation of blood circulation (categorized in circulatory system) is a very common claim in labels of products (52 products) may have different meanings in traditional and conventional medicine. Hence, a mixture of traditional and conventional approaches to the uses (indications) on the label of the same product can cause misunderstanding and confusion especially for consumers who are not familiar with these two systems of medicine.

In a previous study, it was found that most of the consumers shopping at a medical hall in Singapore only did so when there was a specific need (Tan JPT and Freathy P, 2011). It was found that tonic was the most commonly bought product at medical halls in Singapore. Some of the tonics include products with ginseng or Bird's Nest. Besides, prescribed herbs herbal drinks were also popular products to buy and they are often used as preventive medicine.

4.2.5 *Side effects, contraindications, caution and interactions*

Among 188 CPMs studied, 137 products (72.9 %) had comments on their packaging such as "side effects not known", "no contraindication" or "no known side effects". On the other hand, three CPMs (1.6%) had claimed to be "free of side effects". Only one product had reported a potential side effect, which was "impairment of yin and blood by long-term usage of product". The rest of the products (47, 25%) did not provide any information on side effects at all. It is not known whether the products which did not provide relevant information on the external packaging could have provided them in the inserts or on the inner packaging. Use in pregnancy and children were the major contraindications. Among 85 health supplements, the majority (78, 91.8%) had not indicated side effects, three (3.5%) reported potential side effects including transient flushing due to nicotinic acid ingredient and allergic reactions, and four products (4.7%) mentioned, "The side effects are not known".

It is positive that many products do have statements about contraindications. It is important that contraindications, where applicable, are stated. Due to the multi-herbal nature of most of the products, it is difficult for such formulations to clearly specify the contraindication. There might be little scientific evidence from clinical studies since they are not required for the registration of a CPM and trials are usually costly.

In a similar but much smaller study done in the UK, among 7 products containing *P. ginseng*, only one precaution was reported and none of them had reported any side effects or contraindications (Raynor DK *et al.*, 2011). In another study in Brazil, evaluating eight products containing *P. ginseng* regarding their pharmacological claims, there was no homogeneity among products in their indications, adverse effects or interactions. In addition, the claims were not supported enough by available scientific data (Auricchio MT *et al.*, 2007).

Side/adverse effects resulting from the usage of *P. ginseng* had been previously reported e.g., insomnia, diarrhoea, vaginal bleeding, mastalgia, headache, schizophrenia (Ernst E, 2002; Kitts D and Hu C, 2000), systemic allergic reaction (Wiwanitkit V and Taungjaruwinai W, 2004), Steven Johnson's Syndrome (Ernst E, 2002), hypertention, gastrointestinal disorders, nervousness, irritability, hyperestrogenism (Auricchio MT *et al.*, 2007), and hypoglycemia (World Health Organization, 2002). However, according to toxicity studies, *P. ginseng* is a safe plant, rarely with adverse effects (Kitts D and Hu C, 2000).

The therapeutic use of plants is often seen as safe. There are side effects and risks associated directly or indirectly with the use of some of the herbs. The plant-associated health risks (intrinsic adverse effects) arise directly from the active constituents of the plant itself (Wang J *et al.*, 2009). The causes of adverse effects include the presence of undeclared drugs (Koh HL and Woo S, 2000; Yee SK *et al.*, 2005), toxic ingredients, drug–herb interactions, co-existing diseases or overdoses etc. (Wang J *et al.*, 2009). They can be either of type A (dose-dependent and predictable) or type B (non-predictable), the latter occurring as anaphylactic shock or allergy (Drew AK and Myers SP, 1997). Often it is a dose-dependent reaction.

The possibility of drug–food interaction was reported in 38 CPM products (20.1%) and one (1.2%) health supplement. The most common reported interactions with some specific types of foods including raw, sour or cold foods (20 products), pungent or spicy foods (18 products), fried, greasy or oily foods (10 products), sea foods (three products), broad bean, sugary foods and salt (two products each), and peanut and irritant foods (one product each). Two products mentioned possible interactions with alcohol and cigarette while six products had listed other possible interactions with warfarin, *Rhizome et radix veratri, Fructus gleditsiae, Trogopterori faeces* and radish. Since many herbal preparations are not taken solely, drug–herb interactions might occur, affecting the effectiveness and safety of the herb or drug.

In TCM books, *P. ginseng* herb is reported to be incompatible with *Radix Veratri nigri* (commonly known as 藜芦, Li Lu), *Fructus gleditsiae* (commonly known as Zao Jia in TCM)*, or Trogoptrori faeces* (commonly known as 五灵脂, Wu Ling Zhi) (Bensky D *et al.*, 2004. The State Pharmacopoeia Commission of P.R. China, 2010). It has been reported that the most common enzymatic system, cytochrome P450 (CYP) system, affected by *P. ginseng*, can cause several drug–herb interactions (Choi YH *et al.*, 2011), including decreasing the effect of warfarin and some interactions with chemotherapy drugs (imatinib) (Shi S and Klotz U, 2012). More information on drug–herb interactions with *P. ginseng* has been presented in Chapter 2.

4.2.6 *Price*

The most expensive product surveyed was a health supplement (Il Hwa Korean Honeyed Ginseng) costing S$338 for a box, while the cheapest product was a spice (food), named Nature`s Cool JiaJia Herbal Tea-Less Sugar, costing just S$0.70. Due to the differences in package sizes, the retail prices printed on the packages are not representations of their cost per day. Hence, we normalized the prices based on the package sizes and recommended daily doses. Topical products and products without recommended daily doses were excluded from our normalization. As for food products, the cost per day was considered as the cost per suggested serving unit. Based on this, the maximum cost per day was S$45.60 and the lowest was S$0.24 for CPM products. The average costs per day were S$2.75, S$2.99 and S$3.53 for CPMs, health supplements and food products, respectively.

Price is one of the crucial factors affecting the marketing of a product (Foroncewicz B *et al.*, 2011). There is also a general belief that cheaper products are inferior in terms of quality to expensive ones. It is not known whether the more expensive products are more effective or safer than cheaper products with similar ingredients. Typically, a product which indicates the contents of the active ingredients (e.g. indicating the concentrations or amounts of ginsenosides) shows evidence of attempts at quality control and may command a higher price.

4.3 Conclusion

The survey of 309 products demonstrated that although about half of products had minor errors in their labels, the overall information provided on packages was clear and understandable in about 99% of products. From the guidelines published by HSA and AVA, it was found that more than 96% of CPM products, more than 84% of health supplements and more than 88% of food products comply with the respective regulatory guidelines. The only exception was with regards to information on recommended daily dosage. Only 69.9% of oral health supplements provided such information.

Herbal products are often believed to be free of side effects and safe to use. This is only partially true. Herbs and herbal remedies have complex ingredients and effects. This complexity and the multi-herbal usage are a challenge to quality control. Side/adverse effects and drug–herb or herb-herb interactions are often not known when using different herbs or multi-component herbal products. The majority of the analyzed products in this study had provided information about side effects and contraindication on their packaging. This is positive and important for the safe use of the product. However, many products stated that side effects are "not known" or "no known side effects". Since *P. ginseng* and the other species have a long traditional use as a single herb or in formulations empirically, they may be generally safe but may not be devoid of side effects.

The information provided on a product should be comprehensive and clear to ensure its safe use. Guidelines and regulations help to ensure the safety and quality of a product. Nonetheless, not all of the products were found to have all-embracing information stated on their packaging. Providing enough information and to monitor the usage are therefore essential.

References

Auricchio MT, Batistic-Longatto MA, Nicoletti MA (2007). A comparative analysis of inner wrapping and package inserts for medicines containing *Panax ginseng*. C.A. Meyer. *Cad Saude Publica* **23**(10): 2295–2304.

Ayranci U, Son N, Son O (2005). Prevalence of nonvitamin, nonmineral supplement usage among students in a Turkish university. *BMC Public Health* **5**: 47.

Bensky D, Clavey S, Stöger E (2004). *Chinese Herbal Medicine: Materia Medica*. 3rd ed. Seattle: Eastland Press.

Chai K (2007). *Fundamental Theory of Traditional Chinese Medicine*. 2nd ed. China: People's Medical Publishing House.

Chang HM, But PPH, Yao SC, Wang LL, Yeung SCS (2000). *Pharmacology and Applications of Chinese Materia Medica*. Volume 1. Singapore: World Scientific.

Chen P (2004). *Diagnosis in Traditional Medicine*. China: Complementary Medicine Press.

Choi YH, Chin YW, Kim YG (2011). Herb–drug interactions: focus on metabolic enzymes and transporters. *Arch Pharm Res* **34**(11): 1843–1863.

Drew AK, Myers SP (1997). Safety issues in herbal medicine: implications for the health professions. *Med J Aust* **66**(10): 538–541.

Ernst E (2002). The risk-benefit profile of commonly used herbal therapies: Ginkgo, St. John's Wort, Ginseng, Echinacea, Saw Palmetto, and Kava. *Ann Intern Med* **136**(1): 42–53.

Foroncewicz B, Mucha K, Gryszkiewicz J, Florczak M, Mulka M, Chmura A, Szmidt J, Patkowski W, Pączek L (2011). Dietary supplements and herbal preparations in renal and liver transplant recipients. *Transplant Proc* **43**(8): 2935–2937.

Froiland K, Koszewski W, Hingst J, Kopecky L (2004). Nutritional supplement use among college athletes and their sources of information. *Int J Sport Nutr Exerc Metab* **14**(1): 104–120.

Hijikata Y (2006). Analgesic treatment with Kampo prescription. *Expert Rev Neurother* **6**(5): 795–802.

Kang E, Yang EJ, Kim SM, Chung IY, Han SA, Ku DH, Nam SJ, Yang JH, Kim SW (2012). Complementary and alternative medicine use and assessment of quality of life in Korean breast cancer patients: a descriptive study. *Support Care Cancer* **20**(3): 461–473.

Kitts D, Hu C (2000). Efficacy and safety of ginseng. *Public Health Nutr* **3**(4A): 473–485.

Koh HL, Woo S, (2000). Chinese proprietary medicine in Singapore: regulatory control of toxic heavy metals and undeclared drugs. *Drug Saf* **23**(5): 351–362.

Pifferi G, Restani P (2003). The safety of pharmaceutical excipients. *Farmac* **58**(8): 541–550.

Raynor DK, Dickinson R, Knapp P, Long AF, Nicolson DJ (2011). Buyer beware? Does the information provided with herbal products available over the counter enable safe use? *BMC Med* **9**: 94.

Shi S, Klotz U (2012). Drug interactions with herbal medicines. *Clin Pharmacokinet* **51**(2): 77–104.

Smith L, Ernst E, PaulEwings, Myers P, Smith C (2004). Co-ingestion of herbal medicines and warfarin. *Br J Gen Pract* **54**(503): 439–441.

Tan JPT, Freathy P (2011). Consumer decision making and store patronage behavior in Traditional Chinese Medicine (TCM) halls in Singapore. *J Retailing Consum Serv* **18**(4): 285–292.

The *New York Times* (2015). *Retailers Are Warned Over Herbal Supplements*. Retrieved 8 Feb 2015, from http://www.nytimes.com/interactive/2015/02/02/health/herbal_supplement_letters.html?_r=1

The State Pharmacopoeia Commission of P.R. China (2010a: p210; 2010b: p211; 2010c: p310; 2010d: p311; 2010e: p299; 2010f: p6). *Pharmacopoeia of the People's Republic of China*. Beijing: China Medical Science Press [English version].

The State Pharmacopoeia Commission of P.R. China (2000). *Pharmacopoeia of the People's Republic of China*. Volume 1. Beijing: Beijing Chemical Industry Press, p. 184 [Chinese version].

Wang J, van der Heijden R, Spruit S, Hankermeier T, Chan K, van der Greef J, Xu G, Wang M (2009). Quality and Safety of Chinese herbal medicines guided by a systems biology perspective. *J Ethnopharmacol* **126**(1): 31–41.

World Health Organization. *WHO Monographs on Selected Medicinal Plants*. World Health Organization, Retrieved from http://apps.who.int/medicinedocs/en/d/Js2200e

Wiwanitkit V, Taungjaruwinai W (2004). A case report of suspect ginseng allergy. *MedGenMed* **6**(3): 9.

Yee SK, Chu SS, Xu YM, Choo PL (2005). Regulatory control of Chinese proprietary medicines in Singapore. *Health Policy* **71**(2): 133–149.

Yuen JWM, Sonny H, Yung JYK (2012). Traditional Chinese medicine — East meets West in validation and therapeutic application. In: Kuang H, ed. *Recent Advances in Theories and Practice of Chinese Medicine*. Intech, pp. 239–266.

Zhao Z, Hong Kong Baptist University. School of Chinese Medicine (2004). *An Illustrated Chinese Materia Medica in Hong Kong [Xianggang Zhong Yao Cai Tu Jian]*. 1st ed. Hong Kong: School of Chinese Medicine, Hong Kong Baptist University.

Conclusions

Many people have been involved in the production of this book. From an undergraduate student doing her final year project, to graduate students working on their projects, to research staff and academics, to the editorial team at World Scientific and the marketing team. We thank everyone from the bottom of our hearts!

This book does not provide all the answers to your health queries, as every individual is different, and research is on-going. It is challenging to fully understand everything about all the herbs and products covered in this book. This is the beauty and ingenuity of natural products. There are so many components in each herb that exactly how each phytoconstituent works with the rest remains elusive. Is it synergistic (effects more than the mere summation) or is it antagonistic resulting in reduced effects? Different phytoconstituents in the same herb may have opposite effects, e.g. some ginsenosides. Very often, herbs may be used together in a decoction, instead of a single herb being used. Whether it is used in combination with other herbs or used alone, the many components present even in the single herb may act like a cocktail therapy, targeting at different receptors or sites of actions, resulting in the desired biological effects. For most work, researchers are still at the stage of identifying and understanding the effects of one phytoconstituent, e.g. Rg1 and Rb1, and wherever possible, the mechanisms of actions. The many different grades and prices for the same herb can be baffling especially to the general public. Eventually, it is a personal choice with recommendations from qualified practitioners and reputable suppliers.

TCM and herbal medicine have been used since time immemorial, saving lives, improving health and maintaining good health. With increasing healthcare costs, cheaper alternatives are becoming more popular. The physical, social-psychological and mental health are closely inter-related. Healthy lifestyle, healthy diet, plenty of rest and sleep, some exercise (suitable for the individual) as well as mindfulness are recipes for good health and happiness. At this juncture, it is appropriate to reiterate the importance of making informed choices and to consult qualified practitioners.

Wishing one and all great joy and happiness in the lifelong learning journey, in pursuit of better health and to maintain good health!

Glossary

Acupoints 穴位: (TCM concept) specific points on the body that have been traditionally used in acupuncture therapy.

Adjuvant: a pharmacological agent that modifies the effect of other agents, such as enhancing the effects of vaccines.

Analgesic: pain-killing.

Anepithymia: loss of normal appetite.

Anti-angiogenic: inhibits the growth of new blood vessels. This property has been utilised in anti-cancer treatment.

Anti-pica: pica is an eating disorder characterized by persistent and compulsive cravings to eat nonfood items, e.g. paper, clay, metal, chalk, soil, glass or sand. Anti-pica means to alleviate or treat this eating disorder.

Anti-platelet activity: decreases platelet aggregation and inhibits thrombus formation. Drugs with such a property are used to reduce blood clotting in an artery, a vein or the heart, which may otherwise increase the risks of diseases such as heart attack and strokes.

Anti-remodeling: changes in size, shape, structure and physiology of the heart after injury to the myocardium.

Anxiolytic: inhibits anxiety.

Atopic dermatitis: chronic, itchy inflammation of the upper layers of the skin that often develops in people who have hay fever or asthma and in people who have family members with these conditions.

Attention-deficit/hyperactivity disorder (ADHD): a behavioural disorder characterised by poor or short attention span and/or excessive activity and impulsiveness inappropriate for the child's age that interferes with the functioning or development of the child.

Blood Stasis 血瘀: (TCM concept) It literally means stagnation of blood circulation. It represents a collection of signs and symptoms that include stabbing pain, bluish purple skin and presence of hard masses at a localised area.

Channels: *see* Meridians

Chronic myelogenous leukemia: a disease in which cells that normally would develop into neutrophils, basophils, eosinophils, and monocytes become cancerous. In the early stage, people have non-specific signs and symptoms such as tiredness, loss of appetite, and weight loss. As the disease progresses, the lymph nodes and spleen enlarge, and people may also be pale and bruise or bleed easily.

Cold hypersensitivity: the unusual discomfort felt by some people when in a cool environment.

Collaterals 络: (TCM concept) These are imaginary lines that map out the location of acupoints with respect to their therapeutic usage. These lines symbolise passages through which Blood and Qi flow. More specifically, collaterals refer to branches of the Meridians that run horizontally to the axis of the body.

Convalescence: the recovery stage of an infectious disease or illness where the patient gradually returns to health, but may continue to be a source of infection even if feeling better.

Chronic obstructive pulmonary disease: persistent narrowing (obstruction) of the airways occurring with emphysema, chronic obstructive bronchitis, or both disorders. Signs and symptoms include cough and shortness of breath.

Debility: physical weakness, especially as a result of illness.

Decoction: the process of boiling herbs in water to extract the active chemicals from the herbal materials.

Deficiency 虚**:** (TCM concept) It refers to conditions characterized by weakness and insufficiency of the body's resistance.

Dyspnea: shortness of breath.

Emesis: vomiting.

Endotoxic shock: a life-threatening condition in which blood pressure is too low to sustain life due to severe bacterial infection.

Epistaxis: nosebleeds.

Erectile dysfunction or **impotence:** a disorder in which a man is unable to achieve an erection, or achieves erection briefly but not long enough for intercourse, or achieves effective erection inconsistently.

Excipients: substances other than the active principle ingredients added intentionally to the medicinal formulations.

Functional asthenia: weakness without any identified cause.

Haematemesis: vomitting of blood.

Haemopoiesis: formation of blood cellular components.

Haemorrhagic stroke: a life-threatening condition in which an artery to the brain ruptures, resulting in death of an area of brain tissue due to loss of its blood supply. Signs and symptoms include severe headache, paralysis and numbness of usually one side of the body, nausea, vomiting, seizures, and loss of consciousness.

Haemoptysis: coughing up of blood or of blood-stained sputum from the bronchi, larynx, trachea, or lungs.

Haematochezia: blood in the stool.

Hepatoprotective: prevents damage to the liver.

Hepatotoxicity: chemical-driven liver damage.

Hyperanalgesia: increased sensitivity to pain.

Immunomodulatory: modifies or regulates one or more immune functions.

Ischemia: a restriction in blood supply to tissues, causing a shortage of oxygen and glucose needed to keep tissue alive.

Jaundice: a condition in which the skin and whites of the eyes take on a yellowish tinge, as a result of too much bilirubin (a yellow pigment) in the blood.

Mammary involution: the process by which the mammary gland returns to its non-lactating state.

Manic-like symptoms: excessive physical activity and feelings of elation that are greatly out of proportion to the situation. For example, the person may feel exuberant, elated, acts extravagantly, sleeps little, talks excessively, gets easily distracted and pursues dangerous activity, without thinking about the consequences.

Menorrhagia or **Flooding:** excessive or prolonged menstrual blood flow.

Meridians 经**:** (TCM concept) These are imaginary lines that map out the location of acupoints with respect to their therapeutic usage. These lines symbolise passages through which Blood and Qi flow. More specifically, meridians refer to main trunks that run longitudinally to the axis of the body.

Myelopoiesis: regulated formation of myeloid cells, including eosinophilic granulocytes, basophilic granulocytes, neutrophilic granulocytes and monocytes.

Neuroprotective: protects neurons from injury or degeneration.

Palpitation: the awareness of one's own heartbeats. The sensation may feel like pounding, fluttering, racing, or skipping beats.

Phases: Also known as elements, by which their movement and mutation result in all phenomena in the Universe. They consist of Wood (木), Fire (火), Earth (土), Metal (金) and Water (水).

Qi 气: (TCM concept) vital energy.

Renoprotective: refers to the property of a substance or treatment that protects the kidneys from injury.

Spotting: bleeding that is light and is occurring at a time when a woman's period is not expected.

Stagnation 气滞: (TCM concept) Impeded flow of Qi.

Teratogenicity: tendency to cause birth defects.

Tonic: (TCM concept) restores and invigorates systems in the body or promotes general health and well-being.

Topical application: a medication that is applied to body surfaces such as the skin or mucous membranes to treat ailments via a large range of classes including but not limited to creams, foams, gels, lotions, and ointments.

Yang 阳: (TCM concept) Together with Yin, it is the symbolic representation of the polar nature of all things. It refers to the aspect of things that more closely resembles fire, and bears attributes such as dynamic, active and expansive.

Yin 阴: (TCM concept) Together with Yang, it is the symbolic representation of the polar nature of all things. It refers to the aspect of things that more closely resembles water, and bears attributes such as quiescent, static and contracting.

Zang-Fu 脏腑: These refer to the five organ networks 脏 (viscera) (namely, heart, liver, spleen, lung and kidney) and six bowels 腑 (namely, stomach, small intestine, large intestine, bladder, gallbladder and triple burner).

References

Beinfield H, Korngold E (1991). *Between Heaven and Earth: A Guide to Chinese Medicine*. 1st ed. New York: Ballantine Books.

Chai K (2007). *Fundamental Theory of Traditional Chinese Medicine*. 2nd ed. China: People's Medical Publishing House.

Merck Sharp & Dohme Corp. (2014). *The Merck Manual Home Edition*. Retrieved 1 Nov 2014, from: http://www.merckmanuals.com/home

Merriam-Webster, Inc. (2014). *Merriam-Webster*. Retrieved 1 Nov 2014, from http://www.merriam-webster.com/

Wikipedia (2014). *Wikipedia, The Free Encyclopedia*. Retrieved 1 Nov 2014, from http://en.wikipedia.org/wiki/Main_Page

APPENDIX **2**

In this section, we seek to explain some of the TCM terminologies that are mentioned in this book within the context of sickness and treatment. The TCM concepts introduced here are brief and by no means comprehensive, but we hope it can help to convey a more complete picture of how *P. ginseng, P. quinquefolius, P. notoginseng* and *E. senticosus* have been used therapeutically throughout history. Interested readers can refer to the references for Appendix 2 [Beinfield H and Korngold E (1991); Chen P (2004), Chen SY *et al.*, (2003); Chai K (2007); Li GD *et al.* (2003); Wang XH *et al.* (2003); Wang Y (2006); Wiseman N and Ellis A (1994); Wu JN (2005); Xu L and Wang W (2002) and Zhao Z (2004)] for more information.

Yin-Yang Theory 阴阳

The ancient Chinese observed that all phenomenon in the world is characterised by Yin-Yang and the five phases (elements). In particular, they occur as opposites. Time is divided into day and night, season into summer and winter, gender into male and female, temperature into hot and cold. Yin and Yang are the abstract representations of the two opposing aspects of things (Beinfield H and Korngold E, 1991). If Yang is day, Yin will be night. If Yang is summer, Yin will be winter. If Yang is male, Yin will be female. If Yang is hot, Yin will be cold. The aspect which resembles more closely to fire is designated Yang. The aspect which resembles more closely to water is designated Yin. Therefore, in the context of TCM, Yang refers to the aspect of human body that warms, excites, invigorates, dries, expands and generates, while Yin refers to the aspect of human body that cools, inhibits, nourishes, moistens, contracts and stores (Chai K, 2007). Table 2.1 shows the applications of Yin–Yang theory in TCM.

Table A2.1 Applications of Yin–Yang theory in TCM therapy.

Terminology	Definition	Syndrome	Clinical manifestations	Herbs to address the condition
Yang 阳	Yang literally means "the sunny side of the mountain". In TCM, it refers to the aspect of human body that warms, excites, invigorates, dries, expands and generates (Chai K, 2007).	Yang Deficiency 阳虚	The patient complains of a feeling of coldness that lessens when he covers himself with blanket or wears warm clothing. His face appears pale. He prefers warm limbs are cold. He prefers warm drinks or does not feel thirsty at all. He complains of fatigue and lethargy. He suffers from sexual dysfunction. His urine is clear. He has loose stool. He has a moist, pale, fat tongue with white coating and a slow, weak pulse (Chen P, 2004; Wang Y, 2006).	Morinda root, Deer velvet (Zhao Z, 2004)
Yin 阴	Yin literally means "the shady side of the mountain".	Yin Deficiency 阴虚	The patient complains of low grade fever. His cheeks appear red. His palms, soles and chest feel warm.	*P. quinquefolius* Action: "tonify qi and nourish yin"

(*Continued*)

Table A2.1 *(Continued)*

Terminology	Definition	Syndrome	Clinical manifestations	Herbs to address the condition
	In TCM, it refers to the aspect of human body that cools, inhibits, nourishes, moistens, contracts and stores (Chai K, 2007).		He prefers cool drinks. His mouth and throat feels dry, and he may even cough up blood-tinged phlegm. He complains of sleeplessness and feels agitated easily. He has frequent night sweats. His urine is yellow and low in volume. He has dry stool. He has a dry, red tongue with scanty coating and a thready, rapid pulse (Chen P, 2004; Wang Y, 2006).	Indication: "Deficiency of qi and yin", "deficiency heat with vexation and fatigue, panting and coughing with blood in phlegm"
		Wasting-thirst disorder (an example of Yin Deficiency syndrome) 消渴	The patient complains of extreme thirst, excessive appetite and excessive urination. He has lost much weight and appears thin. His mouth and throat feel dry constantly. He complains of low grade fever. His cheeks appear red. His palms, soles and chest feel warm. He complains of sleeplessness. He has frequent night sweats. He has dry stool. He has a dry, red tongue with scanty coating and a thready, rapid pulse (Chen P, 2004; Wang Y, 2006).	*P. ginseng* Indication: "interior heat and wasting-thirst" *P. quinquefolius* Action: "clear heat" Indication: "interior heat wasting thirst, dry mouth and throat"

Qi, Blood and Body Fluids 气血津液

The Chinese believed that life cannot be separated from the way it manifests. When the heart beats and the breath is warm, it is understood that the life force or Qi exists within the body (Beinfield H and Korngold E, 1991). When the heart stops beating and the body becomes cold, Qi is no longer present. When a person's hair is thick and his cheeks have a pink glow, his body is believed to be well nourished by Blood. When the face loses its lustre and the cheeks become sunken, there is not enough Blood to nourish the Body (Beinfield H and Korngold E, 1991). When Body Fluids are well distributed, the body functions like a well-watered garden. When Body Fluids stagnate, phlegm collects in the throat and edema forms in the body (Chai K, 2007). Through their experience with health and disease, the Chinese have sketched out a unique picture of the human body based on the intangible concepts of Qi, Blood and Body Fluids. Table 2.2 shows the applications of Qi, Blood and Body Fluids theory in TCM.

Five Organ Networks (Five Viscera) 五脏

In Chinese medicine, each organ network does not refer to a discrete anatomical structure. Rather, each is understood to be a complete set of functions — physiological and psychological — that have come to be grouped together for the purpose of therapeutic practice (Beinfield H and Korngold E, 1991). Being as abstract as the Chinese's ideas of Qi and Blood, they are defined by the functions abscribed to them in ancient text. For this reason, we shall refer to them as Organ Networks rather than simply organs, so as not to be confused with the actual structures studied in modern biomedicine. The Five Organ Networks are often applied in conjunction with Qi, Blood and Body Fluids theory to paint a more accurate picture of the patient's condition (Chai K, 2007). For example, a patient with Lung Qi deficiency and a patient with Spleen Qi deficiency may

Table A2.2 Applications of Qi, Blood and Body Fluids concepts in TCM therapy.

Terminology	Definition	Syndrome	Clinical manifestations	Herbs to address the condition
Qi 气	That which animates life and maintains its activity (Chai K, 2007).	Qi deficiency 气虚	The patient complains of persistant fatigue and weakness. He feels a lack of energy in exercising, or even talking to people. He becomes short of breath easily. He tends to sweat uncontrollably throughout the day. His symptoms worsen on physical exertion. His condition may be associated with a history of chronic disease or malnutrition or simply a result of old age. He has a pale tongue and a weak pulse (Chen P, 2004; Wang Y, 2006).	***P. ginseng*** Indication: "Deficiency of qi and blood" "frail caused by long-term illness" **Red ginseng** "Tonify Qi" ***P. quinquefolius*** Action: "To tonify qi and nourish yin" Indication: "Deficiency of qi and yin" ***E. senticosus*** Action: "To reinforce qi" Indication: "Spleen-lung qi deficiency, weak constitution and lack of strength, anepithymia"
		Qi stagnation 气滞	The patient experiences a feeling of fullness and discomfort in certain parts of the body, such as bloating in the abdomen, pressure in the chest, tightness along both flanks or a heaviness of the head. The discomfort	Bupleurum, Nut Grass Rhizome (Zhao Z, 2004; Wu JN, 2005)

(Continued)

Table A2.2 (*Continued*)

Terminology	Definition	Syndrome	Clinical manifestations	Herbs to address the condition
			comes and goes and it is difficult to pinpoint an exact location. These symptoms are often relieved by belching or passing of gas. There is little change to the tongue. He has a tense and erratic pulse (Chen P, 2004; Wang Y, 2006).	
		Collapse of Qi 气脱	The patient experiences a decrease in consciousness. Breathing is rapid and weak. He sweats profusely. His face looks pale. His limbs feel cold and clammy. He is extremely weak. He might even have lost control of his bowel and bladder, resulting in involuntary urination or defecation. He has an extremely weak pulse. (Chen P, 2004; Wang Y, 2006)	***P. ginseng*** Action: "To tonify the original qi greatly, resume pulse and secure collapse" Indication: "Being just going to collapse caused by body deficiency, cold limbs and faint pulse" ***Red ginseng*** Action: "To greatly tonify the original qi, regain pulse and secure collapse" Indication: "Tending to collapse caused by body deficiency, coldness of limbs and faint pulse"

(*Continued*)

Table A2.2 (*Continued*)

Terminology	Definition	Syndrome	Clinical manifestations	Herbs to address the condition
Blood 血	That which nourishes and builds up the body's material substance (Chai K, 2007).	Blood deficiency 血虛	The patient presents with paleness of the face, eyelids, lips, finger nails and tongue and has a sallow and lusterless complexion. She gets light-headed and dizzy from time to time, as though she is about to faint. She experiences numbness of both the hands and feet. Sometimes, she becomes aware of her heart beating rapidly. Her menstrual flow is pale in colour, light in volume and her menstrual cycle is often delayed. She has a pale tongue and a thready pulse (Chen P, 2004; Wang Y, 2006).	*P. ginseng* Action: "Nourish blood" Indication: "Deficiency of qi and blood"

(*Continued*)

Table A2.2   (*Continued*)

Terminology	Definition	Syndrome	Clinical manifestations	Herbs to address the condition
		Blood stasis 血瘀	The patient experiences a stabbing pain in a fixed location that worsens at night. The skin may appear bluish purple and sometimes, hard masses may be felt in that particular location. There may be repeated bleeding, the blood of which appears dark purple and contains blood clots. He may have a history of physical injury. He has a purple tongue, with dark spots and a thready and hesitant pulse (Chen P, 2004; Wang Y, 2006).	***P. notoginseng*** Action: "To dissipate stasis and stanch bleeding, disperse swelling and relive pain" Indication: "Hemoptysis, hematemesis, epistaxis, hematochezia, flooding and spotting, traumatic bleeding, stabbing pain in chest and abdomen, swelling and pain caused by injuries from falls"

(*Continued*)

Table A2.2 *(Continued)*

Terminology	Definition	Syndrome	Clinical manifestations	Herbs to address the condition
Body Fluids 津液	That which moisturises and lubricates different parts of the body (Chai K, 2007).	Deficiency in Body Fluids 津液亏虚	The patient complains of dryness in various parts of the body. The eyes feels itchy and gritty, as if there is sand in them. Her mouth feels dry and thirsty, and she might have difficulty in swallowing. Her skin feels dry and cracks easily. Vaginal dryness can sometimes lead to painful intercourse. There is little urine and the stool is in the form of hard, dry, small, round pellets that are painful or difficult to pass. She has a dry, red tongue and a thread, rapid pulse (Chen P, 2004; Wang Y, 2006).	***P. ginseng*** Action: "Engender fluid" Indication: "Thirsty caused by fluid damage" ***P. quinquefolius*** Action: "Engender fluid"

both experience symptoms typical of Qi deficiency, such as persistant fatigue and lethargy (Wang Y, 2006). However, the main complaint of the patient with Lung Qi deficiency will be shortness of breath and coughing, whereas the main complaint of the patient with Spleen Qi deficiency will be reduced appetite, abdominal bloatedness and loose stool. Table 2.3 shows the applications of five organ networks in TCM.

Table A2.3 Applications of Five Organ Networks in TCM therapy (Chai K, 2007; Chen P, 2004; Wang Y, 2006; Wu JN, 2005; Zhao Z, 2004).

Terminology	Definition	Associated signs and symptoms	Herbs to address the condition
Heart Network 心	That which propels the blood.	Abnormalities in the heart beat, such as palpitations. Abnormalities in the rhythm of the pulse, such as irregular or abrupt pulse.	***P. ginseng*** Indication: "Fright palpitations"
	That which houses the mind.	Abnormalities in mental states, cognition and consciousness, such as restlessness, sleeplessness, poor memory, confusion, or even the loss of consciousness.	***P. ginseng*** Action: "Tranquilize the mind and replenish wisdom" Indication: "Insomnia" ***E. senticosus*** Action: "To calm the mind" Indication: "Insomnia and dream-disturbed sleep"
Lung Network 肺	That which governs Qi and controls breathing.	Abnormalities in breathing, such as shortness of breath, weak breathing. Coughing. Fatigue and lethargy. Weak voice.	***P. ginseng*** Indication: "Dyspnea and cough caused by lung deficiency"
	That which disperses Body Fluids to all parts of the body.	If Body Fluids accumulate in the upper body, it manifests as edema of the face and puffiness beneath the eyes.	Descurainia seeds, ephedra

(Continued)

Table A2.3 (*Continued*)

Terminology	Definition	Associated signs and symptoms	Herbs to address the condition
		If Body Fluids accumulate in the lower body, it manifests as edema in the legs and feet. If Body Fluids accumulate in the Lung, it manifests as phlegm in the throat.	Cinnamon twig
	That which assists the Heart.	The symptoms of Lungs and Heart may both appear in the later stage of the illness. For example, a patient with palpitations and chest pain may develop fatigue, shortness of breath and edema of the legs and feet as the illness progresses. Conversely, a patient with long-term breathing difficulties may develop palpitations and chest pain as the illness progresses.	
Spleen Network 脾	That which absorbs and distributes nutrients from food and water.	Reduced appetite. Abdominal bloatedness that occurs after meals. Loose stool or even diarrhea.	***P. ginseng*** Action "Tonify spleen" Indication: "Low appetite caused by spleen deficiency" ***A. senticosus*** Action: "To invigorate the function of the spleen" Indication: "Spleen-lung qi deficiency, weak constitution and lack of strength, anepithymia"

(*Continued*)

Table A2.3 *(Continued)*

Terminology	Definition	Associated signs and symptoms	Herbs to address the condition
	That which transports Water.	Water retention may result in edema and low amount of urine.	Areca peel
	That which controls Blood.	All kinds of bleeding, including: Nose bleeds Blood in the urine Blood in the stool Bleeding under the surface of the skin.	*Red ginseng* Action: "Control the blood" Indication: " Qi failing to control the blood, flooding and spotting"
Liver Network 肝	That which spreads Qi.	Emotionally depressed. Fullness and discomfort in various parts of the body, such as: Pressure in the chest. Tightness along the flanks.	Bupleurum, nut grass rhizome
	That which stores Blood.	Paleness of the face, eyelids, lips, finger nails and tongue. Light-headedness and dizziness. Numbness of both hands and feet. Pale menstrual flow that is low in volume. Delayed menstrual cycle.	White peony root, Chinese angelica root

(Continued)

Table A2.3   (*Continued*)

Terminology	Definition	Associated signs and symptoms	Herbs to address the condition
Kidney Network 肾	That which governs Water.	Water retention may result in edema and low amount of urine.	Plantago seeds
	That which governs growth and reproduction.	Stunted growth. Poor physical and mental development. Delayed puberty. Impotence. Infertility.	*Ginseng* Action: "Replenish kidney" Indication: "Impotence and uterine coldness"
	That which anchors Qi.	Shortness of breath that occurs on the slightest exertion or even on rest. Prolonged exhalation.	*A. senticosus* Action: "[To invigorate the function of] the kidney", "Dual deficiency of lung and kidney, chronic cough and dyspnea of deficiency type, limp aching in lower back and knees caused by kidney deficiency"

References

Beinfield H, Korngold E (1991). *Between Heaven and Earth: A Guide to Chinese Medicine.* 1st ed. New York: Ballantine Books.

Chen P (2004). *Diagnosis in Traditional Medicine.* China: Complementary Medicine Press.

Chen SY, Tang DC, Yao YZ, Yuan Y (2003). "Science of Chinese Materia Medica." A newly compiled practical English-Chinese library of traditional Chinese medicine Vol. 3. Shanghai, China: Publishing house of Shanghai University of Traditional Chinese Medicine.

Chai K (2007). *Fundamental Theory of Traditional Chinese Medicine.* 2nd ed. China: People's Medical Publishing House.

Li GD, Wang LF, Yue PP, Tang CJ (2003). "Diagnostics of Traditional Chinese Medicine." A newly compiled practical English-Chinese library of traditional Chinese medicine Vol. 2. Shanghai, China: Publishing house of Shanghai University of Traditional Chinese medicine.

Wang XH, Wu CG, Mei XY (2003). "Basic Theory of Traditional Chinese Medicine." A newly compiled practical English-Chinese library of traditional Chinese medicine Vol. 1. Shanghai, China: Publishing house of Shanghai University of Traditional Chinese medicine.

Wang Y (2006). *Diagnostics of Traditional Chinese Medicine.* Beijing: Higher Education Press.

Wiseman N, Ellis A (1994). "Fundamentals of Chinese Medicine, Revised edition (translated and amended from Zhong Yi Xue Ji Chu by Nigel Wiseman)." Brookline, Massachusetts, USA: Paradigm Publications.

Wu JN (2005). *An Illustrated Chinese Materia Medica.* 1st ed. Oxford: Oxford University Press.

Xu L, Wang W (2002). *Chinese Materia Medica.* UK: Donica Publishing Ltd.

Zhao Z, Hong Kong Baptist University, School of Chinese Medicine (2004). *An Illustrated Chinese Materia Medica in Hong Kong [Xianggang Zhong Yao Cai Tu Jian].* 1st ed. Hong Kong: School of Chinese Medicine, Hong Kong Baptist University.

Pharmacological Activities and Herb–Drug Interactions

Table A3 Summary of pharmacological activities and herb–drug interactions

Herb	Pharmacological activities	Herb–drug interactions
Chinese Ginseng and Korean Ginseng	Anti-Alzheimer's Anti-depressant Anti-asthmatic Anti-diabetic Anti-fatigue Anti-hyperlipidemic Anti-inflammatory Anti-malarial Anti-microbial Anti-neoplastic Anti-obesity Anti-osteoporotic Anti-oxidative Anti-Parkinson's Anti-pica Anti-remodeling Anti-spasmodic Anti-trypanosomal Anti-ulcer Anti-viral Cardioprotective Chemoprotective Fertility-enhancing	1. Enhances effects of anti-cancer drugs such as 5-fluorouracil, irinotecan, mitomycin C, docetaxel, cisplatin 2. Decreases the anti-coagulant effects of warfarin 3. Decreases blood concentration and effects of alcohol 4. Reduces absorption and increases the elimination of Midazolam from the body 5. Interacts with caffeine, increasing blood pressure 6. Interacts with phenelzine, producing manic-like symptoms

(Continued)

Table A3 (*Continued*)

Herb	Pharmacological activities	Herb–drug interactions
	Hepatoprotective Immunomodulatory Memory-enhancing Neuroprotective Radioprotective Renoprotective Wound healing Improves Chronic Obstructive Pulmonary Diseases (COPD) Improves Erectile Dysfunction (ED) Improves Menopausal symptoms Improves Morphine-withdrawal symptoms Improves Multiple Sclerosis Enhances mammary involution Enhances physical performance	7. Interacts with raltegravir, resulting in an acute elevation of liver enzymes, marked jaundice and significant weight loss 8. Interacts with imatinib, resulting in imatinib-induced hepatotoxicity in a patient with chronic myelogenous leukemia
Red Ginseng and Korean Red Ginseng	Anti-allergy Anti-Alzheimer's Anti-arthritic Anti-bacterial Anti-depressant Anti-diabetic Anti-hyperlipidemic Anti-hypertensive Anti-inflammatory Anti-neoplastic Anti-obesity Anti-osteoporotic Anti-oxidative Anti-ulcer Anti-viral Fertility-enhancing	Similar to *P. ginseng*

(*Continued*)

Table A3   (*Continued*)

Herb	Pharmacological activities	Herb–drug interactions
	Hepatoprotective Hypoglycemic Immunomodulatory Memory-enhancing Cardioprotective Radioprotective Renoprotective Skin-whitening Improves Attention Deficit Hyperactivity Disorder (ADHD) Improves Atopic Dermatitis Improves Benign Prostate Hyperplasia (BPH) Improves Cold hypersensitivity Improves Drug-induced hearing loss Improves Erectile Dysfunction (ED) Improves Menopausal symptoms Improves Pancreatic injury Improves Polycystic Ovarian Syndrome (PCOS) Enhances visual process Protects against certain toxic compounds found in cigarette smoke	
American Ginseng	Anti-Alzheimer's Anti-atherosclerotic Anti-depressant Anti-diabetic Anti-fatigue Anti-hypertensive Anti-inflammatory Anti-neoplastic	1. Enhances antioxidative effect of vitamin C 2. Reduces the anti-coagulant effect of warfarin, thereby increasing the risk of severe bleeding.

(*Continued*)

Table A3 (*Continued*)

Herb	Pharmacological activities	Herb–drug interactions
	Anti-obesity Anti-oxidative Anti-Parkinson's Anti-ulcer Anti-ulcerative collitis Anxiolytic Cardioprotective Cardioregulatory Hypoglycemic Immunomodulatory Memory-enhancing Neuroprotective Radioprotective Improves Multiple Sclerosis (MS) Improves Common cold Improves Menopausal symptoms Improves Premature ovarian failure	
San Qi	Angiogenic Anti-atherosclerotic Anti-diabetic Anti-fatigue Anti-hyperlipidemic Anti-inflammatory Anti-neoplastic Anti-osteoporotic Anti-oxidative Anti-platelet Anti-ulcer Cardioprotective Hypoglycemic Immunomodulatory Neuroprotective	1. Enhances effects of anti-cancer drugs such as cisplatin and 5-fluorouracil 2. Decreases the effects of caffeine by increasing its elimination from the body

(*Continued*)

Table A3   (*Continued*)

Herb	Pharmacological activities	Herb–drug interactions
	Improves Acute Lung Injury (ALI) Improves Erectile Dysfunction (ED) Improves Haemorrhagic shock Improves Pulmonary fibrosis Improves Stroke Enhances the strength of repairing ligament	
Siberian Ginseng	Anti-Alzheimer's Anti-arthritic Anti-depressant Anti-diabetic Anti-fatigue Anti-inflammatory Anti-neoplastic Anti-obesity Anti-osteoporotic Anti-oxidative Anti-Parkinson's Anti-ulcer Anti-viral Anxiolytic Hepatoprotective Immunomodulatory Neuroprotective Protects against Cadmium poisoning Protects against Endotoxic shock	1. Increases the transport of digoxin and decreases the transport of cephalexin *in vitro* (across human intestinal cells)
Five-leaf ginseng	Anti-Alzheimer's Anti-asthmatic Anti-bacterial Anti-diabetic Anti-fungal Anti-hyperlipidemic	1. Gypenosides inhibit drug metabolism of dextromethorphan, paclitaxel, midazolam, testosterone and tolbutamide

(*Continued*)

Table A3 *(Continued)*

Herb	Pharmacological activities	Herb–drug interactions
	Anti-inflammatory	
	Anti-neoplastic	
	Anti-obesity	
	Anti-Parkinson's	
	Anti-oxidative	
	Anti-ulcer	
	Anxiolytic	
	Cardioprotective	
	Hepatoprotective	
	Immunostimulatory	
	Neuroprotective	
	Radioprotective	

Major Chemical Components and Their Pharmacological Activities

Table A4 Major chemical components present in *P. ginseng, P. quinquefolius, P. notoginseng, E. senticocus* and *G. pentaphyllum* and their pharmacological activities.

Chemical class	Chemical components	Major activities	References
Saponins	Ginsenoside F2	Anti-neoplastic	Mai TT *et al.*, 2012; Shin JY *et al.*, 2012
	An intestinal metabolite of Rb1 (Shin HS *et al.*, 2014a)	Anti-obesity Reduction of hair loss	Siraj FM *et al.*, 2014 Shin HS *et al.*, 2014a; Shin HS *et al.*, 2014b
	Ginsenoside F4	Anti-neoplastic	Chen B *et al.*, 2013
	Obtained through steaming (Kim WY *et al.*, 2000)	Prevention of cartilage degradation	Lee JH *et al.*, 2014
	Ginsenoside M1	Anti-Alzheimer's	Tohda C *et al.*, 2004
	Intestinal metabolite of ginsenoside Rb1 (Tohda C *et al.*, 2004)		
	Ginsenoside Rb1	Anti-Alzheimer's	Tohda C *et al.*, 2004; Wang Y *et al.*, 2013a
		Anti-depressant	Yamada N *et al.*, 2011

(Continued)

Table A4 (*Continued*)

Chemical class	Chemical components	Major activities	References
Saponins		Anti-diabetic	Park S *et al.*, 2008; Shang W *et al.*, 2008
		Anti-fatigue	Tan S *et al.*, 2013
		Anti-inflammatory	Tan S *et al.*, 2014; Zhang Y *et al.*, 2014
		Anti-neoplastic	Lee DG *et al.*, 2014
		Anti-oxidative	Liu ZQ *et al.*, 2003
		Anti-osteoporosis	Cheng B *et al.*, 2012
		Anti-remodeling	Jiang QS *et al.*, 2007
		Anti-viral	Jeong JJ *et al.*, 2014
		Cardioprotective	Wang Z *et al.*, 2008; Wu Y *et al.*, 2011
		Oestrogen-like activity	Cho J *et al.*, 2004
		Hepatoprotective	Hou YL *et al.*, 2014; Shen L *et al.*, 2013; Wu LL *et al.*, 2014
		Immunomodulatory	Sun J *et al.*, 2007
		Immunosuppressive	Samimi R *et al.*, 2014
		Inhibitory effect on intestinal contraction	Xu L and Huang SP, 2012
		Neuroprotective	Cheng Y *et al.*, 2005; Kim YC *et al.*, 1998; Liu D *et al.*, 2014; Ni N *et al.*, 2014; Wu J *et al.*, 2009; Zeng XS *et al.*, 2014

(*Continued*)

Table A4   *(Continued)*

Chemical class	Chemical components	Major activities	References
Saponins		Promotion of hair growth	Li Z *et al.*, 2013
		Protection against gentamicin-induced hearing dysfunction	Tian CJ *et al.*, 2013
		Protection against lung injury	Wang J *et al.*, 2013; Wu LL *et al.*, 2014
		Renoprotective	Sun Q *et al.*, 2013
		Skin-whitening	Wang L *et al.*, 2014a
		Stimulation of luteinising hormone secretion	Tsai SC *et al.*, 2003
	Ginsenoside Rb2	Anti-diabetic	Lee KT *et al.*, 2011
		Anti-neoplastic	Fujimoto J *et al.*, 2001; Lee DG *et al.*, 2014
		Anti-osteoporosis	Gao B *et al.*, 2014b; Huang Q *et al.*, 2014
	Ginsenoside Rb3	Anti-depressant	Cui J *et al.*, 2012
		Anti-hypertensive	Wang Y *et al.*, 2014a
		Anti-neoplastic	He F *et al.*, 2014
		Anti-oxidative	Liu ZQ *et al.*, 2003
		Cardioprotective	Ma L *et al.*, 2014; Shi Y *et al.*, 2011; Wang T *et al.*, 2010
		Hypoglycemic	Bu QT *et al.*, 2012
		Neuroprotective	Peng LL *et al.*, 2009

(Continued)

Table A4   (*Continued*)

Chemical class	Chemical components	Major activities	References
Saponins	Ginsenoside Rc	Anti-diabetic	Lee MS *et al.*, 2010
		Anti-oxidative	Kim DH *et al.*, 2014; Liu ZQ *et al.*, 2003
		Fertility-enhancing	Chen JC *et al.*, 2001
		Neuroprotective	Wu J *et al.*, 2009
	Ginsenoside Rd	Anti-Alzheimer's	Liu J *et al.*, 2012
		Anti-atherosclerosis	Li J *et al.*, 2011
		Anti-inflammatory	Kim DH *et al.*, 2013; Zhang YX *et al.*, 2013
		Anti-neoplastic	Chang TL *et al.*, 2008; Kim BJ, 2013; Yoon JH *et al.*, 2012a
		Anti-osteoporosis	Kim DY *et al.*, 2012
		Anti-oxidative	Liu ZQ *et al.*, 2003
		Anti-Parkinson's	Lin WM *et al.*, 2007
		Cardioprotective	Wang Y *et al.*, 2013b
		Immunomodulatory	Han Y and Rhew KY, 2013
		Neuroprotective	Wang B *et al.*, 2013; Zhang X *et al.*, 2013; Zhang X *et al.*, 2014
		Protection against Stroke	Cai BX *et al.*, 2009; Liu X *et al.*, 2012; Ye R *et al.*, 2013
		Promotion of hair growth	Li Z *et al.*, 2013

(*Continued*)

Table A4   (*Continued*)

Chemical class	Chemical components	Major activities	References
Saponins		Renoprotective	Yokozawa T and Liu ZW, 2000; Yokozawa T *et al.*, 1998
		therapeutic effect on Multiple Sclerosis	Zhu D *et al.*, 2014
		Wound-healing	Kim WK *et al.*, 2013
	Ginsenoside Re	Angiogenic	Huang YC *et al.*, 2005
		Anti-Alzheimer's	Chen F *et al.*, 2006; Kim MS *et al.*, 2014
		Anti-inflammatory	Bae HM *et al.*, 2012
		Anti-oxidative	Liu ZQ *et al.*, 2003
		Anti-ulcer	Lee S *et al.*, 2014
		Cardioprotective	Bai CX *et al.*, 2004; Lim KH *et al.*, 2013; Wang YG *et al.*, 2008; Xie JT *et al.*, 2006
		Fertility-enhancing	Zhang H *et al.*, 2007
		Hypoglycemic	Attele AS *et al.*, 2002; Cho WC *et al.*, 2006; Gao Y *et al.*, 2013; Quan HY *et al.*, 2012
		Immunomodulatory	Kim J *et al.*, 2012; Qu D *et al.*, 2013; Su X *et al.*, 2014; Sun J *et al.*, 2007

(*Continued*)

Table A4 (*Continued*)

Chemical class	Chemical components	Major activities	References
Saponins		Neuroprotective	Lee KW *et al.*, 2012; Shin EJ *et al.*, 2014
		Protection against opiod-induced hyperalgesia	Li P *et al.*, 2014
		Renoprotective	Kim JH *et al.*, 2014
		Stimulatory effect on gastric contractility	Xiong Y *et al.*, 2014
		Vasorelaxing effect	Sukrittanon S *et al.*, 2014
	Ginsenoside Rf	Analgesic	Mogil JS *et al.*, 1998; Nemmani KV and Ramarao P, 2003
		Anti-neoplastic	Shangguan WJ *et al.*, 2014
	Ginsenoside Rg1	Angiogenic	Leung KW *et al.*, 2011; Zheng Y *et al.*, 2013
		Anti-allergic	Oh HA *et al.*, 2013
		Anti-Alzheimer's and its related complications	Chen F *et al.*, 2006; Cheng Y *et al.*, 2005; He Y *et al.*, 2014; Quan Q *et al.*, 2013; Song XY *et al.*, 2013; Wang Y *et al.*, 2014b
		Anti-arrhythmia	Wu W *et al.*, 1995
		Anti-arthritic	Gu Y *et al.*, 2014
		Anti-depressant	Jiang B *et al.*, 2012
		Anti-diabetic	Park S *et al.*, 2008

(*Continued*)

Table A4   (*Continued*)

Chemical class	Chemical components	Major activities	References
Saponins		Anti-hypertensive	Pan C *et al.*, 2012
		Anti-inflammatory	Rhule A *et al.*, 2008; Song Y *et al.*, 2013
		Anti-neoplastic	Gao QG *et al.*, 2014; Lee DG *et al.*, 2014; Li J *et al.*, 2014b; Li L *et al.*, 2014
		Antioxidative	Liu ZQ *et al.*, 2003
		Anti-Parkinson's	Chen XC *et al.*, 2005
		Anti-platelet activity	Zhou Q *et al.*, 2014
		Anti-remodeling	Deng J *et al.*, 2010; Li CY *et al.*, 2013; Zhang YJ *et al.*, 2013
		Cardioprotective	Zhu D *et al.*, 2009
		Enhancement of sex drive	Yoshimura H *et al.*, 1998
		Oestrogen-like effect	Chan RY *et al.*, 2002
		Glucocorticoid-like effect	Lee YJ *et al.*, 1997
		Hepatoprotective	Cao L *et al.*, 2013; Li JP *et al.*, 2014
		Immunomodulatory	Lee EJ *et al.*, 2004; Lee JH and Han Y, 2006; Sun J *et al.*, 2007; Wang Y *et al.*, 2014c
		Improves Erectile Dysfunction	Wang X *et al.*, 2010

(*Continued*)

Table A4 *(Continued)*

Chemical class	Chemical components	Major activities	References
Saponins		Improves Haemopoiesis	Xu SF *et al.*, 2012
		Neuroprotective	He Q *et al.*, 2014; Huang SL *et al.*, 2014; Zeng XS *et al.*, 2014; Zhou Y *et al.*, 2014; Zhu J *et al.*, 2014
		Protection against complications related to diabetes	Yang N *et al.*, 2012
		Protection against podocyte injury	Mao N *et al.*, 2014;
		Protection against Sepsis	Zou Y *et al.*, 2013
		Protection from UV radiation	Chen C *et al.*, 2014; Lou JS *et al.*, 2013
		Renoprotective	Xie XS *et al.*, 2010
	Ginsenoside Rg2	Anti-coagulation effect	Li CT *et al.*, 2013
		Anti-diabetic	Yuan HD *et al.*, 2012
		Anti-inflammatory	Cho YS *et al.*, 2013
		Anti-oxidative	Samukawa K *et al.*, 2008
		Immunomodulatory	Sun J *et al.*, 2007
		Neuroprotective	Li N *et al.*, 2007; Shuangyan W *et al.*, 2012; Zhang G *et al.*, 2008;

(Continued)

Table A4   (*Continued*)

Chemical class	Chemical components	Major activities	References
Saponins		Prevention against UV	Ha SE *et al.*, 2010
	Ginsenoside 20(S)-Rg3 obtained through steaming (Kim WY *et al.*, 2000)	Anti-Alzheimer's	Chen F *et al.*, 2006
		Anti-diabetic	Park MW *et al.*, 2008
		Anti-fatigue	Xu Y *et al.*, 2013
		Anti-inflammatory	Kim SS *et al.*, 2014
		Anti-neoplastic	Chang L *et al.*, 2014; Guo JQ *et al.*, 2014; Kim BM *et al.*, 2014; Kim DG *et al.*, 2014; Lee YJ *et al.*, 2014; Liu T *et al.*, 2014; Park EH *et al.*, 2014; Qiu XM *et al.*, 2014; Wang JH *et al.*, 2014; Zhang YH *et al.*, 2014
		Anti-platelet activity	Lee WM *et al.*, 2008
		Anti-viral	Kang LJ *et al.*, 2013
		Immunomodulatory	Sun J *et al.*, 2007
		Prevention of cartilage degradation	Lee JH *et al.*, 2014
		Promotion of hair growth	Shin DH *et al.*, 2014

(*Continued*)

Table A4 (*Continued*)

Chemical class	Chemical components	Major activities	References
Saponins		Neuroprotective	Kim JH *et al.*, 2007; Kim YC *et al.*, 1998; Peña ID *et al.*, 2014
		Wound-healing effects	Sun X *et al.*, 2014
	Ginsenoside 20(R)-Rg3, obtained from steaming (Kim WY *et al.*, 2000)	Anti-neoplastic	Kim YJ *et al.*, 2014
		Neuroprotective	He B *et al.*, 2012
	Ginsenoside Rg5 Steamed (Kim WY *et al.*, 2000)	Anti-Alzheimer's	Chu S *et al.*, 2014
		Anti-inflammatory	Kim TW *et al.*, 2012; Lee YY *et al.*, 2013
		Anti-neoplastic	Lee KY and Lee SK, 1997; Yun TK *et al.*, 2001
		Neuroprotective	Kim EJ *et al.*, 2013; Wu J *et al.*, 2009
		Protection effects against dermatitis	Shin YW *et al.*, 2006a
	Ginsenoside Rh1, Intestinal metabolite of Re (Shin YW *et al.*, 2006b)	Anti-inflammatory	Choi YJ *et al.*, 2011; Li J *et al.*, 2014a; Park EK *et al.*, 2004
		Anti-neoplastic	Jung JS *et al.*, 2013; Yoon JH *et al.*, 2012b
		Anti-obesity	Gu W *et al.*, 2013
		Anti-osteoporotic	Siddiqi MH *et al.*, 2014

(*Continued*)

Table A4   (*Continued*)

Chemical class	Chemical components	Major activities	References
Saponins		Anti-oxidative	Liu ZQ *et al.*, 2003
		Cardioprotective	Gai Y *et al.*, 2012
		Oestrogenic effects	Lee Y *et al.*, 2003
		Memory-enhancing	Hou J *et al.*, 2014; Wang YZ *et al.*, 2009
		Neuroprotective	Jung JS *et al.*, 2010a; Jung JS *et al.*, 2010b
		Protection against Atopic Dermatitis	Shin YW *et al.*, 2006b; Zheng H *et al.*, 2011
	Ginsenoside 20(S)-Rh2, Intestinal metabolite of ginsenoside Rg3 (Wee JJ *et al.*, 2011)	Anti-Alzheimer's	Qiu J *et al.*, 2014; Shieh PC *et al.*, 2008
		Anti-neoplastic	Bae EA *et al.* 2002; Guo XX *et al.*, 2014; Jia WW *et al.*, 2004; Kim HS *et al.*, 2004; Kim MJ *et al.*, 2014; Shi Q *et al.*, 2014; Tang XP *et al.*, 2013; You ZM *et al.*, 2014
		Anti-obesity	Hwang JT *et al.*, 2007
		Cardioprotective	Wang H *et al.*, 2012
		Hypoglycemic	Fatmawati S *et al.*, 2014; Lee WK *et al.*, 2006
		Immunomodulatory	Lian LH *et al.*, 2013

(*Continued*)

Table A4 *(Continued)*

Chemical class	Chemical components	Major activities	References
Saponins		improves Stress Urinary Incontinence	Chen YH *et al.*, 2014
		Memory-enhancing	Hou J *et al.*, 2013a
		Neuroprotective	Bae EA *et al.*, 2006b
		Protection against ulcerative colitis	Ye H *et al.*, 2014
		Protection against UV radiation	Oh SJ *et al.*, 2014
	Ginsenoside 20(R)-Rh2, Intestinal metabolite of ginsenoside Rg3 (Wee JJ *et al.*, 2011)	Anti-inflammatory	Choi WY *et al.*, 2013
		Anti-osteoporotic	Liu J *et al.*, 2009
	Ginsenoside Rh3, Intestinal metabolite of ginsenoside Rg5 (Shin YW *et al.*, 2006a)	Neuroprotective	Kim EJ *et al.*, 2013
		Protects against Chronic Dermatitis	Shin YW *et al.*, 2006a
	Ginsenoside Rk1 obtained from steaming (Park IH *et al.*, 2002b)	Anti-neoplastic	Kim JS *et al.*, 2012; Kim YJ *et al.*, 2008
		Anti-platelet activity	Ju HK *et al.*, 2012
		Blocking effect on vascular leakage	Maeng YS *et al.*, 2013
	Ginsenoside Ro	Hepatoprotective	Matsuda H *et al.*, 1991
		Immunomodulatory	Yu JL *et al.*, 2005
		Promotion of hair growth	Murata K *et al.*, 2012

(Continued)

Table A4   (*Continued*)

Chemical class	Chemical components	Major activities	References
Saponins	Ginsenoside Rs4 obtained from steaming (Park IH *et al.*, 2002a)	Anti-neoplastic	Kim SE *et al.*, 1999
	Ginsenoside R1	Antioxidative	Liu ZQ *et al.*, 2003
	Gypenoside XVII	Anti-Alzheimer's disease	Meng X *et al.*, 2014a
	Gypenoside TN2	Improves learning impairment	Hong XW *et al.*, 2011
	Gypenoside LXXIV	improves learning impairment	Joh EW *et al.*, 2010
	Gypenoside XLIX	Anti-inflammatory	Huang TH *et al.* 2006; Huang TH *et al.*, 2007
	Gypenoside III	Bronchodilatory	Circosta C *et al.*, 2005
	Gypenoside VII	Bronchodilatory	Circosta C *et al.*, 2005
	Malonylginsenoside Rb1	Potentiates neurite outgrowth	Abe K *et al.*, 1994; Nishiyama N *et al.*, 1994
	Phanoside Compound K, Intestinal metabolite of protopanaxadiol ginsenosides (Wee JJ *et al.*, 2011)	Anti-diabetic	Hoa NK *et al.*, 2007
		Anti-Alzheimer's	Guo J *et al.*, 2014
		Anti-angiogenic	Shin KO *et al.*, 2014
		Anti-arthritic	Chen J *et al.*, 2014; Choi YS *et al.*, 2013; Liu KK *et al.*, 2014
		Anti-atherosclerotic	Park ES *et al.*, 2013

(*Continued*)

Table A4 *(Continued)*

Chemical class	Chemical components	Major activities	References
Saponins		Anti-diabetic	Gu J *et al.*, 2013; Guan FY *et al.*, 2014; Han CG *et al.*, 2007; Jiang S *et al.*, 2014; Yoon SH *et al.*, 2007
		Anti-inflammatory	Li J *et al.*, 2014c; Park JS *et al.*, 2012
		Anti-depression	Yamada N *et al.*, 2011
		Anti-neoplastic	Chen Y *et al.*, 2013; Kim AD *et al.*, 2013; Law CK *et al.*, 2014; Zheng ZZ *et al.*, 2014
		Hepatoprotective	Kim MS *et al.*, 2013
		Neuroprotective	Hou JG *et al.*, 2013b
	Pseudoginsenoside F11	Anti-Alzheimer's	Wang CM *et al.*, 2013
		Anti-obesity	Wu G *et al.*, 2014
		Anti-Parkinson's	Wang JY *et al.*, 2013
		Neuroprotective	Li Z *et al.*, 1999; Wang X *et al.*, 2014; Wu CF *et al.*, 2003
		Protection against cisplatin-induced renotoxicity	Wang H *et al.*, 2014

(Continued)

Table A4   (*Continued*)

Chemical class	Chemical components	Major activities	References
Saponins		Protection against morphine-induced behavioural changes	Hao Y *et al.*, 2007; Li Z *et al.*, 2000; Li Z *et al.*, 2001
	Notoginsenoside Ft1	Angiogenic	Shen K *et al.*, 2012
		Anti-neoplastic	Gao B *et al.*, 2014c
		Haemostatic	Gao B *et al.*, 2014a
		Vasorelaxing effects	Shen K *et al.*, 2014
	Notoginsenoside R1	Anti-Alzheimer's	Ma B *et al.*, 2014; Yan S *et al.*, 2014
		Anti-atherosclerotic	Jia C *et al.*, 2014; Zhang WJ *et al.*, 1997
		Anti-inflammatory	Sun K *et al.*, 2007
		Anti-remodeling	Zhang HS and Wang SQ, 2006
		Anti-oxidative	Meng X *et al.*, 2014
		Cardioprotective	He K *et al.* 2014; Sun B *et al.*, 2013
		Hepatoprotective	Chen WX *et al.*, 2008
		Immunomodulatory	Sun HX *et al.*, 2006
		Neuroprotective	Gu B *et al.*, 2009; Meng X *et al.*, 2014a; Meng X *et al.*, 2014b
		Protection against intestinal Ischaemic-Reperfusion	Li C *et al.*, 2014a

(*Continued*)

Table A4 (*Continued*)

Chemical class	Chemical components	Major activities	References
Saponins		Protection against Pulmonary Arterial Hypertension	Xu Y *et al.*, 2014
		Renoprotective	Liu WJ *et al.*, 2010
	Notoginsenoside R2	Anti-Parkinson's	Meng XB *et al.*, 2013
	Notoginsenoside Rb1	Anti-Alzheimer's	Wang Y *et al.*, 2013a
	Notoginsenoside ST-4	Anti-viral	Pei Y *et al.*, 2011
	Compound Mx Intestinal metabolite of ginsenoside Rb3 (He K *et al.*, 2005)	Anti-neoplastic	He K *et al.*, 2005
	20(S)-25-methoxyl-dammarane-3β, 12β, 20-triol (a ginsenoside)	Anti-neoplastic	Bi X *et al.*, 2009; Wang W *et al.*, 2012; Wu YL *et al.*, 2011
	20S-dihydroproto-panaxadiol	Immunomodulatory	Kim MY *et al.*, 2013
Lignans	Sesamin	Anti-neoplastic	Hibasami H *et al.*, 2000
		Anti-Parkinson's	Fujikawa T *et al.*, 2005
Polysac-charide	American Ginseng Polysaccharides	Immunomodulatory	Azike CG *et al.*, 2014
	Acidic polysaccharide	Anti-depressant	Wang J *et al.*, 2010a
Polysac-charides		Anti-diabetic	Sun C *et al.*, 2014
		Immunomodulatory	Wang Z *et al.*, 2013
		Radioprotective	Bing SJ *et al.*, 2014; Park E *et al.*, 2011
		Therapeutic effect against Influenza Viral infection	Yoo DG *et al.*, 2012

(*Continued*)

Table A4   (*Continued*)

Chemical class	Chemical components	Major activities	References
Polysac-charides	Alkali-extractable polysaccharide	Immunomodulatory	Yu X *et al.*, 2014
	E. senticosus polysaccharides	Anti-diabetic	Fu J *et al.*, 2012
		Anti-oxidant	Chen R *et al.*, 2011
		Immunomodulatory	Chen R *et al.*, 2011 Han J *et al.*, 2014
		Neuroprotective	Xie U *et al.*, 2015
	G. pentaphyllum	Anti-fatigue	Shan LN and Shi YX, 2014
	polysaccharide	Anti-neoplastic	Liu J *et al.*, 2014
		Anti-oxidant	Chi A *et al.*, 2012
		Anti-Parkinson's	Deng Q and Yang Y, 2014
		Immunomodulatory	Yang X *et al.*, 2008
	Ginsan	Immunomodulatory	Shim JY *et al.*, 2007
	Ginseng Polysaccharides	Anti-fatigue	Wang J *et al.*, 2014
		Anti-neoplastic	Cheng H *et al.*, 2011; Wang J *et al.*, 2010b; Zhou X *et al.*, 2014
		Immunomodulatory	Zhang SD *et al.*, 2010
	Ginseng neutral polysaccharides	Anti-neoplastic	Ni W *et al.*, 2010
	GP-B1	Anti-neoplastic	Li XL *et al.*, 2012a
	GP-I	Therapeutic effects on Psioriasis	Li XL *et al.*, 2012b
	GP50-dHR	Anti-viral	Baek SH *et al.*, 2010
	GP50-eHR	Anti-viral	Baek SH *et al.*, 2010
	Panaxane A	Hypoglycemic	Konno C *et al.*, 1984

(*Continued*)

Table A4 (*Continued*)

Chemical class	Chemical components	Major activities	References
Polysac-charides	Panaxane B	Hypoglycemic	Konno C *et al.*, 1984
	Panaxane C	Hypoglycemic	Konno C *et al.*, 1984
	Panaxane D	Hypoglycemic	Konno C *et al.*, 1984
	Panaxane E	Hypoglycemic	Konno C *et al.*, 1984
	Panaxane I	Hypoglycemic	Oshima Y *et al.*, 1985
	Panaxane J	Hypoglycemic	Oshima Y *et al.*, 1985
	Panaxane K	Hypoglycemic	Oshima Y *et al.*, 1985
	Panaxane L	Hypoglycemic	Oshima Y *et al.*, 1985
	Panaxane Q	Hypoglycemic	Konno C *et al.* 1985
	Panaxane R	Hypoglycemic	Konno C *et al.* 1985
	Panaxane S	Hypoglycemic	Konno C *et al.* 1985
	Panaxane T	Hypoglycemic	Konno C *et al.* 1985
	Panaxane U	Hypoglycemic	Konno C *et al.* 1985
	PBGA11	Immunostimulatory	Gao H *et al.*, 1996
	PBGA12	Immunostimulatory	Gao H *et al.*, 1996
	PF3111	Immunostimulatory	Gao H *et al.*, 1996
	PF3112	Immunostimulatory	Gao H *et al.*, 1996
	PG-F2	Protective effects against Bacterial Infection	Lee JH *et al.*, 2009
	PG-HMW	Protective effects against Bacterial Infection	Lee JH *et al.*, 2009
	PGPW1	Anti-neoplastic	Cai JP *et al.*, 2013; Li C *et al.*, 2012
	PGP2a	Anti-neoplastic	Li C *et al.*, 2014b
	PPQN	Anti-inflammatory	Wang L *et al.*, 2014b
	Red ginseng acidic polysaccharide	Anti-hyperlipidemic	Kwak YS *et al.*, 2010
		Immunomodulatory	Byeon SE *et al.*, 2012

(*Continued*)

Table A4   (*Continued*)

Chemical class	Chemical components	Major activities	References
Polyace- tylenes	Falacrinol (panaxynol)	Anti-neoplastic	Matsunaga H *et al.*, 1990; Purup S *et al.*, 2009; Yan Z *et al.*, 2011
		Anti-platelet	Teng CM *et al.*, 1989
		Induces neurite outgrowth	Wang ZJ *et al.*, 2006
		Anti-Alzheimer's	Hao W *et al.*, 2005
	Panaxydol	Anti-neoplastic	Guo L *et al.*, 2009; Hai J *et al.*, 2009; Matsunaga H *et al.*, 1990; Moon J *et al.*, 2000; Purup S *et al.*, 2009; Yan Z *et al.*, 2011
	Falcarintriol (panaxytriol)	Anti-bacterial	Bae EA *et al.*, 2001
		Anti-neoplastic	Kim JY *et al.*, 2002; Matsunaga H *et al.*, 1990; Matsunaga H *et al.*, 1994; Matsunaga H *et al.*, 1995; Ng F *et al.*, 2008
Flavonol glycosides	Kaempferol-3-O- sophoroside	Anti-inflammatory	Kim TH *et al.*, 2012a; Kim TH *et al.*, 2012b
	Quercetin 3-O-β-D- xylopyranosyl-β-D- galactopyranoside	Anti-Alzheimer's	Choi RC *et al.*, 2010
Glycosides	Eleutheroside E	Anti-Alzheimer's	Bai Y *et al.*, 2011

(*Continued*)

Table A4 (*Continued*)

Chemical class	Chemical components	Major activities	References
Glycosides		Anti-arthritic	He C *et al.*, 2014
		Anti-diabetic	Ahn J *et al.*, 2013
		Memory-enhancing	Huang D *et al.*, 2013
		Reduce behavioural alteration arising from sleep deprivation	Huang LZ *et al.*, 2011
	Eleutheroside B	Anti-diabetic	Liu KY *et al.*, 2008; Niu HS *et al.*, 2007; Niu HS *et al.*, 2008
		Hepatoprotective	Gong X *et al.*, 2014
		Immunomodulatory	Cho JY *et al.*, 2001
		Memory-enhancing	Huang D *et al.*, 2013
G protein-coupled lysophos-phatidic acid (LPA) receptor ligand	Gintonin	Affects cardiac rhythmicity	Choi SH *et al.*, 2014
		Anti-Alzheimer's	Hwang SH *et al.* 2012
		Anti-neoplastic	Hwang SH *et al.*, 2013
		Memory-enhancing	Shin TJ *et al.*, 2012
		Regulates neuronal activities	Lee JH *et al.*, 2013
		Stimulate gastrointestinal motility	Kim BJ *et al.*, 2014
		Vaso-relaxing effects	Choi SH *et al.*, 2013
Amino acids	Dencichine	Haemostatic	Huang LF *et al.*, 2014

References

Abe K, Cho SI, Kitagawa I, Nishiyama N, Saito H (1994). Differential effects of ginsenoside Rb1 and malonylginsenoside Rb1 on long-term potentiation in the dentate gyrus of rats. *Brain Res* **649**(1–2): 7–11.

Ahn J, Um MY, Lee H, Jung CH, Heo SH, Ha TY (2013). Eleutheroside E, an active component of *Eleutherococcus senticosus*, ameliorates insulin resistance in type 2 diabetic db/db mice. *Evid Based Complement Alternat Med* 934183.

Attele AS, Zhou YP, Xie JT, Wu JA, Zhang L, Dey L, Pugh W, Rue PA, Polonsky KS, Yuan CS (2002). Antidiabetic effects of *Panax ginseng* berry extract and the identification of an effective component. *Diabetes* **51**: 1851–1858.

Azike CG, Charpentier PA, Lui EM (2014). Stimulation and suppression of innate immune function by american ginseng polysaccharides: biological relevance and identification of bioactives. *Pharm Res* [Epub ahead of print].

Bae EA, Han MJ, Baek NI, Kim DH (2001). *In vitro* anti-*Helicobacter pylori* activity of panaxytriol isolated from ginseng. *Arch Pharm Res* **24**(4): 297–299.

Bae EA, Han MJ, Choo MK, Park SY, Kim DH (2002). Metabolism of 20(S)- and 20(R)-ginsenoside Rg3 by human intestinal bacteria and its relation to *in vivo* biological activities. *Biol Pharm Bull* **25**: 58–63.

Bae EA, Han MJ, Shin YW, Kim DH (2006a). Inhibitory effects of Korean red ginseng and its genuine constituents ginsenosides Rg3, Rf, and Rh2 in mouse passive cutaneous anaphylaxis reaction and contact dermatitis models. *Biol Pharm Bull.* **29**(9): 1862–1867.

Bae EA, Kim EJ, Park JS, Kim HS, Ryu JH, Kim DH (2006b). Ginsenosides Rg3 and Rh2 inhibit the activation of AP-1 and protein kinase A pathway in lipopolysaccharide/interferon-gamma-stimulated BV-2 microglial cells. *Planta Med* **72**: 627–633.

Bae HM, Cho OS, Kim SJ, Im BO, Cho SH, Lee S, Kim MG, Kim KT, Leem KH, Ko SK (2012). Inhibitory effects of ginsenoside Re isolated from ginseng berry on histamine and cytokine release in human mast cells and human alveolar epithelial cells. *J Ginseng Res* **36**(4): 369–374.

Baek SH, Lee JG, Park SY, Bae ON, Kim DH, Park JH (2010). Pectic polysaccharides from Panax ginseng as the antirotavirus principals in ginseng. *Biomacromolecules* **11**(8): 2044–2052.

Bai CX, Takahashi K, Masumiya H, Sawanobori T, Furukawa T (2004). Nitric oxide-dependent modulation of the delayed rectifier K^+ current and the L-type Ca^{2+} current by ginsenoside Re, an ingredient of *Panax ginseng*, in guinea-pig cardiomyocytes. *Br J Pharmacol* **142**: 567–575.

Bai Y, Tohda C, Zhu S, Hattori M, Komatsu K (2011). Active components from Siberian ginseng (*Eleutherococcus senticosus*) for protection of amyloid β(25-35)-induced neuritic atrophy in cultured rat cortical neurons. *J Nat Med* **65**(3–4): 417–423.

Bi X, Zhao Y, Fang W, Yang W (2009). Anticancer activity of *Panax notoginseng* extract 20(S)-25-OCH3-PPD: targeting beta-catenin signalling. *Clin Exp Pharmacol Physiol* **36**(11): 1074–1078.

Bing SJ, Kim MJ, Ahn G, Im J, Kim DS, Ha D, Cho J, Kim A, Jee Y (2014). Acidic polysaccharide of Panax ginseng regulates the mitochondria/caspase-dependent apoptotic pathway in radiation-induced damage to the jejunum in mice. *Acta Histochem* **116**(3): 514–521.

Bu QT, Zhang WY, Chen QC, Zhang CZ, Gong XJ, Liu WC, Li W, Zheng YN (2012). Anti-diabetic effect of ginsenoside Rb(3) in alloxan-induced diabetic mice. *Med Chem* **8**(5): 934–941.

Byeon SE, Lee J, Kim JH, Yang WS, Kwak YH, Kim SY, Choung ES, Rhee MH, Choi JY (2012). Molecular mechanism of macrophage activation by red ginseng acidic polysaccharide from Korean red ginseng. *Mediators Inflamm* **2012**: 1–7.

Cai BX, Li XY, Chen JH, Tang YB, Wang GL, Zhou JG, Qui QY, Guan YY (2009). Ginsenoside-Rd, a new voltage-independent Ca^{2+} entry blocker, reverses basilar hypertrophic remodeling in stroke-prone renovascular hypertensive rats. *Eur J Pharmacol* **606**: 142–149.

Cai JP, Wu YJ, Li C, Feng MY, Shi QT, Li R, Wang ZY, Geng JS (2013). Panax ginseng polysaccharide suppresses metastasis via modulating Twist expression in gastric cancer. *Int J Biol Macromol* **57**: 22–25.

Cao L, Zou Y, Zhu J, Fan X, Li J (2013). Ginsenoside Rg1 attenuates concanavalin A-induced hepatitis in mice through inhibition of cytokine secretion and lymphocyte infiltration. *Mol Cell Biochem* **380**(1–2): 203–210.

Chan RY, Chen WF, Dong A, Guo D, Wong MS (2002). Estrogen-like activity of ginsenoside Rg1 derived from Panax notoginseng. *J Clin Endocrinol Metab* **87**: 3691–3695.

Chang L, Huo B, Lv Y, Wang Y, Liu W (2014). Ginsenoside Rg3 enhances the inhibitory effects of chemotherapy on esophageal squamous cell carcinoma in mice. *Mol Clin Oncol* **2**(6): 1043–1046.

Chang TL, Ding HY, Kao YW (2008). Role of ginsenoside Rd in inhibiting 26S proteasome activity. *J Agric Food Chem* **56**(24): 12011–12015.

Chen B, Shen YP, Zhang DF, Cheng J, Jia XB (2013). The apoptosis-inducing effect of ginsenoside F4 from steamed notoginseng on human lymphocytoma JK cells. *Nat Prod Res* **27**(24): 2351–2354.

Chen C, Mu XY, Zhou Y, Shun K, Geng S, Liu J, Wang JW, Chen J, Li TY, Wang YP (2014). Ginsenoside Rg1 enhances the resistance of hematopoietic stem/progenitor cells to radiation-induced aging in mice. *Acta Pharmacol Sin* **35**(1): 143–150.

Chen F, Eckman EA, Eckman CB (2006). Reductions in levels of the Alzheimer's amyloid betapeptide after oral administration of ginsenosides. *FASEB J* **20**: 1269–1271.

Chen J, Wu H, Wang Q, Chang Y, Liu K, Song S, Yuan P, Fu J, Sun W, Huang Q, Liu L, Wu Y, Zhang Y, Zhou A, Wei W (2014). Ginsenoside metabolite compound k alleviates adjuvant-induced arthritis by suppressing T cell activation. *Inflammation* **37**(5): 1608–1615.

Chen JC, Chen LD, Tsauer W, Tsai CC, Chen BC, Chen YJ (2001). Effects of ginsenoside Rb2 and Rc on inferior human sperm motility *in vitro*. *Am J Chin Med* **29**: 155–160.

Chen R, Liu Z, Zhao J, Chen R, Meng F, Zhang M, Ge W (2011). Antioxidant and immunobiological activity of water-soluble polysaccharide fractions purified from *Acanthopanax senticosu*. *Food Chem* **127**(2): 434–440.

Chen WX, Wang F, Liu YY, Zeng QJ, Sun K, Xue X, Li X, Yang JY, An LH, Hu BH, Yang JH, Wang CS, Li ZX, Liu LY, Li Y, Zheng J, Liao FL, Han D, Fan JY, Han JY (2008). Effect of notoginsenoside R1 on hepatic microcirculation disturbance induced by gut ischemia and reperfusion. *World J Gastroenterol* **14**(1): 29–37.

Chen XC, Zhou YC, Chen Y, Zhu YG, Fang F, Chen LM (2005). Ginsenoside Rg1 reduces MPTP-induced substantia nigra neuron loss by suppressing oxidative stress. *Acta Pharmacol Sin* **26**: 56–62.

Chen Y, Xu Y, Zhu Y, Li X (2013). Anti-cancer effects of ginsenoside compound K on pediatric acute myeloid leukemia cells. *Cancer Cell Int* **13**(1): 24.

Chen YH, Lin YN, Chen WC, Hsieh WT, Chen HY (2014). Treatment of stress urinary incontinence by ginsenoside Rh2. *Am J Chin Med* **42**(4): 817–831.

Cheng B, Li J, Du J, Lv X, Weng L, Ling C (2012). Ginsenoside Rb1 inhibits osteoclastogenesis by modulating NF-κB and MAPK pathways. *Food Chem Toxicol* **50**: 1610–1615.

Cheng H, Li S, Fan Y, Gao X, Hao M, Wang J, Zhang X, Tai G, Zhou Y (2011). Comparative studies of the antiproliferative effects of ginseng polysaccharides on HT-29 human colon cancer cells. *Med Oncol* **28**(1): 175–181.

Cheng Y, Shen LH, Zhang JT (2005). Anti-amnestic and anti-aging effects of ginsenoside Rg1 and Rb1 and its mechanism of action. *Acta Pharmacol Sin* **26**: 143–149.

Chi A, Tang L, Zhang J, Zhang K (2012). Chemical composition of three polysaccharides from *Gynostemma pentaphyllum* and their antioxidant activity in skeletal muscle of exercised mice. *Int J Sport Nutr Exerc Metab* **22**(6): 479–485.

Cho J, Park W, Lee S, Ahn W, Lee Y (2004) Ginsenoside-Rb1 from *Panax ginseng* C.A. Meyer activates estrogen receptor-alpha and -beta, independent of ligand binding. *J Clin Endocrinol Metab* **89**: 3510–3515.

Cho JY, Nam KH, Kim AR, Park J, Yoo ES, Baik KU, Yu YH, Park MH (2001). *In-vitro* and *in-vivo* immunomodulatory effects of syringin. *J Pharm Pharmacol* **53**(9): 1287–1294.

Cho WC, Chung WS, Lee SK, Leung AW, Cheng CH, Yue KK (2006). Ginsenoside Re of *Panax ginseng* possesses significant antioxidant and antihyperlipidemic efficacies in streptozotocin-induced diabetic rats. *Eur J Pharmacol* **550**: 173–179.

Cho YS, Kim CH, Ha TS, Lee SJ, Ahn HY (2013). Ginsenoside Rg2 inhibits lipopolysaccharide-induced adhesion molecule expression in human umbilical vein endothelial cell. *Korean J Physiol Pharmacol* **17**(2): 133–137.

Choi RC, Zhu JT, Leung KW, Chu GK, Xie HQ, Chen VP, Zheng KY, Lau DT, Dong TT, Chow PC, Han YF, Wang ZT, Tsim KW (2010).

A flavonol glycoside, isolated from roots of *Panax notoginseng*, reduces amyloid-beta-induced neurotoxicity in cultured neurons: signaling transduction and drug development for Alzheimer's disease. *J Alzheimers Dis* **19**(3): 795–811.

Choi SH, Lee BH, Hwang SH, Kim HJ, Lee SM, Kim HC, Rhim HW, Nah SY (2013). Molecular mechanisms of large-conductance Ca(2+)-activated potassium channel activation by ginseng gintonin. *Evid Based Complement Alternat Med* 323709.

Choi SH, Lee BH, Kim HJ, Jung SW, Kim HS, Shin HC, Lee JH, Kim HC, Rhim H, Hwang SH, Ha TS, Kim HJ, Cho H, Nah SY (2014). Ginseng gintonin activates the human cardiac delayed rectifier K(+) channel: involvement of Ca(2+)/calmodulin binding sites. *Mol Cells* **37**(9): 656–663.

Choi WY, Lim HW, Lim CJ (2013). Anti-inflammatory, antioxidative and matrix metalloproteinase inhibitory properties of 20(R)-ginsenoside Rh2 in cultured macrophages and keratinocytes. *J Pharm Pharmacol* **65**(2): 310–316.

Choi YJ, Yoon JH, Cha SW, Lee SG (2011). Ginsenoside Rh1 inhibits the invasion and migration of THP-1 acute monocytic leukemia cells via inactivation of the MAPK signaling pathway. *Fitoterapia* **82**(6): 911–919.

Choi YS, Kang EH, Lee EY, Gong HS, Kang HS, Shin K, Lee EB, Song YW, Lee YJ (2013). Joint-protective effects of compound K, a major ginsenoside metabolite, in rheumatoid arthritis: *in vitro* evidence. *Rheumatol Int* **33**(8): 1981–1990.

Chu S, Gu J, Feng L, Liu J, Zhang M, Jia X, Liu M, Yao D (2014). Ginsenoside Rg5 improves cognitive dysfunction and beta-amyloid deposition in STZ-induced memory impaired rats via attenuating neuroinflammatory responses. *Int Immunopharmacol* **19**(2): 317–326.

Circosta C, De Pasquale R, Palumbo DR, Occhiuto F (2005). Bronchodilatory effects of the aqueous extract of *Gynostemma pentaphyllum* and gypenosides III and VIII in anaesthetized guinea-pigs. *J Pharm Pharmacol* **57**(8): 1053–1058.

Cui J, Jiang L, Xiang H (2012). Ginsenoside Rb3 exerts antidepressant-like effects in several animal models. *J Psychopharmacol* **26**(5): 697–713.

Deng J, Wang YW, Chen WM, Wu Q, Huang XN (2010). Role of nitric oxide in ginsenoside Rg(1)-induced protection against left ventricular hypertrophy produced by abdominal aorta coarctation in rats. *Biol Pharm Bull* **33**: 631–635.

Deng Q, Yang X (2014). Protective effects of Gynostemma pentaphyllum polysaccharides on PC12 cells impaired by MPP(+). *Int J Biol Macromol* **69**: 171–175.

Fatmawati S, Ersam T, Yu H, Zhang C, Jin F, Shimizu K (2014). 20(S)-Ginsenoside Rh2 as aldose reductase inhibitor from *Panax ginseng*. *Bioorg Med Chem Lett* **24**(18): 4407–4409.

Fu J, Fu J, Yuan J, Zhang N, Gao B, Fu G, Tu Y, Zhang Y (2012). Anti-diabetic activities of *Acanthopanax senticosus* polysaccharide (ASP) in combination with metformin. *Int J Biol Macromol* **50**(3): 619–623.

Fujikawa T, Kanada N, Shimada A, Ogata M, Suzuki I, Hayashi I, Nakashima K (2005). Effect of sesamin in *Acanthopanax senticosus* HARMS on behavioral dysfunction in rotenone-induced parkinsonian rats. *Biol Pharm Bull* **28**(1): 169–172.

Fujimoto J, Sakaguchi H, Aoki I, Toyoki H, Khatun S, Tamaya T (2001). Inhibitory effect of ginsenoside-Rb2 on invasiveness of uterine endometrial cancer cells to the basement membrane. *Eur J Gynaecol Oncol* **22**: 339–341.

Gai Y, Ma Z, Yu X, Qu S, Sui D (2012). Effect of ginsenoside Rh1 on myocardial injury and heart function in isoproterenol-induced cardiotoxicity in rats. *Toxicol Mech Methods* **22**(8): 584–591.

Gao B, Huang L, Liu H, Wu H, Zhang E, Yang L, Wu X, Wang Z (2014a). Platelet $P2Y_{12}$ receptors are involved in the haemostatic effect of notoginsenoside Ft1, a saponin isolated from *Panax notoginseng*. *Br J Pharmacol* **171**(1): 214–223.

Gao B, Huang Q, Jie Q, Zhang HY, Wang L, Guo YS, Sun Z, Wei BY, Han YH, Liu J, Yang L, Luo ZJ (2014b). Ginsenoside-Rb2 inhibits dexamethasone-induced apoptosis through promotion of GPR120 induction in bone marrow-derived mesenchymal stem cells. *Stem Cells Dev* [Epub ahead of print].

Gao B, Shi HL, Li X, Qiu SP, Wu H, Zhang BB, Wu XJ, Wang ZT (2014c). p38 MAPK and ERK1/2 pathways are involved in the pro-apoptotic effect of notoginsenoside Ft1 on human neuroblastoma SH-SY5Y cells. *Life Sci* **108**(2): 63–70.

Gao H, Wang F, Lien EJ, Trousdale MD (1996). Immunostimulating poly-saccharides from *Panax notoginseng*. *Pharm Res* **13**: 1196–1200.

Gao QG, Chan HY, Man CW, Wong MS (2014). Differential ERα-mediated rapid estrogenic actions of ginsenoside Rg1 and estren in human breast cancer MCF-7 cells. *J Steroid Biochem Mol Biol* **141**: 104–112.

Gao Y, Yang MF, Su YP, Jiang HM, You XJ, Yang YJ, Zhang HL (2013). Ginsenoside Re reduces insulin resistance through activation of PPAR-γ pathway and inhibition of TNF-α production. *J Ethnophar-macol* **147**(2): 509–516.

Gong X, Zhang L, Jiang R, Wang CD, Yin XR, Wan JY (2014). Hepatoprotective effects of syringin on fulminant hepatic failure induced by D-galactosamine and lipopolysaccharide in mice. *J Appl Toxicol* **34**(3): 265–271.

Gu B, Nakamichi N, Zhang WS, Nakamura Y, Kambe Y, Fukumori R, Takuma K, Yamada K, Takarada T, Taniura H, Yoneda Y (2009). Possible protection by notoginsenoside R1 against glutamate neuro-toxicity mediated by N-methyl-D-aspartate receptors composed of an NR1/NR2B subunit assembly. *J Neurosci Res* **87**(9): 2145–2156.

Gu J, Li W, Xiao D, Wei S, Cui W, Chen W, Hu Y, Bi X, Kim Y, Li J, Du H, Zhang M, Chen L (2013). Compound K, a final intestinal metabolite of ginsenosides, enhances insulin secretion in MIN6 pancreatic β-cells by upregulation of GLUT2. *Fitoterapia* **87**: 84–88.

Gu W, Kim KA, Kim DH (2013). Ginsenoside Rh1 ameliorates high fat diet-induced obesity in mice by inhibiting adipocyte differentiation. *Biol Pharm Bull* **36**(1): 102–107.

Gu Y, Fan W, Yin G (2014). The study of mechanisms of protective effect of Rg1 against arthritis by inhibiting osteoclast differentiation and maturation in CIA mice. *Mediators Inflamm* 305071.

Guan FY, Gu J, Li W, Zhang M, Ji Y, Li J, Chen L, Hatch GM (2014). Compound K protects pancreatic islet cells against apoptosis through inhibition of the AMPK/JNK pathway in type 2 diabetic mice and in MIN6 β-cells. *Life Sci* **107**(1–2): 42–49.

Guo J, Chang L, Zhang X, Pei S, Yu M, Gao J (2014). Ginsenoside com-pound K promotes β-amyloid peptide clearance in primary astrocytes via autophagy enhancement. *Exp Ther Med* **8**(4): 1271–1274.

Guo JQ, Zheng QH, Chen H, Chen L, Xu JB, Chen MY, Lu D, Wang ZH, Tong HF, Lin S (2014). Ginsenoside Rg3 inhibition of vasculogenic mimicry in pancreatic cancer through downregulation of VE cadherin/EphA2/MMP9/MMP2 expression. *Int J Oncol* **45**(3): 1065–1072.

Guo L, Song L, Wang Z, Zhao W, Mao W, Yin M (2009). Panaxydol inhibits the proliferation and induces the differentiation of human hepato-carcinoma cell line HepG2. *Chem Biol Interact* **181**(1): 138–143.

Guo XX, Li Y, Sun C, Jiang D, Lin YJ, Jin FX, Lee SK, Jin YH (2014). p53-dependent Fas expression is critical for Ginsenoside Rh2 trig-gered caspase-8 activation in HeLa cells. *Protein Cell* **5**(3): 224–234.

Ha SE, Shin DH, Kim HD, Shim SM, Kim HS, Kim BH, Lee JS, Park JK (2010). Effects of ginsenoside Rg2 on the ultraviolet B-induced DNA damage responses in HaCaT cells. *Naunyn Schmiedebergs Arch Pharmacol* **382**(1): 89–101.

Hai J, Lin Q, Lu Y (2009). Phosphatidylinositol 3-kinase activity is required for the induction of differentiation in C6 glioma cells by panaxydol. *J Clin Neurosci* **16**(3): 444–448.

Han CG, Ko SK, Sung JH, Chung SH (2007). Compound K enhances insulin secretion with beneficial metabolic effects in db/db mice. *J Agric Food Chem* **55**: 10641–10648.

Han J, Bian L, Liu X, Zhang F, Zhang Y, Yu N (2014). Effects of *Acantho-panax senticosus* polysaccharide supplementation on growth performance, immunity, blood parameters and expression of pro-inflammatory cytokines genes in challenged weaned piglets. *Asian-Australas J Anim Sci* **27**(7): 1035–1043.

Han Y, Rhew KY (2013). Ginsenoside Rd induces protective anti-*Candida albicans* antibody through immunological adjuvant activity. *Int Immunopharmacol* **17**(3): 651–657.

Hao W, Xing-Jun W, Yong-Yao C, Liang Z, Yang L, Hong-Zhuan C (2005). Up-regulation of M1 muscarinic receptors expressed in CHOm1 cells by panaxynol via cAMP pathway. *Neurosci Lett* **383**(1–2): 121–126.

Hao Y, Yang JY, Wu CF, Wu MF (2007). Pseudoginsenoside-F11 decreases morphine-induced behavioral sensitization and extracellular glutamate levels in the medial prefrontal cortex in mice. *Pharmacol Biochem Behav* **86**(4): 660–666.

He B, Chen P, Yang J, Yun Y, Zhang X, Yang R, Shen Z (2012). Neuroprotective effect of 20(R)-ginsenoside Rg(3) against transient focal cerebral ischemia in rats. *Neurosci Lett* **526**(2): 106–111.

He C, Chen X, Zhao C, Qie Y, Yan Z, Zhu X (2014). Eleutheroside E ameliorates arthritis severity in collagen-induced arthritis mice model by suppressing inflammatory cytokine release. *Inflammation* **37**(5): 1533–1543.

He F, Ding Y, Liang C, Song SB, Dou DQ1, Song GY, Kim YH (2014). Antitumor effects of dammarane-type saponins from steamed notoginseng. *Pharmacogn Mag* **10**(39): 314–317.

He K, Liu Y, Yang Y, Li P, Yang L (2005). A dammarane glycoside derived from ginsenoside Rb3. *Chem Pharm Bull* **53**: 177–179.

He K, Yan L, Pan CS, Liu YY, Cui YC, Hu BH, Chang X, Li Q, Sun K, Mao XW, Fan JY, Han JY (2014). ROCK-dependent ATP5D modulation contributes to the protection of notoginsenoside NR1 against ischemia/reperfusion-induced myocardial injury. *Am J Physiol Heart Circ Physiol* **307**(12): H1764–H1776.

He Q, Sun J, Wang Q, Wang W, He B (2014). Neuroprotective effects of ginsenoside Rg1 against oxygen-glucose deprivation in cultured hippocampal neurons. *J Chin Med Assoc* **77**(3): 142–149.

He Y, Zhao H, Su G (2014). Ginsenoside Rg1 decreases neurofibrillary tangles accumulation in retina by regulating activities of neprilysin and PKA in retinal cells of AD mice model. *J Mol Neurosci* **52**(1): 101–106.

Hibasami H, Fujikawa T, Takeda H, Nishibe S, Satoh T, Fujisawa T, Nakashima K (2000). Induction of apoptosis by *Acanthopanax senticosus* HARMS and its component, sesamin in human stomach cancer KATO III cells. *Oncol Rep* **7**(6): 1213–1216.

Hoa NK, Norberg A, Sillard R, Van Phan D, Thuan ND, Dzung DT, Jörnvall H, Ostenson CG (2007). The possible mechanisms by which phanoside stimulates insulin secretion from rat islets. *J Endocrinol* **192**(2): 389–394.

Hong SW, Yang JH, Joh EH, Kim HJ, Kim DH (2011). Gypenoside TN-2 ameliorates scopolamine-induced learning deficit in mice. *J Ethnopharmacol* **134**(3): 1010–1013.

Hou J, Xue J, Lee M, Liu L, Zhang D, Sun M, Zheng Y, Sung C (2013a). Ginsenoside Rh2 improves learning and memory in mice. *J Med Food* **16**(8): 772–776.

Hou J, Xue J, Lee M, Sun MQ, Zhao XH, Zheng YN, Sung CK (2013b). Compound K is able to ameliorate the impaired cognitive function and hippocampal neurogenesis following chemotherapy treatment. *Biochem Biophys Res Commun* **436**(1): 104–109.

Hou J, Xue J, Lee M, Yu J, Sung C (2014). Long-term administration of ginsenoside Rh1 enhances learning and memory by promoting cell survival in the mouse hippocampus. *Int J Mol Med* **33**(1): 234–240.

Hou YL, Tsai YH, Lin YH, Chao JC (2014). Ginseng extract and ginsenoside Rb1 attenuate carbon tetrachloride-induced liver fibrosis in rats. *BMC Complement Alternat Med* **14**(1): 415.

Huang D, Hu Z, Yu Z (2013). Eleutheroside B or E enhances learning and memory in experimentally aged rats. *Neural Regen Res* **8**(12): 1103–1112.

Huang LF, Shi HL, Gao B, Wu H, Yang L, Wu XJ, Wang ZT (2014). Decichine enhances hemostasis of activated platelets via AMPA receptors. *Thromb Res* **133**(5): 848–854.

Huang LZ, Wei L, Zhao HF, Huang BK, Rahman K, Qin LP (2011). The effect of Eleutheroside E on behavioral alterations in murine sleep deprivation stress model. *Eur J Pharmacol* **658**(2–3): 150–155.

Huang Q, Gao B, Jie Q, Wei BY, Fan J, Zhang HY, Zhang JK, Li XJ, Shi J, Luo ZJ, Yang L, Liu J (2014). Ginsenoside-Rb2 displays anti-osteoporosis effects through reducing oxidative damage and bone-resorbing cytokines during osteogenesis. *Bone* **66**: 306–314.

Huang SL, He XJ, Li ZF, Lin L, Cheng B (2014). Neuroprotective effects of ginsenoside Rg1 on oxygen-glucose deprivation reperfusion in PC12 cells. *Pharmazie* **69**(3): 208–211.

Huang TH, Li Y, Razmovski-Naumovski V, Tran VH, Li GQ, Duke CC, Roufogalis BD (2006). Gypenoside XLIX isolated from *Gynostemma pentaphyllum* inhibits nuclear factor-kappaB activation via a PPAR-alpha-dependent pathway. *J Biomed Sci* **13**(4): 535–548.

Huang TH, Tran VH, Roufogalis BD, Li Y (2007). Gypenoside XLIX, a naturally occurring PPAR-alpha activator, inhibits cytokine-induced vascular cell adhesion molecule-1 expression and activity in human endothelial cells. *Eur J Pharmacol* **565**(1–3): 158–165.

Huang YC, Chen CT, Chen SC, Lai PH, Liang HC, Chang Y, Yu LC, Sung HW (2005). A natural compound (ginsenoside Re) isolated from *Panax ginseng* as a novel angiogenic agent for tissue regeneration. *Pharm Res* **22**: 636–646.

Hwang JT, Kim SH, Lee MS, Kim SH, Yang HJ, Kim MJ, Kim HS, Ha J, Kim MS, Kwon DY (2007). Anti-obesity effects of ginsenoside Rh2 are associated with the activation of AMPK signaling pathway in 3T3-L1 adipocyte. *Biochem Biophys Res Commun* **364**: 1002–1008.

Hwang SH, Lee BH, Kim HJ, Cho HJ, Shin HC, Im KS, Choi SH, Shin TJ, Lee SM, Nam SW, Kim HC, Rhim H, Nah SY (2013). Suppression of metastasis of intravenously-inoculated B16/F10 melanoma cells by the novel ginseng-derived ingredient, gintonin: involvement of auto-taxin inhibition. *Int J Oncol* **42**: 317–326.

Hwang SH, Shin EJ, Shin TJ, Lee BH, Choi SH, Kang J, Kim HJ, Kwon SH, Jang CG, Lee JH, Kim HC, Nah SY (2012). Gintonin, a ginseng-derived lysophosphatidic acid receptor ligand, attenuates Alzheimer's disease-related neuropathies: involvement of non-amyloidogenic processing. *J Alzheimers Dis* **31**: 207–223.

Jeong JJ, Kim B, Kim DH (2014). Ginsenoside Rb1 eliminates HIV-1 (D3)-transduced cytoprotective human macrophages by inhibiting the AKT pathway. *J Med Food* **17**(8): 849–854.

Jia C, Xiong M, Wang P, Cui J, Du X, Yang Q, Wang W, Chen Y, Zhang T (2014). Notoginsenoside R1 attenuates atherosclerotic lesions in ApoE deficient mouse model. *PLoS One* **9**(6): e99849.

Jia WW, Bu X, Philips D, Yan H, Liu G, Chen X, Bush JA, Li G (2004). Rh2, a compound extracted from ginseng, hypersensitizes multidrug-resistance tumor cells to chemotherapy. *Can J Physiol Pharmacol* **82**: 431–437.

Jiang B, Xiong Z, Yang J, Wang W, Wang Y, Hu ZL, Wang F, Chen JG (2012). Antidepressant-like effects of ginsenoside Rg1 are due to activation of the BDNF signalling pathway and neurogenesis in the hippocampus. *Br J Pharmacol* **166**: 1872–1887.

Jiang QS, Huang XN, Dai ZK, Yang GZ, Zhou QX, Shi JS, Wu Q (2007). Inhibitory effect of ginsenoside Rb1 on cardiac hypertrophy induced by monocrotaline in rat. *J Ethnopharmacol* **111**: 567–572.

Jiang S, Ren D, Li J, Yuan G, Li H, Xu G, Han X, Du P, An L (2014). Effects of compound K on hyperglycemia and insulin resistance in rats with type 2 diabetes mellitus. *Fitoterapia* **95**: 58–64.

Joh EH, Yang JW, Kim DH (2010). Gypenoside LXXIV ameliorates sco-polamine-induced learning deficit in mice. *Planta Med* **76**(8): 793–795.

Ju HK, Lee JG, Park MK, Park SJ, Lee CH, Park JH, Kwon SW (2012). Metabolomic investigation of the anti-platelet aggregation activity of ginsenoside Rk_1 reveals attenuated 12-HETE production. *J Proteome Res* **11**(10): 4939–4946.

Jung JS, Ahn JH, Le TK, Kim DH, Kim HS (2013). Protopanaxatriol ginsenoside Rh1 inhibits the expression of matrix metalloproteinases and the *in vitro* invasion/migration of human astroglioma cells. *Neurochem Int* **63**(2): 80–86.

Jung JS, Kim DH, Kim HS (2010a). Ginsenoside Rh1 suppresses inducible nitric oxide synthase gene expression in IFN-gamma-stimulated microglia via modulation of JAK/STAT and ERK signaling pathways. *Biochem Biophys Res Commun* **397**: 323–328.

Jung JS, Shin JA, Park EM, Lee JE, Kang YS, Min SW, Kim DH, Hyun JW, Shin CY, Kim HS (2010b). Anti-inflammatory mechanism of ginsenoside Rh1 in lipopolysaccharide-stimulated microglia: critical role of the protein kinase A pathway and hemeoxygenase-1 expression. *J Neurochem* **115**: 1668–1680.

Kang LJ, Choi YJ, Lee SG (2013). Stimulation of TRAF6/TAK1 degradation and inhibition of JNK/AP-1 signalling by ginsenoside Rg3 attenuates hepatitis B virus replication. *Int J Biochem Cell Biol* **45**(11): 2612–2621.

Kim AD, Kang KA, Kim HS, Kim DH, Choi YH, Lee SJ, Kim HS, Hyun JW (2013). A ginseng metabolite, compound K, induces autophagy and apoptosis via generation of reactive oxygen species and activation of JNK in human colon cancer cells. *Cell Death Dis* **4**: e750.

Kim BJ (2013). Involvement of melastatin type transient receptor potential 7 channels in ginsenoside Rd-induced apoptosis in gastric and breast cancer cells. *J Ginseng Res.* **37**(2): 201–209.

Kim BJ, Nam JH, Kim KH, Joo M, Ha TS, Weon KY, Choi S, Jun JY, Park EJ, Wie J, So I, Nah SY (2014). Characteristics of gintonin-mediated membrane depolarization of pacemaker activity in cultured interstitial cells of Cajal. *Cell Physiol Biochem* **34**(3): 873–890.

Kim BM, Kim DH, Park JH, Surh YJ, Na HK (2014). Ginsenoside Rg3 inhibits constitutive activation of NF-κB signaling in human breast cancer (MDA-MB-231) cells: ERK and Akt as potential upstream targets. *J Cancer Prev* **19**(1): 23–30.

Kim DG, Jung KH, Lee DG, Yoon JH, Choi KS, Kwon SW, Shen HM, Morgan MJ, Hong SS, Kim YS (2014). 20(S)-Ginsenoside Rg3 is a novel inhibitor of autophagy and sensitizes hepatocellular carcinoma to doxorubicin. *Oncotarget* **5**(12): 4438–4451.

Kim DH, Chung JH, Yoon JS, Ha YM, Bae S, Lee EK, Jung KJ, Kim MS, Kim YJ, Kim MK, Chung HY (2013). Ginsenoside Rd inhibits the expressions of iNOS and COX-2 by suppressing NF-κB in LPS-stimulated RAW264.7 cells and mouse liver. *J Ginseng Res* **37**(1): 54–63.

Kim DH, Park CH, Park D, Choi YJ, Park MH, Chung KW, Kim SR, Lee JS, Chung HY (2014). Ginsenoside Rc modulates Akt/FoxO1 pathways and suppresses oxidative stress. *Arch Pharm Res* **37**(6): 813–820.

Kim DY, Park YG, Quan HY, Kim SJ, Jung MS, Chung SH (2012). Ginsenoside Rd stimulates the differentiation and mineralization of osteoblastic MC3T3-E1 cells by activating AMP-activated protein kinase via the BMP-2 signaling pathway. *Fitoterapia* **83**(1): 215–222.

Kim EJ, Jung IH, Van Le TK, Jeong JJ, Kim NJ, Kim DH (2013). Ginsenosides Rg5 and Rh3 protect scopolamine-induced memory deficits in mice. *J Ethnopharmacol* **146**(1): 294–299.

Kim HS, Lee EH, Ko SR, Choi KJ, Park JH, Im DS (2004). Effects of ginsenosides Rg3 and Rh2 on the proliferation of prostate cancer cells. *Arch Pharm Res* **27**: 429–435.

Kim J, Han BJ, Kim H, Lee JY, Joo I, Omer S, Kim YS, Han Y (2012). Th1 immunity induction by ginsenoside Re involves in protection of mice against disseminated candidiasis due to *Candida albicans*. *Int Immunopharmacol* **14**(4): 481–486.

Kim JH, Cho SY, Lee JH, Jeong SM, Yoon IS, Lee BH, Lee JH, Pyo MK, Lee SM, Chung JM, Kim S, Rhim H, Oh JW, Nah SY (2007). Neuroprotective effects of ginsenoside Rg3 against homocysteine-induced excitotoxicity in rat hippocampus. *Brain Res* **1136**: 190–199.

Kim JH, Han IH, Yamabe N, Kim YJ, Lee W, Eom DW, Choi P, Cheon GJ, Jang HJ, Kim SN, Ham J, Kang KS (2014). Renoprotective effects of Maillard reaction products generated during heat treatment of ginsenoside Re with leucine. *Food Chem* **143**: 114–121.

Kim JS, Joo EJ, Chun J, Ha YW, Lee JH, Han Y, Kim YS (2012). Induction of apoptosis by ginsenoside Rk1 in SK-MEL-2-human melanoma. *Arch Pharm Res* **35**(4): 717–722.

Kim JY, Lee KW, Kim SH, Wee JJ, Kim YS, Lee HJ (2002). Inhibitory effect of tumor cell proliferation and induction of G2/M cell cycle arrest by panaxytriol. *Planta Med* **68**(2): 119–122.

Kim MJ, Yun H, Kim DH, Kang I, Choe W, Kim SS, Ha J (2014). AMP-activated protein kinase determines apoptotic sensitivity of cancer cells to ginsenoside-Rh2. *J Ginseng Res* **38**(1): 16–21.

Kim MS, Lee KT, Iseli TJ, Hoy AJ, George J, Grewal T, Roufogalis BD (2013). Compound K modulates fatty acid-induced lipid droplet formation and expression of proteins involved in lipid metabolism in hepatocytes. *Liver Int* **33**(10): 1583–1593.

Kim MS, Yu JM, Kim HJ, Kim HB, Kim ST, Jang SK, Choi YW, Lee do I, Joo SS (2014). Ginsenoside Re and Rd enhance the expression of cholinergic markers and neuronal differentiation in Neuro-2a cells. *Biol Pharm Bull* **37**(5): 826–833.

Kim MY, Cho JY (2013). 20S-dihydroprotopanaxadiol, a ginsenoside derivative, boosts innate immune responses of monocytes and macrophages. *J Ginseng Res* **37**(3): 293–299.

Kim SE, Lee YH, Park JH, Lee SK (1999). Ginsenoside-Rs4, a new type of ginseng saponin concurrently induces apoptosis and selectively elevates protein levels of p53 and p21WAF1 in human hepatoma SK-HEP-1 cells. *Eur J Cancer* **35**(3): 507–511.

Kim SS, Jang HJ, Oh MY, Eom DW, Kang KS, Kim YJ, Lee JH, Ham JY, Choi SY, Wee YM, Kim YH, Han DJ (2014). Ginsenoside Rg3 enhances islet cell function and attenuates apoptosis in mouse islets. *Transplant Proc* **46**(4): 1150–1155.

Kim TH, Ku SK, Bae JS (2012a). Inhibitory effects of kaempferol-3-O-sophoroside on HMGB1-mediated proinflammatory responses. *Food Chem Toxicol* **50**(3–4): 1118–1123.

Kim TH, Ku SK, Lee IC, Bae JS (2012b). Anti-inflammatory effects of kaempferol-3-O-sophoroside in human endothelial cells. *Inflamm Res* **61**(3): 217–224.

Kim TW, Joh EH, Kim B, Kim DH, (2012). Ginsenoside Rg5 ameliorates lung inflammation in mice by inhibiting the binding of LPS to Toll-like receptor-4 on macrophages. *Int Immunopharmacol* **12**(1): 110–116.

Kim WK, Song SY, Oh WK, Kaewsuwan S, Tran TL, Kim WS, Sung JH (2013). Wound-healing effect of ginsenoside Rd from leaves of *Panax ginseng* via cyclic AMP-dependent protein kinase pathway. *Eur J Pharmacol* **702**(1–3): 285–293.

Kim WY, Kim JM, Han SB, Lee SK, Kim ND, Park MK, Kim CK, Park JH (2000). Steaming of ginseng at high temperature enhances biological activity. *J Nat Prod* **63**(12): 1702–1704.

Kim YC, Kim SR, Markelonis GJ, Oh Th (1998). Ginsenosides Rb1 and Rg3 protect cultured rat cortical cells from glutamate-induced neurodegeneration. *J Neurosci Res* **4**: 426–432.

Kim YJ, Choi WI, Jeon BN, Choi KC, Kim K, Kim TJ, Ham J, Jang HJ, Kang KS, Ko H (2014). Stereospecific effects of ginsenoside 20-Rg3 inhibits TGF-β1-induced epithelial–mesenchymal transition and suppresses lung cancer migration, invasion and anoikis resistance. *Toxicology* **322**: 23–33.

Kim YJ, Kwon HC, Ko H, Park JH, Kim HY, Yoo JH, Yang HO (2008). Anti-tumor activity of the ginsenoside Rk1 in human hepatocellular carcinoma cells through inhibition of telomerase activity and induction of apoptosis. *Biol Pharm Bull* **231**(5): 826–830.

Konno C, Murakami M, Oshima Y, Hikino H (1985). Isolation and hypoglycemic activity of panaxans Q, R, S, T and U, glycans of *Panax ginseng* roots. *J Ethnopharmacol* **14**(1): 69–74.

Konno C, Sugiyama K, Kano M, Takahashi M, Hikino H (1984). Isolation and hypoglycemic activity of panaxans A, B, C, D and E, glycans of *Panax ginseng* roots. *Planta Med* **50**(5): 434–436.

Kwak YS, Kyung JS, Kim JS, Cho JY, Rhee MH (2010). Anti-hyperlipidemic effects of red ginseng acidic polysaccharide from Korean red ginseng. *Biol Pharm Bull* **33**(3): 468–472.

Law CK, Kwok HH, Poon PY, Lau CC, Jiang ZH, Tai WC, Hsiao WW, Mak NK, Yue PY, Wong RN (2014). Ginsenoside compound K induces apoptosis in nasopharyngeal carcinoma cells via activation of apoptosis-inducing factor. *Chin Med* **9**(1): 11.

Lee DG, Jang SI, Kim YR, Yang KE, Yoon SJ, Lee ZW, An HJ, Jang IS, Choi JS, Yoo HS (2014). Anti-proliferative effects of ginsenosides extracted from mountain ginseng on lung cancer. *Chin J Integr Med* [Epub ahead of print].

Lee EJ, Ko E, Lee J, Rho S, Ko S, Shin MK, Min BI, Hong MC, Kim SY, Bae H (2004). Ginsenoside Rg1 enhances CD4(+) T-cell activities and modulates Th1/Th2 differentiation. *Int Immunopharmacol* **4**: 235–244.

Lee JH, Choi SH, Lee BH, Hwang SH, Kim HJ, Rhee J, Chung C, Nah SY (2013). Activation of lysophosphatidic acid receptor by gintonin inhibits Kv1.2 channel activity: involvement of tyrosine kinase and receptor protein tyrosine phosphatase α. *Neurosci Lett* **548**: 143–148.

Lee JH, Han Y (2006). Ginsenoside Rg1 helps mice resist to disseminated candidiasis by Th1 type differentiation of CD4+ T cell. *Int Immunopharmacol* **6**: 1424–1430.

Lee JH, Lim H, Shehzad O, Kim YS, Kim HP (2014). Ginsenosides from Korean red ginseng inhibit matrix metalloproteinase-13 expression in articular chondrocytes and prevent cartilage degradation. *Eur J Pharmacol* **724**: 145–151.

Lee JH, Shim JS, Chung MS, Lim ST, Kim KH (2009). Inhibition of pathogen adhesion to host cells by polysaccharides from Panax ginseng. *Biosci Biotechnol Biochem* **73**(1): 209–212.

Lee KT, Jung TW, Lee HJ, Kim SG, Shin YS, Whang WK (2011). The antidiabetic effect of ginsenoside Rb2 via activation of AMPK. *Arch Pharm Res* **34**: 1201–1208.

Lee KW, Jung SY, Choi SM, Yang EJ (2012). Effects of ginsenoside Re on LPS-induced inflammatory mediators in BV2 microglial cells. *BMC Complement Alternat Med* **12**: 196.

Lee KY, Lee SK (1997). Ginsenoside-Rg5 supresses cyclin E-dependent protein kinase activity via up-regulation of p21Waf1 with concomitant down-regulation of cdc25A in SK-HEP-1 Cells. *Anticancer Res* **17**: 1067–1072.

Lee MS, Hwang JT, Kim SH, Yoon S, Kim MS, Yang HJ, Kwon DY (2010). Ginsenoside Rc, an active component of *Panax ginseng*, stimulates glucose uptake in C2C12 myotubes through an AMPK-dependent mechanism. *J Ethnopharmacol* **127**: 771–776.

Lee S, Kim MG, Ko SK, Kim HK, Leem KH, Kim YJ (2014). Protective effect of ginsenoside Re on acute gastric mucosal lesion induced by compound 48/80. *J Ginseng Res* **38**(2): 89–96.

Lee WK, Kao ST, Liu IM, Cheng JT (2006). Increase of insulin secretion by ginsenoside Rh2 to lower plasma glucose in Wistar rats. *Clin Exp Pharmacol Physiol* **33**: 27–32.

Lee WM, Kim SD, Park MH, Cho JY, Park HJ, Seo GS, Rhee MH (2008). Inhibitory mechanisms of dihydroginsenoside Rg3 in platelet aggregation: critical roles of ERK2 and cAMP. *J Pharm Pharmacol* **60**: 1531–1536.

Lee Y, Jin Y, Lim W, Ji S, Choi S, Jang S, Lee S (2003). Ginsenoside-Rh1, a component of ginseng saponin, activates estrogen receptor in human breast carcinoma MCF-7 cells. *J Steroid Biochem Mol Biol* **84**: 463–468.

Lee YJ, Chung E, Lee KY, Lee YH, Huh B, Lee SK (1997). Ginsenoside-Rg1, one of the major active molecules from *Panax ginseng*, is a functional ligand of glucocorticoid receptor. *Mol Cell Endocrinol* **133**: 135–140.

Lee YJ, Lee S, Ho JN, Byun SS, Hong SK, Lee SE, Lee E (2014). Synergistic antitumor effect of ginsenoside Rg3 and cisplatin in cisplatin-resistant bladder tumor cell line. *Oncol Rep* **32**(5): 1803–1808.

Lee YY, Park JS, Jung JS, Kim DH, Kim HS (2013). Anti-inflammatory effect of ginsenoside Rg5 in lipopolysaccharide-stimulated BV2 microglial cells. *Int J Mol Sci* **14**(5): 9820–9833.

Leung KW, Ng HM, Tang MKS, Wong CCK, Wong RNS, Wong AST (2011). Ginsenoside-Rg1 mediates a hypoxia-independent upregulation of hypoxia-inducible factor-1α to promote angiogenesis. *Angiogenesis* **14**(4): 515–522.

Li C, Cai J, Geng J, Li Y, Wang Z, Li R (2012). Purification, characterization and anticancer activity of a polysaccharide from Panax ginseng. *Int J Biol Macromol* **51**(5): 968–973.

Li C, Li Q, Liu YY, Wang MX, Pan CS, Yan L, Chen YY, Fan JY, Han JY (2014a). Protective effects of notoginsenoside R1 on intestinal ischemia-reperfusion injury in rats. *Am J Physiol Gastrointest Liver Physiol* **306**(2): G111–G122.

Li C, Tian ZN, Cai JP, Chen KX, Zhang B, Feng MY, Shi QT, Li R, Qin Y, Geng JS (2014b). *Panax ginseng* polysaccharide induces apoptosis by targeting Twist/AKR1C2/NF-1 pathway in human gastric cancer. *Carbohydr Polym* **102**: 103–109.

Li CT, Wang HB, Xu BJ (2013). A comparative study on anticoagulant activities of three Chinese herbal medicines from the genus *Panax* and anticoagulant activities of ginsenosides Rg1 and Rg2. *Pharm Biol* **51**(8): 1077–1080.

Li CY, Deng W, Liao XQ, Deng J, Zhang YK, Wang DX (2013). The effects and mechanism of ginsenoside Rg1 on myocardial remodeling in an animal model of chronic thromboembolic pulmonary hypertension. *Eur J Med Res* **18**: 16.

Li J, Du J, Liu D, Cheng B, Fang F, Weng L, Wang C, Ling C (2014a). Ginsenoside Rh1 potentiates dexamethasone's anti-inflammatory effects for chronic inflammatory disease by reversing dexamethasone-induced resistance. *Arthritis Res Ther* **16**(3): R106.

Li J, Wei Q, Zuo GW, Xia J, You ZM, Li CL, Chen DL (2014b). Ginsenoside Rg1 induces apoptosis through inhibition of the EpoR-mediated JAK2/STAT5 signalling pathway in the TF-1/ Epo human leukemia cell line. *Asian Pac J Cancer Prev* **15**(6): 2453–2459.

Li J, Xie ZZ, Tang YB, Zhou JG, Guan YY (2011). Ginsenoside-Rd, a purified component from *Panax notoginseng* saponins, prevents atherosclerosis in apoE knockout mice. *Eur J Pharmacol* **652**: 104–110.

Li J, Zhong W, Wang W, Hu S, Yuan J, Zhang B, Hu T, Song G (2014c). Ginsenoside metabolite compound K promotes recovery of dextran sulfate sodium-induced colitis and inhibits inflammatory responses by suppressing NF-κB activation. *PLoS One* **9**(2): e87810.

Li JP, Gao Y, Chu SF, Zhang Z, Xia CY, Mou Z, Song XY, He WB, Guo XF, Chen NH (2014). Nrf2 pathway activation contributes to anti-fibrosis effects of ginsenoside Rg1 in a rat model of alcohol- and CCl4-induced hepatic fibrosis. *Acta Pharmacol Sin* **35**(8): 1031–1044.

Li L, Wang Y, Qi B, Yuan D, Dong S, Guo D, Zhang C, Yu M (2014). Suppression of PMA-induced tumor cell invasion and migration by ginsenoside Rg1 via the inhibition of NF-κB-dependent MMP-9 expression. *Oncol Rep* **32**(5): 1779–1786.

Li N, Liu B, Dluzen DE, Jin Y (2007). Protective effects of ginsenoside Rg2 against glutamate-induced neurotoxicity in PC12 cells. *J Ethnopharmacol* **111**: 458–463.

Li P, Tang M, Li H, Huang X, Chen L, Zhai H (2014). Effects of ginsenosides on opioid-induced hyperalgesia in mice. *Neuroreport* **25**(10): 749–752.

Li XL, Wang ZH, Zhao YX, Luo SJ, Zhang DW, Xiao SX, Peng ZH (2012a). Isolation and antitumor activities of acidic polysaccharide from Gynostemma pentaphyllum Makino. *Carbohydr Polym* **89**(3): 942–947.

Li XL, Wang ZH, Zhao YX, Luo SJ, Zhang DW, Xiao SX, Peng ZH (2012b). Purification of a polysaccharide from Gynostemma pentaphyllum Makino and its therapeutic advantages for psoriasis. *Carbohydr Polym* **89**(4): 1232–1237.

Li Z, Guo YY, Wu CF, Li X, Wang JH (1999). Protective effects of pseudoginsenoside-F11 on scopolamine-induced memory impairment in mice and rats. *J Pharm Pharmacol* **51**(4): 435–440.

Li Z, Li JJ, Gu LJ, Zhang DL, Wang YB, Sung CK (2013). Ginsenosides Rb_1 and Rd regulate proliferation of mature keratinocytes through induction of p63 expression in hair follicles. *Phytother Res* **27**(7): 1095–1101.

Li Z, Wu CF, Pei G, Guo YY, Li X (2000). Antagonistic effect of pseudoginsenoside-F11 on the behavioral actions of morphine in mice. *Pharmacol Biochem Behav* **66**(3): 595–601.

Li Z, Xu NJ, Wu CF, Xiong Y, Fan HP, Zhang WB, Sun Y, Pei G (2001). Pseudoginsenoside-F11 attenuates morphine-induced signalling in Chinese hamster ovary-mu cells. *Neuroreport* **12**(7): 1453–1456.

Lian LH, Jin Q, Song SZ, Wu YL, Bai T, Jiang S, Li Q, Yang N, Nan JX (2013). Ginsenoside Rh2 downregulates LPS-induced NF-κB activation through inhibition of tak1 phosphorylation in RAW 264.7 murine macrophage. *Evid Based Complement Alternat Med* 646728.

Lim KH, Lim DJ, Kim JH (2013). Ginsenoside-Re ameliorates ischemia and reperfusion injury in the heart: a hemodynamics approach. *J Ginseng Res* **37**(3): 283–292.

Lin WM, Zhang YM, Moldzio R, Rausch WD (2007). Ginsenoside Rd attenuates neuroinflammation of dopaminergic cells in culture. *J Neural Transm Suppl* (72): 105–112.

Liu D, Zhang H, Gu W, Liu Y, Zhang M (2014). Ginsenoside Rb1 protects hippocampal neurons from high glucose-induced neurotoxicity by inhibiting GSK3β-mediated CHOP induction. *Mol Med Rep* **9**(4): 1434–1438.

Liu J, Shiono J, Shimizu K, Yu H, Zhang C, Jin F, Kondo R (2009). 20(R)-ginsenoside Rh2, not 20(S), is a selective osteoclastgenesis inhibitor without any cytotoxicity. *Bioorg Med Chem Lett* **19**: 3320–3323.

Liu J, Yan X, Li L, Zhu Y, Qin K, Zhou L, Sun D, Zhang X, Ye R, Zhao G (2012). Ginsenoside Rd attenuates cognitive dysfunction in a rat model of Alzheimer's disease. *Neurochem Res* **37**(12): 2738–2747.

Liu J, Zhang L, Ren Y, Gao Y, Kang L, Qiao Q (2014). Anticancer and immunoregulatory activity of *Gynostemma pentaphyllum* polysaccharides in H22 tumor-bearing mice. *Int J Biol Macromol* **69**: 1–4.

Liu KK, Wang QT, Yang SM, Chen JY, Wu HX, Wei W (2014). Ginsenoside compound K suppresses the abnormal activation of T lymphocytes in mice with collagen-induced arthritis. *Acta Pharmacol Sin* **35**(5): 599–612.

Liu KY, Wu YC, Liu IM, Yu WC, Cheng JT (2008). Release of acetylcholine by syringin, an active principle of *Eleutherococcus senticosus*, to raise insulin secretion in Wistar rats. *Neurosci Lett* **434**(2): 195–199.

Liu T, Zhao L, Zhang Y, Chen W, Liu D, Hou H, Ding L, Li X (2014). Ginsenoside 20(S)-Rg3 targets HIF-1α to block hypoxia-induced epithelial-mesenchymal transition in ovarian cancer cells. *PLoS One* **9**(9): e103887.

Liu WJ, Tang HT, Jia YT, Ma B, Fu JF, Wang Y, Lv KY, Xia ZF (2010). Notoginsenoside R1 attenuates renal ischemia-reperfusion injury in rats. *Shock* **34**(3): 314–320.

Liu X, Wang L, Wen A, Yang J, Yan Y, Song Y, Liu X, Ren H, Wu Y, Li Z, Chen W, Xu Y, Li L, Xia J, Zhao G (2012). Ginsenoside-Rd improves outcome of acute ischaemic stroke — a randomized, double-blind, placebo-controlled, multicenter trial. *Eur J Neurol* **19**(6): 855–863.

Liu ZQ, Luo XY, Liu GZ, Chen YP, Wang ZC, Sun YX (2003). *In vitro* study of the relationship between the structure of ginsenoside and its antioxidative or prooxidative activity in free radical induced hemolysis of human erythrocytes. *J Agric Food Chem* **51**: 2555–2558.

Lou JS, Chen XE, Zhang Y, Gao ZW, Chen TP, Zhang GQ, Ji C (2013). Photoprotective and immunoregulatory capacity of ginsenoside Rg1 in chronic ultraviolet B-irradiated BALB/c mouse skin. *Exp Ther Med* **6**(4): 1022–1028.

Ma B, Meng X, Wang J, Sun J, Ren X, Qin M, Sun J, Sun G, Sun X (2014). Notoginsenoside R1 attenuates amyloid-β-induced damage in neurons by inhibiting reactive oxygen species and modulating MAPK activation. *Int Immunopharmacol* **22**(1): 151–159.

Ma L, Liu H, Xie Z, Yang S, Xu W, Hou J, Yu B (2014). Ginsenoside Rb3 protects cardiomyocytes against ischemia-reperfusion injury via the inhibition of JNK-mediated NF-κB pathway: a mouse cardiomyocyte model. *PLoS One* **9**(8): e103628.

Maeng YS, Maharjan S, Kim JH, Park JH, Suk Yu Y, Kim YM, Kwon YG (2013). Rk1, a ginsenoside, is a new blocker of vascular leakage acting through actin structure remodeling. *PLoS One* **8**(7): e68659.

Mai TT, Moon J, Song Y, Viet PQ, Phuc PV, Lee JM, Yi TH, Cho M, Cho SK (2012). Ginsenoside F2 induces apoptosis accompanied by protective autophagy in breast cancer stem cells. *Cancer Lett* **321**(2): 144–153.

Mao N, Cheng Y, Shi XL, Wang L, Wen J, Zhang Q, Hu QD, Fan JM (2014). Ginsenoside Rg1 protects mouse podocytes from aldosterone-induced injury *in vitro*. *Acta Pharmacol Sin* **35**(4): 513–522.

Matsuda H, Samukawa K, Kubo M (1991). Anti-hepatitic activity of ginsenoside Ro. *Planta Med* **57**(6): 523–526.

Matsunaga H, Katano M, Saita T, Yamamoto H, Mori M (1994). Potentiation of cytotoxicity of mitomycin C by a polyacetylenic alcohol, panaxytriol. *Cancer Chemother Pharmacol* **33**(4): 291–297.

Matsunaga H, Katano M, Yamamoto H, Fujito H, Mori M, Takata K (1990). Cytotoxic activity of polyacetylene compounds in *Panax ginseng* C. A. Meyer. *Chem Pharm Bull (Tokyo)* **38**(12): 3480–3482.

Matsunaga H, Saita T, Nagumo F, Mori M, Katano M (1995). A possible mechanism for the cytotoxicity of a polyacetylenic alcohol, panaxytriol: inhibition of mitochondrial respiration. *Cancer Chemother Pharmacol* **35**(4): 291–296.

Meng X, Sun G, Ye J, Xu H, Wang H, Sun X (2014a). Notoginsenoside R1-mediated neuroprotection involves estrogen receptor-dependent crosstalk between Akt and ERK1/2 pathways: a novel mechanism of Nrf2/ARE signaling activation. *Free Radic Res* **48**(4): 445–460.

Meng X, Wang M, Sun G, Ye J, Zhou Y, Dong X, Wang T, Lu S, Sun X (2014b). Attenuation of Aβ25-35-induced parallel autophagic and apoptotic cell death by gypenoside XVII through the estrogen receptor-dependent activation of Nrf2/ARE pathways. *Toxicol Appl Pharmacol* **279**(1): 63–75.

Meng X, Wang M, Wang X, Sun G, Ye J, Xu H, Sun X (2014c). Suppression of NADPH oxidase- and mitochondrion-derived superoxide by Notoginsenoside R1 protects against cerebral ischemia-reperfusion injury through estrogen receptor-dependent activation of Akt/Nrf2 pathways. *Free Radic Res* **48**(7): 823–838.

Meng XB, Sun GB, Wang M, Sun J, Qin M, Sun XB (2013). P90RSK and Nrf2 activation via MEK1/2-ERK1/2 pathways mediated by notoginsenoside R2 to prevent 6-hydroxydopamine-induced apoptotic death in SH-SY5Y cells. *Evid Based Complement Alternat Med* 971712.

Mogil JS, Shin YH, McCleskey EW, Kim SC, Nah SY (1998). Ginsenoside Rf, a trace component of ginseng root, produces antinociception in mice. *Brain Res* **792**(2): 218–228.

Moon J, Yu SJ, Kim HS, Sohn J (2000). Induction of G(1) cell cycle arrest and p27(KIP1) increase by panaxydol isolated from Panax ginseng. *Biochem Pharmacol* **59**(9): 1109–1116.

Murata K, Takeshita F, Samukawa K, Tani T, Matsuda H (2012). Effects of ginseng rhizome and ginsenoside Ro on testosterone 5α-reductase and hair re-growth in testosterone-treated mice. *Phytother Res* **26**(1): 48–53.

Nemmani KV, Ramarao P (2003). Ginsenoside Rf potentiates U-50,488H-induced analgesia and inhibits tolerance to its analgesia in mice. *Life Sci* **72**(7): 759–768.

Ng F, Yun H, Lei X, Danishefsky SJ, Fahey J, Stephenson K, Flexner C, Lee L (2008). (3R, 9R, 10R)-panaxytriol: a molecular-based nutraceutical with possible application to cancer prevention and treatment. *Tetrahedron Lett* **49**(50): 7178–7179.

Ni N, Liu Q, Ren H, Wu D, Luo C, Li P, Wan JB, Su H (2014). Ginsenoside Rb1 protects rat neural progenitor cells against oxidative injury. *Molecules* **19**(3): 3012–3024.

Ni W, Zhang X, Wang B, Chen Y, Han H, Fan Y, Zhou Y, Tai G (2010). Antitumor activities and immunomodulatory effects of ginseng neutral polysaccharides in combination with 5-fluorouracil. *J Med Food* **13**(2): 270–277.

Nishiyama N, Cho SI, Kitagawa I, Saito H (1994). Malonylginsenoside Rb1 potentiates nerve growth factor (NGF)-induced neurite outgrowth of cultured chick embryonic dorsal root ganglia. *Biol Pharm Bull* **17**: 509–513.

Niu HS, Hsu FL, Liu IM, Cheng JT (2007). Increase of beta-endorphin secretion by syringin, an active principle of *Eleutherococcus senticosus*, to produce antihyperglycemic action in type 1-like diabetic rats. *Horm Metab Res* **39**(12): 894–898.

Niu HS, Liu IM, Cheng JT, Lin CL, Hsu FL (2008). Hypoglycemic effect of syringin from *Eleutherococcus senticosus* in streptozotocin-induced diabetic rats. *Planta Med* **74**(2): 109–113.

Oh HA, Seo JY, Jeong HJ, Kim HM (2013). Ginsenoside Rg1 inhibits the TSLP production in allergic rhinitis mice. *Immunopharmacol Immunotoxicol* **35**(6): 678–686.

Oh SJ, Lee S, Choi WY, Lim CJ (2014). Skin anti-photoaging properties of ginsenoside Rh2 epimers in UV-B-irradiated human keratinocyte cells. *J Biosci* **39**(4): 673–682.

Oshima Y, Konno C, Hikino H (1985). Isolation and hypoglycemic activity of panaxans I, J, K and L, glycans of *Panax ginseng* roots. *J Ethnopharmacol* **14**(2–3): 255–259.

Pan C, Huo Y, An X, Singh G, Chen M, Yang Z, Pu J, Li J (2012). *Panax notoginseng* and its components decreased hypertension via stimulation of endothelial-dependent vessel dilatation. *Vasc Pharmacol* **56**(3–4): 150–158.

Park E, Hwang I, Song JY, Jee Y (2011). Acidic polysaccharide of Panax ginseng as a defense against small intestinal damage by whole-body gamma irradiation of mice. *Acta Histochem* **113**(1): 19–23.

Park EH, Kim YJ, Yamabe N, Park SH, Kim HK, Jang HJ, Kim JH, Cheon GJ, Ham J, Kang KS (2014). Stereospecific anticancer effects of ginsenoside Rg3 epimers isolated from heat-processed American ginseng on human gastric cancer cell. *J Ginseng Res* **38**(1): 22–27.

Park EK, Choo MK, Han MJ, Kim DH (2004). Ginsenoside Rh1 possesses antiallergic and anti-inflammatory activities. *Int Arch Allergy Immunol* **133**(2): 113–120.

Park ES, Lee KP, Jung SH, Lee DY, Won KJ, Yun YP, Kim B (2013). Compound K, an intestinal metabolite of ginsenosides, inhibits PDGF-BB-induced VSMC proliferation and migration through G1 arrest and attenuates neointimal hyperplasia after arterial injury. *Atherosclerosis* **228**(1): 53–60.

Park IH, Han SB, Kim JM, Piao L, Kwon SW, Kim NY, Kang TL, Park MK, Park JH (2002a). Four new acetylated ginsenosides from processed ginseng (sun ginseng). *Arch Pharm Res* **25**(6): 837–841.

Park IH, Kim NY, Han SB, Kim JM, Kwon SW, Kim HJ, Park MK, Park JH (2002b). Three new dammarane glycosides from heat processed ginseng. *Arch Pharm Res* **25**(4): 428–432.

Park JS, Shin JA, Jung JS, Hyun JW, Van Le TK, Kim DH, Park EM, Kim HS (2012). Anti-inflammatory mechanism of compound K in activated microglia and its neuroprotective effect on experimental stroke in mice. *J Pharmacol Exp Ther* **341**: 59–67.

Park MW, Ha J, Chung SH (2008). 20(S)-ginsenoside Rg3 enhances glucose-stimulated insulin secretion and activates AMPK. *Biol Pharm Bull* **31**(4): 748–751.

Park S, Ahn IS, Kwon DY, Ko BS, Jun WK (2008). Ginsenosides Rb1 and Rg1 suppress triglyceride accumulation in 3T3-L1 adipocytes and enhance beta-cell insulin secretion and viability in Min6 cells via PKA-dependent pathways. *Biosci Biotechnol Biochem* **72**: 2815–2823, doi: 10.1271/bbb.80205

Pei Y, Du Q, Liao PY, Chen ZP, Wang D, Yang CR, Kitazato K, Wang YF, Zhang YJ (2011). Notoginsenoside ST-4 inhibits virus penetration of herpes simplex virus *in vitro*. *J Asian Nat Prod Res* **13**(6): 498–504.

Peña ID, Yoon SY, Kim HJ, Park S, Hong EY, Ryu JH, Park IH, Cheong JH (2014). Effects of ginseol k-g3, an Rg3-enriched fraction, on scopolamine-induced memory impairment and learning deficit in mice. *J Ginseng Res* **38**(1): 1–7.

Peng LL, Shen HM, Jiang ZL, Li X, Wang GH, Zhang YF, Ke KF (2009). Inhibition of NMDA receptors underlies the neuroprotective effect of ginsenoside Rb3. *Am J Chin Med* **37**(4): 759–770.

Purup S, Larsen E, Christensen LP (2009). Differential effects of falcarinol and related aliphatic C(17)-polyacetylenes on intestinal cell proliferation. *J Agric Food Chem* **57**(18): 8290–8296.

Qiu J, Li W, Feng SH, Wang M, He ZY (2014). Ginsenoside Rh2 promotes nonamyloidgenic cleavage of amyloid precursor protein via a cholesterol-dependent pathway. *Genet Mol Res* **13**(2): 3586–3598.

Qiu XM, Bai X, Jiang HF, He P, Wang JH (2014). 20-(s)-ginsenoside Rg3 induces apoptotic cell death in human leukemic U937 and HL-60 cells through PI3K/Akt pathways. *Anticancer Drugs* **25**(9): 1072–1080.

Qu D, Han J, Du A (2013). Enhancement of protective immune response to recombinant *Toxoplasma gondii* ROP18 antigen by ginsenoside Re. *Exp Parasitol* **135**(2): 234–239.

Quan HY, Yuan HD, Jung MS, Ko SK, Park YG, Chung SH (2012). Ginsenoside Re lowers blood glucose and lipid levels via activation of AMP-activated protein kinase in HepG2 cells and high-fat diet fed mice. *Int J Mol Med* **29**: 73–80.

Quan Q, Wang J, Li X, Wang Y (2013). Ginsenoside Rg1 decreases Aβ(1-42) level by upregulating PPARγ and IDE expression in the hippocampus of a rat model of Alzheimer's disease. *PLoS One* **8**(3): e59155.

Rhule A, Rase B, Smith JR, Shepherd DM (2008). Toll-like receptor ligand-induced activation of murine DC2.4 cells is attenuated by *Panax notoginseng*. *J Ethnopharmacol* **116**(1): 179–186.

Samimi R, Xu WZ, Lui EM, Charpentier PA (2014). Isolation and immunosuppressive effects of 6″-O-acetylginsenoside Rb1 extracted from North American ginseng. *Planta Med* **80**(6): 509–516.

Samukawa K, Suzuki Y, Ohkubo N, Aoto M, Sakanaka M, Mitsuda N (2008). Protective effect of ginsenosides Rg(2) and Rh(1) on oxidation-induced impairment of erythrocyte membrane properties. *Biorheology* **45**: 689–700.

Shan LN, Shi YX (2014). Effects of polysaccharides from Gynostemma pentaphyllum (thunb.), makino on physical fatigue. *Afr J Tradit Complement Alternat Med* **11**(3): 112–117.

Shang W, Yang Y, Zhou L, Jiang B, Jin H, Chen M (2008). Ginsenoside Rb1 stimulates glucose uptake through insulin-like signaling pathway in 3T3-L1 adipocytes. *J Endocrinol* **198**: 561–569.

Shangguan WJ, Li H, Zhang YH (2014). Induction of G2/M phase cell cycle arrest and apoptosis by ginsenoside Rf in human osteosarcoma MG 63 cells through the mitochondrial pathway. *Oncol Rep* **31**(1): 305–313.

Shen K, Ji L, Gong C, Ma Y, Yang L, Fan Y, Hou M, Wang Z (2012). Notoginsenoside Ft1 promotes angiogenesis via HIF-1α-mediated VEGF secretion and the regulation of PI3K/AKT and Raf/MEK/ERK signaling pathways. *Biochem Pharmacol* **84**(6): 784–792.

Shen K, Leung SW, Ji L, Huang Y, Hou M, Xu A, Wang Z, Vanhoutte PM (2014). Notoginsenoside Ft1 activates both glucocorticoid and estrogen receptors to induce endothelium-dependent, nitric oxide-mediated relaxations in rat mesenteric arteries. *Biochem Pharmacol* **88**(1): 66–74.

Shen L, Xiong Y, Wang DQ, Howles P, Basford JE, Wang J, Xiong YQ, Hui DY, Woods SC, Liu M (2013). Ginsenoside Rb1 reduces fatty liver by activating AMP-activated protein kinase in obese rats. *J Lipid Res* **54**(5): 1430–1438.

Shi Q, Li J, Feng Z, Zhao L, Luo L, You Z, Li D, Xia J, Zuo G, Chen D (2014). Effect of ginsenoside Rh2 on the migratory ability of HepG2 liver carcinoma cells: recruiting histone deacetylase and inhibiting activator protein 1 transcription factors. *Mol Med Rep* **10**(4): 1779–1785.

Shi Y, Han B, Yu X, Qu S, Sui D (2011). Ginsenoside Rb3 ameliorates myocardial ischemia-reperfusion injury in rats. *Pharm Biol* **49**(9): 900–906.

Shieh PC, Tsao CW, Li JS, Wu HT, Wen YJ, Kou DH, Cheng JT (2008). Role of pituitary adenylate cyclase-activating polypeptide (PACAP) in the action of ginsenoside Rh2 against beta-amyloid-induced inhibition of rat brain astrocytes. *Neurosci Lett* **434**: 1–5.

Shim JY, Han Y, Ahn JY, Yun YS, Song JY (2007). Chemoprotective and adjuvant effects of immunomodulator ginsan in cyclophosphamide-treated normal and tumor-bearing mice. *Int J Immunopathol Pharmacol* **20**: 487–497.

Shin DH, Cha YJ, Yang KE, Jang IS, Son CG, Kim BH, Kim JM (2014). Ginsenoside Rg3 up-regulates the expression of vascular endothelial growth factor in human dermal papilla cells and mouse hair follicles. *Phytother Res* **28**(7): 1088–1095.

Shin EJ, Shin SW, Nguyen TT, Park DH, Wie MB, Jang CG, Nah SY, Yang BW, Ko SK, Nabeshima T, Kim HC (2014). Ginsenoside Re rescues methamphetamine-induced oxidative damage, mitochondrial dysfunction, microglial activation, and dopaminergic degeneration by inhibiting the protein kinase Cδ gene. *Mol Neurobiol* **49**(3): 1400–1421.

Shin HS, Park SY, Hwang ES, Lee DG, Mavlonov GT, Yi TH (2014a). Ginsenoside F2 reduces hair loss by controlling apoptosis through the sterol regulatory element-binding protein cleavage activating protein and transforming growth factor-β pathways in a dihydrotestosterone-induced mouse model. *Biol Pharm Bull* **37**(5): 755–763.

Shin HS, Park SY, Hwang ES, Lee DG, Song HG, Mavlonov GT, Yi TH (2014b). The inductive effect of ginsenoside F2 on hair growth by altering the WNT signal pathway in telogen mouse skin. *Eur J Pharmacol* **730**: 82–89.

Shin JY, Lee JM, Shin HS, Park SY, Yang JE, Cho SK, Yi TH (2012). Anticancer effect of ginsenoside F2 against glioblastoma multiforme in xenograft model in SD rats. *J Ginseng Res* **36**(1): 86–92.

Shin KO, Seo CH, Cho HH, Oh S, Hong SP, Yoo HS, Hong JT, Oh KW, Lee YM (2014). Ginsenoside compound K inhibits angiogenesis via regulation of sphingosine kinase-1 in human umbilical vein endothelial cells. *Arch Pharm Res* **37**(9): 1183–1192.

Shin TJ, Kim HJ, Kwon BJ, Choi SH, Kim HB, Hwang SH, Lee BH, Lee SM, Zukin RS, Park JH, Kim HC, Rhim H, Lee JH, Nah SY (2012). Gintonin, a ginseng-derived novel ingredient, evokes long-term potentiation through N-methyl-D-aspartic acid receptor activation: involvement of LPA receptors. *Mol Cells* **34**(6): 563–572.

Shin YW, Bae EA, Kim DH (2006a). Inhibitory effect of ginsenoside Rg5 and its metabolite ginsenoside Rh3 in an oxazolone-induced mouse chronic dermatitis model. *Arch Pharm Res* **29**(8): 685–690.

Shin YW, Bae EA, Kim SS, Lee YC, Lee BY, Kim DH (2006b). The effects of ginsenoside Re and its metabolite, ginsenoside Rh1, on 12-O-tetradecanoylphorbol 13-acetate- and oxazolone-induced mouse dermatitis models. *Planta Med* **72**(4): 376–378.

Shuangyan W, Ruowu S, Hongli N, Bei Z, Yong S (2012). Protective effects of Rg2 on hypoxia-induced neuronal damage in hippocampal neurons. *Artif Cells Blood Substit Immobil Biotechnol* **40**(1–2): 142–145.

Siddiqi MH, Siddiqi MZ, Ahn S, Kim YJ, Yang DC (2014). Ginsenoside Rh1 induces mouse osteoblast growth and differentiation through the bone morphogenetic protein 2/runt-related gene 2 signalling pathway. *J Pharm Pharmacol* [Epub ahead of print].

Siraj FM, Sathishkumar N, Kim YJ, Kim SY, Yang DC (2014). Ginsenoside F2 possesses anti-obesity activity via binding with PPARγ and inhibiting adipocyte differentiation in the 3T3-L1 cell line. *J Enzyme Inhib Med Chem* [Epub ahead of print].

Song XY, Hu JF, Chu SF, Zhang Z, Xu S, Yuan YH, Han N, Liu Y, Niu F, He X, Chen NH (2013). Ginsenoside Rg1 attenuates okadaic acid induced spatial memory impairment by the GSK3β/tau signaling pathway and the Aβ formation prevention in rats. *Eur J Pharmacol* **710**(1–3): 29–38.

Song Y, Zhao F, Zhang L, Du Y, Wang T, Fu F (2013). Ginsenoside Rg1 exerts synergistic anti-inflammatory effects with low doses of glucocorticoids *in vitro*. *Fitoterapia* **91**: 173–179.

Su X, Pei Z, Hu S (2014). Ginsenoside Re as an adjuvant to enhance the immune response to the inactivated rabies virus vaccine in mice. *Int Immunopharmacol* **20**(2): 283–289.

Sukrittanon S, Watanapa WB, Ruamyod K (2014). Ginsenoside Re enhances small-conductance Ca(2+)-activated K(+) current in human coronary artery endothelial cells. *Life Sci.* **115**(1–2): 15–21.

Sun B, Xiao J, Sun XB, Wu Y (2013). Notoginsenoside R1 attenuates cardiac dysfunction in endotoxemic mice: an insight into oestrogen receptor activation and PI3K/Akt signalling. *Br J Pharmacol* **168**(7): 1758–1770.

Sun C, Chen Y, Li X, Tai G, Fan Y, Zhou Y (2014). Anti-hyperglycemic and anti-oxidative activities of ginseng polysaccharides in STZ-induced diabetic mice. *Food Funct* **5**(5): 845–848.

Sun HX, Chen Y, Ye Y (2006). Ginsenoside Re and notoginsenoside R1: immunologic adjuvants with low haemolytic effect. *Chem Biodivers* **3**(7): 718–726.

Sun J, Hu S, Song X (2007). Adjuvant effects of protopanaxadiol and protopanaxatriol saponins from ginseng roots on the immune responses to ovalbumin in mice. *Vaccine* **25**: 1114–1120.

Sun K, Wang CS, Guo J, Horie Y, Fang SP, Wang F, Liu YY, Liu LY, Yang JY, Fan JY, Han JY (2007). Protective effects of ginsenoside Rb1, ginsenoside Rg1, and notoginsenoside R1 on lipopolysaccharide-induced microcirculatory disturbance in rat mesentery. *Life Sci* **81**(6): 509–518.

Sun Q, Meng QT, Jiang Y, Liu HM, Lei SQ, Su WT, Duan WN, Wu Y, Xia ZY, Xia ZY (2013). Protective effect of ginsenoside Rb1 against intestinal ischemia-reperfusion induced acute renal injury in mice. *PLoS One* **8**(12): e80859.

Sun X, Cheng L, Zhu W, Hu C, Jin R, Sun B, Shi Y, Zhang Y, Cui W (2014). Use of ginsenoside Rg3-loaded electrospun PLGA fibrous membranes as wound cover induces healing and inhibits hypertrophic scar formation of the skin. *Colloids Surf B Biointerfaces* **115**: 61–70.

Tan S, Yu W, Lin Z, Chen Q, Shi J, Dong Y, Duan K, Bai X, Xu L, Li J, Li N (2014). Anti-inflammatory effect of ginsenoside Rb1 contributes to the recovery of gastrointestinal motility in the rat model of postoperative ileus. *Biol Pharm Bull* [Epub ahead of print].

Tan S, Zhou F, Li N, Dong Q, Zhang X, Ye X, Guo J, Chen B, Yu Z (2013). Anti-fatigue effect of ginsenoside Rb1 on postoperative fatigue syndrome induced by major small intestinal resection in rat. *Biol Pharm Bull* **36**(10): 1634–1639.

Tang XP, Tang GD, Fang CY, Liang ZH, Zhang LY (2013). Effects of ginsenoside Rh2 on growth and migration of pancreatic cancer cells. *World J Gastroenterol* **19**(10): 1582–1592.

Teng CM, Kuo SC, Ko FN, Lee JC, Lee LG, Chen SC, Huang TF (1989). Antiplatelet actions of panaxynol and ginsenosides isolated from ginseng. *Biochim Biophys Acta* **990**(3): 315–320.

Tian CJ, Kim SW, Kim YJ, Lim HJ, Park R, So HS, Choung YH (2013). Red ginseng protects against gentamicin-induced balance dysfunction and hearing loss in rats through antiapoptotic functions of ginsenoside Rb1. *Food Chem Toxicol* **60**: 369–376.

Tohda C, Matsumoto N, Zou K, Meselhy MR, Komatsu K (2004). Abeta(25–35)-induced memory impairment, axonal atrophy, and synaptic loss are ameliorated by M1, A metabolite of protopanaxadiol-type saponins. *Neuropsychopharmacology* **29**: 860–868.

Tsai SC, Chiao YC, Lu CC, Wang PS (2003). Stimulation of the secretion of luteinizing hormone by ginsenoside-Rb1 in male rats. *Chin J Physiol* **46**: 1–7.

Wang B, Feng G, Tang C, Wang L, Cheng H, Zhang Y, Ma J, Shi M, Zhao G (2013). Ginsenoside Rd maintains adult neural stem cell proliferation during lead-impaired neurogenesis. *Neurol Sci* **34**(7): 1181–1188.

Wang CM, Liu MY, Wang F, Wei MJ, Wang S, Wu CF, Yang JY (2013). Anti-amnesic effect of pseudoginsenoside-F11 in two mouse models of Alzheimer's disease. *Pharmacol Biochem Behav* **106**: 57–67.

Wang H, Kong L, Zhang J, Yu G, Lv G, Zhang F, Chen X, Tian J, Fu F (2014). The pseudoginsenoside F11 ameliorates cisplatin-induced nephrotoxicity without compromising its anti-tumor activity *in vivo*. *Sci Rep* **4**: 4986.

Wang H, Yu P, Gou H, Zhang J, Zhu M, Wang ZH, Tian JW, Jiang YT, Fu FH (2012). Cardioprotective effects of 20(s)-ginsenoside Rh2 against doxorubicin-induced cardiotoxicity *in vitro* and *in vivo*. *Evid Based Complement Alternat Med* 506214.

Wang J, Flaisher-Grinberg S, Li S, Liu H, Sun L, Zhou Y, Einat H (2010a). Antidepressant-like effects of the active acidic polysaccharide portion of ginseng in mice. *J Ethnopharmacol* **132**(1): 65–69.

Wang J, Qiao L, Li S, Yang G (2013). Protective effect of ginsenoside Rb1 against lung injury induced by intestinal ischemia-reperfusion in rats. *Molecules* **18**(1): 1214–1226.

Wang J, Sun C, Zheng Y, Pan H, Zhou Y, Fan Y (2014). The effective mechanism of the polysaccharides from Panax ginseng on chronic fatigue syndrome. *Arch Pharm Res* **37**(4): 530–538.

Wang J, Zuo G, Li J, Guan T, Li C, Jiang R, Xie B, Lin X, Li F, Wang Y, Chen D (2010b). Induction of tumoricidal activity in mouse peritoneal macrophages by ginseng polysaccharide. *Int J Biol Macromol* **46**(4): 389–395.

Wang JH, Nao JF, Zhang M, He P (2014). 20(s)-ginsenoside Rg3 promotes apoptosis in human ovarian cancer HO-8910 cells through PI3K/Akt and XIAP pathways. *Tumour Biol* [Epub ahead of print].

Wang JY, Yang JY, Wang F, Fu SY, Hou Y, Jiang B, Ma J, Song C, Wu CF (2013). Neuroprotective effect of pseudoginsenoside-F11 on a rat model of Parkinson's disease induced by 6-hydroxydopamine. *Evid Based Complement Alternat Med* 152798.

Wang L, Lu AP, Yu ZL, Wong RN, Bian ZX, Kwok HH, Yue PY, Zhou LM, Chen H, Xu M, Yang Z (2014a). The melanogenesis-inhibitory effect and the percutaneous formulation of ginsenoside Rb1. *AAPS PharmSciTech* [Epub ahead of print].

Wang L, Yu X, Yang X, Yao Y, Lui EM, Ren G (2014b). Structural and anti-inflammatory characterization of a novel neutral polysaccharide from North American ginseng (*Panax quinquefolius*). *Int J Biol Macromol* [Epub ahead of print].

Wang T, Yu X, Qu S, Xu H, Han B, Sui D (2010). Effect of ginsenoside Rb3 on myocardial injury and heart function impairment induced by isoproterenol in rats. *Eur J Pharmacol* **636**(1–3): 121–125.

Wang W, Zhang X, Qin JJ, Voruganti S, Nag SA, Wang MH, Wang H, Zhang R (2012). Natural product ginsenoside 25-OCH3-PPD inhibits breast cancer growth and metastasis through down-regulating MDM2. *PLoS One* **7**(7): e41586.

Wang X, Chu S, Qian T, Chen J, Zhang J (2010). Ginsenoside Rg1 improves male copulatory behavior via nitric oxide/cyclic guanosine monophosphate pathway. *J Sex Med* **7**: 743–750.

Wang X, Wang C, Wang J, Zhao S, Zhang K, Wang J, Zhang W, Wu C, Yang J (2014). Pseudoginsenoside-F11 (PF11) exerts anti-neuro-inflammatory effects on LPS-activated microglial cells by inhibiting TLR4-mediated TAK1/IKK/NF-κB, MAPKs and Akt signaling pathways. *Neuropharmacology* **79**: 642–656.

Wang Y, Dong J, Liu P, Lau CW, Gao Z, Zhou D, Tang J, Ng CF, Huang Y (2014a). Ginsenoside Rb3 attenuates oxidative stress and preserves endothelial function in renal arteries from hypertensive rats. *Br J Pharmacol* **171**(13): 3171–3181.

Wang Y, Feng Y, Fu Q, Li L (2013a). Panax notoginsenoside Rb1 ameliorates Alzheimer's disease by upregulating brain-derived neurotrophic factor and downregulating Tau protein expression. *Exp Ther Med* **6**(3): 826–830.

Wang Y, Kan H, Yin Y, Wu W, Hu W, Wang M, Li W, Li W (2014b). Protective effects of ginsenoside Rg1 on chronic restraint stress induced learning and memory impairments in male mice. *Pharmacol Biochem Behav* **120**: 73–81.

Wang Y, Li X, Wang X, Lau W, Wang Y, Xing Y, Zhang X, Ma X, Gao F (2013b). Ginsenoside Rd attenuates myocardial ischemia/reperfusion injury via Akt/GSK-3β signaling and inhibition of the mitochondria-dependent apoptotic pathway. *PLoS One* **8**(8): e70956.

Wang Y, Liu Y, Zhang XY, Xu LH, Ouyang DY, Liu KP, Pan H, He J, He XH (2014c). Ginsenoside Rg1 regulates innate immune responses in macrophages through differentially modulating the NF-κB and PI3K/Akt/mTOR pathways. *Int Immunopharmacol* **23**(1): 77–84.

Wang YG, Zima AV, Ji X, Pabbidi R, Blatter LA, Lipsius SL (2008). Ginsenoside Re suppresses electromechanical alternans in cat and human cardiomyocytes. *Am J Physiol Heart Circ Physiol* **295**: H851–H859.

Wang YZ, Chen J, Chu SF, Wang YS, Wang XY, Chen NH, Zhang JT (2009). Improvement of memory in mice and increase of hippocampal excitability in rats by ginsenoside Rg1's metabolites ginsenoside Rh1 and protopanaxatriol. *J Pharmacol Sci* **109**(4): 504–510.

Wang Z, Meng J, Xia Y, Meng Y, Du L, Zhang Z, Wang E, Shan F (2013). Maturation of murine bone marrow dendritic cells induced by acidic ginseng polysaccharides. *Int J Biol Macromol* **53**: 93–100.

Wang Z, Li M, Wu WK, Tan HM, Geng DF (2008). Ginsenoside Rb1 preconditioning protects against myocardial infarction after regional ischemia and reperfusion by activation of phosphatidylinositol-3-kinase signal transduction. *Cardiovasc Drugs Ther* **22**: 443–452.

Wang ZJ, Nie BM, Chen HZ, Lu Y (2006). Panaxynol induces neurite outgrowth in PC12D cells via cAMP- and MAP kinase-dependent mechanisms. *Chem Biol Interact* **159**(1): 58–64.

Wee JJ, Mee Park K, Chung AS (2011). Biological activities of ginseng and its application to human health. In: Benzie IFF, Wachtel-Galor S (eds.) *Herbal Medicine: Biomolecular and Clinical Aspects*. 2nd ed. Boca Raton: CRC Press, Chapter 8.

Wu CF, Liu YL, Song M, Liu W, Wang JH, Li X, Yang JY (2003). Protective effects of pseudoginsenoside-F11 on methamphetamine-induced neuro-toxicity in mice. *Pharmacol Biochem Behav* **76**: 103–109.

Wu G, Yi J, Liu L, Wang P, Zhang Z, Li Z (2014). Pseudoginsenoside F11, a novel partial PPAR-γ agonist, promotes adiponectin oligomerization and secretion in 3T3-L1 adipocytes. *PPAR Res* 701017.

Wu J, Jeong HK, Bulin SE, Kwon SW, Park JH, Bezprozvanny I (2009). Ginsenosides protect striatal neurons in a cellular model of Huntington's disease. *J Neurosci Res* **87**: 1904–1912.

Wu LL, Jia BH, Sun J, Chen JX, Liu ZY, Liu Y (2014). Protective effects of ginsenoside Rb1 on septic rats and its mechanism. *Biomed Environ Sci* **27**(4): 300–303.

Wu W, Zhang XM, Liu PM, Li JM, Wang JF (1995). Effects of *Panax notoginseng* saponin Rg1 on cardiac electrophysiological properties and ventricular fibrillation threshold in dogs. *Acta Pharmacol Sin* **16**(5): 459–463.

Wu Y, Xia ZY, Dou J, Zhang L, Xu JJ, Zhao B, Lei S, Liu HM (2011). Protective effect of ginsenoside Rb1 against myocardial ischemia/reperfusion injury in streptozotocin-induced diabetic rats. *Mol Biol Rep* **38**: 4327–4335.

Wu YL, Wan Y, Jin XJ, OuYang BQ, Bai T, Zhao YQ, Nan JX (2011). 25-OCH3-PPD induces the apoptosis of activated t-HSC/Cl-6 cells via c-FLIP-mediated NF-κB activation. *Chem Biol Interact* **194**(2–3): 106–112.

Xie JT, Shao ZH, Vanden Hoek TL, Chang WT, Li J, Mehendale S, Wang CZ, Hsu CW, Becker LB, Yin JJ, Yuan CS (2006). Antioxidant effects of ginsenoside Re in cardiomyocytes. *Eur J Pharmacol* **532**: 201–207.

Xie XS, Liu HC, Wang FP, Zhang CL, Zuo C, Deng Y, Fan JM (2010). Ginsenoside Rg1 modulation on thrombospondin-1 and vascular endothelial growth factor expression in early renal fibrogenesis in unilateral obstruction. *Phytother Res* **24**: 1581–1587.

Xie Y, Zhang B, Zhang Y (2015). Protective effects of *Acanthopanax polysaccharides* on cerebral ischemia-reperfusion injury and its mechanisms. *Int J Biol Macromol* **72**: 946–950.

Xiong Y, Chen D, Lv B, Liu F, Yao Q, Tang Z, Lin Y (2014). Effects of ginsenoside Re on rat jejunal contractility. *J Nat Med* **68**(3): 530–538.

Xu L, Huang SP (2012). Effect of the ginsenoside Rb1 on the spontaneous contraction of intestinal smooth muscle in mice. *World J Gastroenterol* **18**(38): 5462–5469.

Xu SF, Yu LM, Fan ZH, Wu Q, Yuan Y, Wei Y, Fang N (2012). Improvement of ginsenoside Rg1 on hematopoietic function in cyclophosphamide-induced myelosuppression mice. *Eur J Pharmacol* **695**(1–3): 7–12.

Xu Y, Lin L, Tang L, Zheng M, Ma Y, Huang L, Meng W, Wang W (2014). Notoginsenoside R1 attenuates hypoxia and hypercapnia-induced vasoconstriction in isolated rat pulmonary arterial rings by reducing the expression of ERK. *Am J Chin Med* **42**(4): 799–816.

Xu Y, Zhang P, Wang C, Shan Y, Wang D, Qian F, Sun M, Zhu C (2013). Effect of ginsenoside Rg3 on tyrosine hydroxylase and related mechanisms in the forced swimming-induced fatigue rats. *J Ethnopharmacol* **150**(1): 138–147.

Yamada N, Araki H, Yoshimura H (2011). Identification of antidepressant-like ingredients in ginseng root (*Panax ginseng* C.A. Meyer) using a menopausal depressive-like state in female mice: participation of 5-HT2A receptors. *Psychopharmacology (Berl)* **216**: 589–599.

Yan S, Li Z, Li H, Arancio O, Zhang W (2014). Notoginsenoside R1 increases neuronal excitability and ameliorates synaptic and memory dysfunction following amyloid elevation. *Sci Rep* **4**: 6352.

Yan Z, Yang R, Jiang Y, Yang Z, Yang J, Zhao Q, Lu Y (2011). Induction of apoptosis in human promyelocytic leukemia HL60 cells by panaxynol and panaxydol. *Molecules* **16**(7): 5561–5573.

Yang N, Chen P, Tao Z, Zhou N, Gong X, Xu Z, Zhang M, Zhang D, Chen B, Tao Z, Yang Z (2012). Beneficial effects of ginsenoside-Rg1 on ischemia-induced angiogenesis in diabetic mice. *Acta Biochim Biophys Sin (Shanghai)* **44**(12): 999–1005.

Yang X, Zhao Y, Yang Y, Ruan Y (2008). Isolation and characterization of immunostimulatory polysaccharide from an herb tea, *Gynostemma pentaphyllum* Makino. *J Agric Food Chem* **56**(16): 6905–6909.

Ye H, Wu Q, Zhu Y, Guo C, Zheng X (2014). Ginsenoside Rh2 alleviates dextran sulfate sodium-induced colitis via augmenting TGFβ signaling. *Mol Biol Rep* **41**(8): 5485–5490.

Ye R, Zhao G, Liu X (2013). Ginsenoside Rd for acute ischemic stroke: translating from bench to bedside. *Expert Rev Neurother* **13**(6): 603–613.

Yokozawa T, Liu ZW (2000). The role of ginsenoside-Rd in cisplatin-induced acute renal failure. *Ren Fail* **22**: 115–127.

Yokozawa T, Liu ZW, Dong E (1998). A study of ginsenoside-Rd in a renal ischemia-reperfusion model. *Nephronology* **78**: 201–206.

Yoo DG, Kim MC, Park MK, Park KM, Quan FS, Song JM, Wee JJ, Wang BZ, Cho YK, Compans RW, Kang SM (2012). Protective effect of ginseng polysaccharides on influenza viral infection. *PLoS One* **7**(3): e33678.

Yoon JH, Choi YJ, Cha SW, Lee SG (2012a). Anti-metastatic effects of ginsenoside Rd via inactivation of MAPK signaling and induction of focal adhesion formation. *Phytomedicine* **19**(3–4): 284–292.

Yoon JH, Choi YJ, Lee SG (2012b). Ginsenoside Rh1 suppresses matrix metalloproteinase-1 expression through inhibition of activator protein-1 and mitogen-activated protein kinase signaling pathway in human hepatocellular carcinoma cells. *Eur J Pharmacol* **679**(1–3): 24–33.

Yoon SH, Han EJ, Sung JH, Chung SH (2007). Anti-diabetic effects of compound K versus metformin versus compound K-metformin combination therapy in diabetic db/db mice. *Biol Pharm Bull* **30**: 2196–2200.

Yoshimura H, Kimura N, Sugiura K (1998). Preventive effects of various ginseng saponins on the development of copulatory disorder induced by prolonged individual housing in male mice. *Methods Find Exp Clin Pharmacol* **20**: 59–64.

You ZM, Zhao L, Xia J, Wei Q, Liu YM, Liu XY, Chen DL, Li J (2014). Down-regulation of phosphoglucose isomerase/autocrine motility factor enhances ginsenoside Rh2 pharmacological action on leukemia KG1α cells. *Asian Pac J Cancer Prev* **15**(3): 1099–1104.

Yu JL, Dou DQ, Chen XH, Yang HZ, Hu XY, Cheng GF (2005). Ginsenoside-Ro enhances cell proliferation and modulates Th1/Th2 cytokines production in murine splenocytes. *Yao Xue Xue Bao* **40**(4): 332–336.

Yu X, Yang X, Cui B, Wang L, Ren G (2014). Antioxidant and immunoregulatory activity of alkali-extractable polysaccharides from North American ginseng. *Int J Biol Macromol* **65**: 357–361.

Yuan HD, Kim do Y, Quan HY, Kim SJ, Jung MS, Chung SH (2012). Ginsenoside Rg2 induces orphan nuclear receptor SHP gene expression and inactivates GSK3β via AMP-activated protein kinase to inhibit hepatic glucose production in HepG2 cells. *Chem Biol Interact* **195**(1): 35–42.

Yun TK, Lee YS, Lee YH (2001). Anticarcinogenic effect of *Panax ginseng* C.A. Meyer and identification of active compounds. *J Korean Med Sci* **16**: S6–S18.

Zeng XS, Zhou XS, Luo FC, Jia JJ, Qi L, Yang ZX, Zhang W, Bai J (2014). Comparative analysis of the neuroprotective effects of ginsenosides Rg1 and Rb1 extracted from *Panax notoginseng* against cerebral ischemia. *Can J Physiol Pharmacol* **92**(2): 102–108.

Zhang G, Liu A, Zhou Y, San X, Jin T, Jin Y (2008). *Panax ginseng* ginsenoside-Rg2 protects memory impairment via anti-apoptosis in a rat model with vascular dementia. *J Ethnopharmacol* **115**: 441–448.

Zhang H, Zhou Q, Li X, Zhao W, Wang Y, Liu H, Li N (2007). Ginsenoside Re promotes human sperm capacitation through nitric oxide-dependent pathway. *Mol Reprod Dev* **74**: 497–501.

Zhang HS, Wang SQ (2006). Notoginsenoside R1 inhibits TNF-alpha-induced fibronectin production in smooth muscle cells via the ROS/ERK pathway. *Free Radic Biol Med* **40**(9): 1664–1674.

Zhang SD, Yin YX, Wei Q (2010). Immunopotentiation on murine spleen lymphocytes induced by polysaccharide fraction of Panax ginseng via upregulating calcineurin activity. *APMIS* **118**(4): 288–296.

Zhang WJ, Wojta J, Binder BR (1997). Effect of notoginsenoside R1 on the synthesis of components of the fibrinolytic system in cultured smooth muscle cells of human pulmonary artery. *Cell Mol Biol* **43**(4): 581–587.

Zhang X, Shi M, Bjørås M, Wang W, Zhang G, Han J, Liu Z, Zhang Y, Wang B, Chen J, Zhu Y, Xiong L, Zhao G (2013). Ginsenoside Rd promotes glutamate clearance by up-regulating glial glutamate transporter GLT-1 via PI3K/AKT and ERK1/2 pathways. *Front Pharmacol* **4**: 152.

Zhang X, Shi M, Ye R, Wang W, Liu X, Zhang G, Han J, Zhang Y, Wang B, Zhao J, Hui J, Xiong L, Zhao G (2014). Ginsenoside Rd attenuates tau protein phosphorylation via the PI3K/AKT/GSK-3β pathway after transient forebrain ischemia. *Neurochem Res* **39**(7): 1363–1373.

Zhang Y, Sun K, Liu YY, Zhang YP, Hu BH, Chang X, Yan L, Pan CS, Li Q, Fan JY, He K, Mao XW, Tu L, Wang CS, Han JY (2014). Ginsenoside Rb1 ameliorates lipopolysaccharide-induced albumin leakage from rat mesenteric venules by intervening in both trans- and paracellular pathway. *Am J Physiol Gastrointest Liver Physiol* **306**(4): G289–G300.

Zhang YH, Li HD, Li B, Jiang SD, Jiang LS (2014). Ginsenoside Rg3 induces DNA damage in human osteosarcoma cells and reduces MNNG-induced DNA damage and apoptosis in normal human cells. *Oncol Rep* **31**(2): 919–925.

Zhang YJ, Zhang XL, Li MH, Iqbal J, Bourantas CV, Li JJ, Su XY, Muramatsu T, Tian NL, Chen SL (2013). The ginsenoside Rg1 prevents transverse aortic constriction-induced left ventricular hypertrophy and cardiac dysfunction by inhibiting fibrosis and enhancing angiogenesis. *J Cardiovasc Pharmacol* **62**(1): 50–57.

Zhang YX, Wang L, Xiao EL, Li SJ, Chen JJ, Gao B, Min GN, Wang ZP, Wu YJ (2013). Ginsenoside-Rd exhibits anti-inflammatory activities through elevation of antioxidant enzyme activities and inhibition of JNK and ERK activation *in vivo*. *Int Immunopharmacol* **17**(4): 1094–1100.

Zheng H, Jeong Y, Song J, Ji G (2011). Oral administration of ginsenoside Rh1 inhibits the development of atopic dermatitis-like skin lesions induced by oxazolone in hairless mice. *Int Immunopharmacol* **11**(4): 511–518.

Zheng Y, Feng Z, You C, Jin Y, Hu X, Wang X, Han C (2013). *In vitro* evaluation of *Panax notoginseng* Rg1 released from collagen/chitosan-gelatin microsphere scaffolds for angiogenesis. *Biomed Eng Online* **12**: 134.

Zheng ZZ, Ming YL, Chen LH, Zheng GH, Liu SS, Chen QX (2014). Compound K-induced apoptosis of human hepatocellular carcinoma MHCC97-H cells *in vitro*. *Oncol Rep* **32**(1): 325–331.

Zhou Q, Jiang L, Xu C, Luo D, Zeng C, Liu P, Yue M, Liu Y, Hu X, Hu H (2014). Ginsenoside Rg1 inhibits platelet activation and arterial thrombosis. *Thromb Res* **133**(1): 57–65.

Zhou X, Shi H, Jiang G, Zhou Y, Xu J (2014). Antitumor activities of ginseng polysaccharide in C57BL/6 mice with Lewis lung carcinoma. *Tumour Biol* [Epub ahead of print].

Zhou Y, Li HQ, Lu L, Fu DL, Liu AJ, Li JH, Zheng GQ (2014). Ginsenoside Rg1 provides neuroprotection against blood brain barrier disruption and neurological injury in a rat model of cerebral ischemia/reperfusion through downregulation of aquaporin 4 expression. *Phytomedicine* **21**(7): 998–1003.

Zhu D, Liu M, Yang Y, Ma L, Jiang Y, Zhou L, Huang Q, Pi R, Chen X (2014). Ginsenoside Rd ameliorates experimental autoimmune encephalomyelitis in C57BL/6 mice. *J Neurosci Res* **92**(9): 1217–1226.

Zhu D, Wu L, Li CR, Wang XW, Ma YJ, Zhong ZY, Zhao HB, Cui J, Xun SF, Huang XL, Zhou Z, Wang SQ (2009). Ginsenoside Rg1 protects rat cardiomyocyte from hypoxia/reoxygenation oxidative injury via anti-oxidant and intracellular calcium homeostasis. *J Cell Biochem* **108**(1): 117–124.

Zhu J, Mu X, Zeng J, Xu C, Liu J, Zhang M, Li C, Chen J, Li T, Wang Y (2014). Ginsenoside Rg1 prevents cognitive impairment and hippocampus senescence in a rat model of D-galactose-induced aging. *PLoS One* **9**(6): e101291.

Zou Y, Tao T, Tian Y, Zhu J, Cao L, Deng X, Li J (2013). Ginsenoside Rg1 improves survival in a murine model of polymicrobial sepsis by suppressing the inflammatory response and apoptosis of lymphocytes. *J Surg Res* **183**(2): 760–766.

Decoction and Dosage

What Does the Dosage Really Mean?

A herb's dosage refers to the recommended quantity to be consumed by an adult per day. Unless stated otherwise, the dosage is measured in terms of the herb's dried weight to be used to prepare the decoction. Children above five years old usually take half the standard dosage. Children below five years old usually take ¼ of the standard dosage.

What Cookware Is Suitable for Brewing Herbs?

The most preferred cookware is a clay or earthenware pot. However, a ceramic pot can also be used. Iron, aluminium and copper pots should be avoided because chemical interaction can occur and affect the therapeutic effects of the ingredients.

How Should One Prepare and Consume the Herbal Decoction?

You may be prescribed a mixture of herbs and the clinic/hospital may prepare the decoction for you in sachets. Often, you may need to prepare the decoction yourself. Herbal formulae are commonly prescribed in packets. Each packet usually represents a single day's usage (一剂). Before boiling, soak the herbs in water for 30–60 min to allow time for the effective contents in herbs to dissolve. The amount of water should be enough to cover the surface of all the herbs. Bring the water to boil quickly, before turning down the heat to allow the decoction to simmer. After straining out the liquid portion, the same set of ingredients can be boiled a second time. The amount of water used in the second boiling should be less than the first (approximately half of the amount used in the first boiling or just enough to cover the herbs). Repeat the brewing process (with less water). After the dregs are removed, the liquid from both boilings are combined and divided into equal doses. The decoction is usually consumed warm or at room temperature, once in the morning and once in the evening. It can be refrigerated and reheated as needed.

Additional Information

The instruction above serves as a general guideline. The actual preparation time may vary for different formulae, herbs and patients. When in doubt, please consult the attending physician.

References

Beinfield H, Korngold E (1992). *Between Heaven and Earth — A Guide to Chinese Medicine*. New York: The Random House Publishing Group.
Gao XM (2008). *Zhong Yao Xue*. Beijing: China Press of Traditional Medicine.
Sheng-Nong Ltd. (2005). *Questions About Taking Chinese Herbs*. Retrived from http://www.shen-nong.com/eng/principles/takingchiherbs.html

Product Information

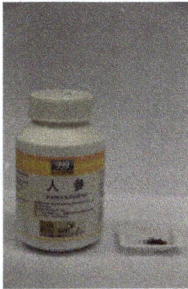

Radix Ginseng (D1960) (Sanjiu Enterprise Group)	Korean Red Ginseng (Korea Ginseng Corp.)	American Ginseng Capsule (ZK)
Raw Tienchi Tablets (Camellia Brand)	Steamed Tienchi Tablets (Camellia Brand)	American Ginseng Plus Notoginseng Capsules (Nature's Green)

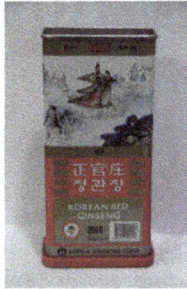

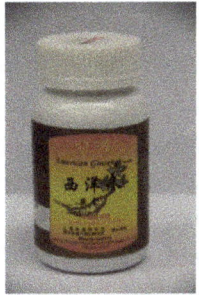

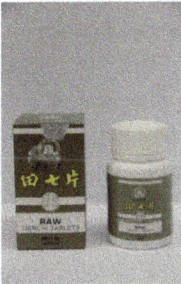

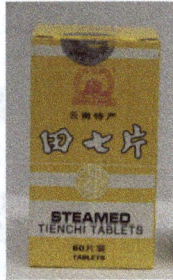

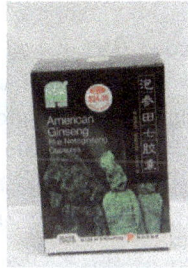

Figure A6 Photographs of selected products.

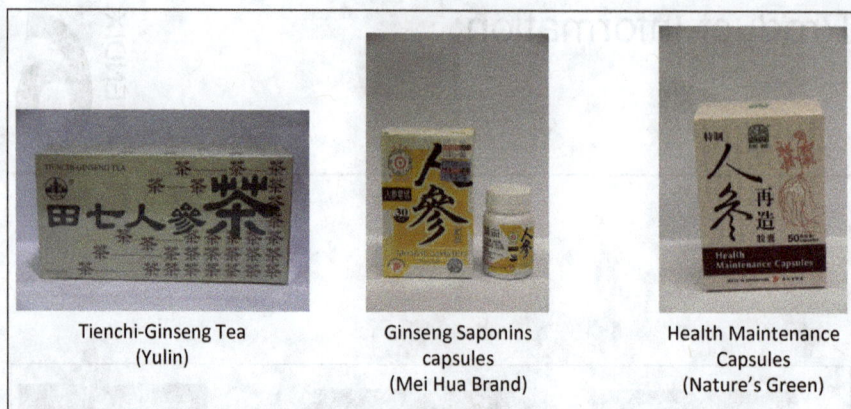

| Tienchi-Ginseng Tea (Yulin) | Ginseng Saponins capsules (Mei Hua Brand) | Health Maintenance Capsules (Nature's Green) |

Figure A6   (*Continued*)

The information on the packaging of 309 products is compiled below, arranged in alphabetical order of the product names. The brand of each product is listed in brackets next to its name.

The product information is listed in the following format wherever possible: **Description**, **Actions**, **Indications**, **Ingredients**, **Instructions/Dosage**, **Safety considerations**, **Price** and **Manufacturer/Importer/Distributor**. **"Description"** outlines the product's general information, such as health claims and marketing messages. **"Actions"** explains how the product is believed to act on the body, usually based on TCM theories. **"Indications"** refers to the various conditions for appropriate use. For products that do not provide information on **Description**, **Actions** and **Indications** on their labels, they are denoted as **"Details:** No information available". **"Ingredients"** specify the ingredients and their quantities. **"Instructions"** refer to specific methods of application or consumption. **"Dosage"** states the prescribed amount or serving size of the product, as well as its frequency of administration. **"Safety considerations"** include side effects, contraindications, caution and interactions associated with the use of the product. **"Price"** indicates the cost, as well as the net amount wherever available. **"Manufacturer/Importer/Distributor"** bears information on the country of origin, address and contacts of the companies responsible for the production and distribution of the product. Unless otherwise stated, all information is collated from the products' packaging. Information that is found on the Product Information Leaflet is designated as "PIL".

1. **Active Plus + Ginseng (Supradyn)**
Description:
Why take Supradyn active plus? With increasing demands from your family and social life, you may find yourself needing to keep up your energy level more than

ever. Supradyn Active Plus is specially formulated to help you achieve just that so that you can stay active all day. Unlike most multivitamins that are simply designed as a supplement to balance out any missing nutrients in your diet, Supradyn Active Plus contains much more. It is specially formulated with standardized root extract of Panax ginseng and extra B vitamins. Ginseng is known to enhance endurance, reduce fatigue and boost immunity. Taken daily, it gives your body the extra vitality it needs. B vitamins support your metabolism by releasing the energy efficiently from the food you take. Ginseng and B vitamins, together with other essential vitamins and minerals in Supradyn Active Plus, help you stay energized and active all day.

Ingredients:
Each tablet contains: GINSENG extract (*Panax Ginseng* C.A. Meyer) 50 mg, 12 vitamins: Vitamin A 1333 I.U, Vitamin B1 2.1 mg, Vitamin B2 2.4 mg, Vitamin B6 3 mg, Vitamin B12 1.5 µg, Vitamin C 90 mg, Vitamin D3 200 I.U, Vitamin E 15 mg, Biotin 75 µg, Pantothenic Acid 6 mg, Folic Acid 0.3 mg, Nicotinamide 18 mg. 9 Minerals and trace elements: Calcium 160 mg, Magnesium 120 mg, Iron 5.6 mg, Manganese 1.4 mg, Copper 1 mg, Zinc 6 mg, Molybdenum 60 µg, Chromium 50 µg, Selenium 28 µg.

Dosage:
Adults: 1 tablet daily or as directed by your doctor.

Instruction:
Tablet to be swallowed with water.

Price: 60 tablets — $37.50 (not sealed)

Manufacturer:
Bayer Consumer Care AQ, Basel Switzerland.

Imported by:
Bayer (SEA) Pte Ltd 9 Benoi Sector Singapore 629844.

2. **American Ginseng & Cordyceps Capsule (SeaGull)**

Actions:
Reinforcing vital energy, invigorate kidney and lungs

Indications:
Premature senility, lumbar and knee weakness, palpitation cough and phlegm, asthma.

Ingredients:
Each capsule (300 mg) contains: *Radix Panacis Quinquefolii* 135 mg, *Cordyceps Sinensis* (Fermented) 165 mg.

Dosage:
2–3 capsules to be taken each time, 2 times per day. Best results when taken regularly.

Safety considerations:
Side effects not known. Not to be taken when having cold or fever.
Price: 80 capsules — $56.00, 3 × 80 capsules — $151.00 (sealed)

Manufacturer:
Union Chemical & Pharmaceutical Pte Ltd No. 113, Eunos Ane 3, #06-06/10. Gordon Industrial Building, Singapore 409838.

Sole Agent:
Sea Gull Trading (Pte) Ltd. Blk 217 Henderson Industrial Park, #03-05 Henderson Road, Singapore 159555. Tel: 6274 1033, Fax: 62724997. Email: sea_gull@pacific. net.sg CPM No: 113996

3. **American Ginseng & Notoginseng capsules (AL)**

    Actions:
    Strengthen the body, promote blood circulation, remove blood stasis, relieve pain, promote health and preserving youth.

    Indications:
    It is effective for the conditions related to coronary arterioscelerosis, hyperlipidae-mia, high cholesterol and menstruation pain. Under long-term administration, the product is able to strengthen physical conditions and prevent cardiac vascular diseases.

    Ingredients:
    Each capsule (0.35 g) contains extract equivalent to raw herbs: *Radix Panacis Quinquefolii* 175 mg, *Radix Notoginseng* 175 mg.

    Dosage:
    2 to 3 capsules each time, twice a day. For health maintenance: Take 2 capsules each time, once a day.

    Safety considerations:
    Side effects not known. Not suitable for pregnant women.

    Price: 60 capsules — $29.40 (sealed)

    Manufacturer and sole distributor in Singapore:
    All link Medical and Health Products Pte Ltd. 10 Kaki Bukit Road 1, #03-27 K B Industrial Building, Singapore 416175 Tel: 68460337 Fax: 68460336

4. **American ginseng and pseudoginseng capsules (Mei Hua Brand)**

Description:
PIL: Pseudo Ginseng, originally known as San Qi, is a special kind of herb and is classified under acanthopanax plants, the common family of Ginseng. Traditionally, Chinese physicians use Pseudo Ginseng against bruises and blood clots caused by sport injuries or accidents, and against thrombosis in certain cases. But from a medical and scientific point of view, Pseudo Ginseng contains the property of dilating coronary arteries, increasing the volume of blood flow in the blood vessels. It also helps effectively to reduce cholesterol and blood stasis. Meihua Brand American Ginseng & Pseudoginseng Capsules is scientifically processed using Pseudo Ginseng with American Ginseng. With its excellent ingredients, this product is effective for combating chest discomfort and angina caused by coronary arteriosclerosis. Regular taking would also lower hyperlipidaemia and cholesterol level, prevent the narrowing of the arteries.

Actions:
Remove blood stasis and promote regeneration of blood tissues, activate blood circulation and unblock channels, invigorate energy and nourish yin.

Indications:
Effective for conditions related to coronary arteriosclerosis. Lower hyperlipidaemia and cholesterol level and improve the circulation in the blood vessels. Helps to prevent angina and arteriosclerosis.

Ingredients:
Each capsule weighted 380 mg. *Radix Notoginseng* 30%, *American Ginseng* 70%

Dosage:
For curative purpose: Take 3 capsules three times daily, with warm water. For prevention, take 2 capsules once a day.

Safety considerations:
PIL: Products no Side Effect.

Price: 30 capsules — $15 (sealed)

Manufacturer:
Science Arts Co Pte Ltd. 150 MacPherson Rd, Science Arts Building Singapore 348524

5. **American Ginseng Candy (Prince of Peace®)**

Description:
This Prince of Peace® American Ginseng Candy (*Panax quinquefolium*) has been carefully formulated and packaged for your enjoyment from what is prized as one of

the highest valued Ginseng in the world. Prince of Peace® American Ginseng Candy are conveniently packaged and conserved individually in a foil wrap to ensure the freshness and quality. Prince of Peace® American Ginseng — an ancient but still sought after natural gift to mankind has long been treasured and safely consumed by millions throughout the world for its exclusive properties — the Rb ginsenosides. The growing number of consumers includes people from all walks of life. It is also the perfect trendy gift to your friends and families. Use 100% Wisconsin American Ginseng.

Ingredients:
Sugar, Glucose, Pure Wisconsin American Ginseng Chunks (*Panax Quinquefolium*), Peppermint and American Ginseng Flavor.

Dosage:
No information available

Price: $6.00

Manufacturer:
Exclusively Made in China for: Prince of Peace Enterprises, Inc.®, 3536 Arden Road, Hayward, CA 94545-3908, U.S.A.; Questions/Comments: 1 (510) 887-1899; Please visit: www.popus.com; www.popsfoundation.org.

Distributor (China, Hong Kong & Macau):
Prince of Peace (Hong Kong) Limited Unit 1, 5/F, Block B, Shatin industrial Centre, 5-7 Yuen Shun Circuit, Shatin, N.T., Hong Kong; Consumer Hotline: (852) 2314-8919; Website: www.princeofpeace.hk

6.   **American Ginseng Capsule (ZK)**

Description:
ZK Brand Amerian Ginseng Capsule is made from ultrafined American Ginseng powder which is easily absorbed by human body. Function experiments prove that this product has the health-care function of anti fatigue.

Actions:
Anti fatigue.

Indications:
People who are prone to fatigue.

Ingredients:
Each capsule contains 250 mg Ultrafined American Ginseng. Active ingredients: 100 g contains saponins 6.3 g.

Dosage:
2–3 capsules each time, twice daily.

Safety considerations:
Side effects not known. Not suitable for children.

Price: 100 capsules — $40 (sealed)

Manufacturer:
Nanjing Zhongke Biochemical Techonology Co., Ltd, Nanjing, China. Importer: ZK Singapore 1 Ubi Crescent #05-01 Number One Bldg Singapore 408563 Tel: 67480266 Fax: 68416477 Email: 08@zk.com.sg www.zk.com.sg. CPM Product Reference No. 110149 (Singapore).

7. **American Ginseng Plus Cordyceps Capsules (Nature's Green)**

Actions:
Invigorates the body, restores and maintains vitality, strengthens the immune system.

Indications:
Indicated for recuperation after illness, lumbago, knee pain, persistent cough, and frequent sweating.

Ingredients:
Each 300 mg capsule contains: *Radix Panacis quinquefolii* 150 mg, *Cordyceps* 100 mg, *Cordyceps Hypha* 50 mg.

Dosage:
For oral administration, take 2–4 capsules, twice daily.

Price: 50 capsules — $28.00, 3 × 50 capsules — $73.00

Manufacturer:
Tong Jum Chew Pte Ltd. 21 Kaki Bukit View Tech Park II Singapore 415957. Tel: 62781134 Fax: 62781246. Singapore Manufacturer Licence No. MLCP 04000400 Singapore CPM Product Reference No.: 112822

8. **American Ginseng Plus Notoginseng Capsules (Nature's Green)**

Actions and indications:
The product is a special tonic that invigorates the body's system by restoring and maintaining vitality, and strengthens the immune system. It can relieve chest pain and palpitation

Ingredients:
Each 300 mg capsule contains: *Radix Panacis Quinquefolii* 60 mg, *Radix Notoginseng* 120 mg, *Radix Salviae Miltiorrhiae* 120 mg

Dosage:
For oral administration, take 2–4 capsules, twice daily.

Price: 50 capsules — $24, 3 × 50 capsules — $63.00 (Sealed)

Manufacturer:
Tong Jum Chew Pte Ltd 21 Kaki Bukit View Tech Park II Singapore 415957 tel: 62781134 Fax: 62781246 Singapore Manufacturer Licence No. MLCP: 04000400 Singapore CPM Product Reference No.: 112822

9. **American Ginseng Slice with Honey (Avalon)**

Description:
American Ginseng Slice with Honey is undoubtedly an excellent tonic for good stamina and vigor. It is pure, natural and does not contain additives. Daily consumption helps to replenish energy, relieve tiredness, enhance overall wellbeing, nourish lungs, maintain youthful looks, improve concentration and memory and support immunity.

Ingredients:
Each packet contains 5 g of honey ginseng. American ginseng, linden honey.

Dosage:
Take 5 to 10 g daily. Chew it as directed.

Price: $68.80 (sealed) $116.00 (25 g × 12 packs + 5 g × 5 packs).

Manufacturer:
Hi-Beau International Pte Ltd. Tel: 65159818 http://www.hibeau.com.sg.

10. **American Ginseng Soup (Yew Chian Haw)**

Details:
No information available

Ingredients:
American ginseng, Rhizoma polygonati odorati, Fructus lycii, Rhizoma dioscorea batatas, Euphoria longan, Fructus ziziphi jujubee

Instruction:
Boil 2000 ml (or 8 rice bowls) water, add in YEW CHIAN HAW 'American Ginseng Soup' ingredients and boil vigorously. Then add in 500 gm of meat (any kind) and simmer. Add salt to taste.

Price: 50 gm +/– 5 gm — $3.90

Manufacturer:
YEW CHIAN HAW (MALAYSIA) SDN. BHD., (Company No. 218632-A) 2, Lingtang Beringin 2, Jalan Permatang Damar Laut, 11960 Batu Maung, Penang, Malaysia. Tel: 604-626 2020 (8 lines): Fax: 604-626 1010: Email: ych@e-ych.com.

Distributed by:
YEW CHIAN HAW (SINGAPORE) PTE. LTD. (Company No. 199200237-N) 7 Fan Yoong Road, Singapore 629785, Email: ych.sg@e-ych.com; YEW CHIAN HAW TAIWAN INTERNATIONAL PTE. LTD, (rest all in chinese).

11. **American Ginseng Tea (Ge Xian Weng)**

Description:
This product is finely made with American ginseng through advanced modern technologies. It is mild in nature and natural in taste, is extremely convenient to carry and suits men and women, and young and old in all seasons. It is an excellent natural nourishment for home and travel.

Ingredients:
American ginseng.

Instruction:
Put 1 or 2 bags into the cup each time and add boiling water and soak for 3–10 minutes. Drink while it is hot. It can be soaked and used repeatedly until it is pale in color.

Price: 2 g × 20 bags — $5.00

Imported by:
Winter Honey Trading Company, 32 Kallang Pudding Road #05-01 Elite Industrial Building 1, Singapore 349313. Made in China. Product standard: Q/GXW24; Sanitation license: GWSZ Zi No. 450331-001318; Food product license code: WS4500 1402 0012; Export sanitation license No.: 4500/11019, Add.: No. 237 Liliu Road, Lipu, Guilin, Guangxi.

12. **American Ginseng Tonic Herbal Tea (Nature's Green)**

Actions and indications:
Adjusts immune system in middle-aged and elderly persons, and restores the vital energy and builds up health.

Ingredients:
Each 3.5 g tea bag contains: Radix Panacis Quinquefolii (1000 mg), Fructus Jujubae (800 mg), Flos Chrysanthemi (600 mg), Radix Angelicae Sinensis (300 mg), Semen Nelumbinis (400 mg), Fructus Mori (400 mg)

Dosage:
Steep tea bag in boiling water and consume the tea 2–3 times a day.

Safety considerations:
Side effects and contraindication not known.

Price: 10 bags × 3.5 g. $12.00

Manufacturer:
Tong Jum Chew Pte Ltd., 21 Kaki Bukit Yiew Tech Park II Singapore 415957; Tel: 6278 1134; Fax: 6278 1246; Singapore Manufacturer Licence: MLCCP0400040; Singapore CPM Product Referenc No.: 116229.

13. **American Ginseng Tonic Soup (Eu Yan Sang)**

Description:
Good for people with a stressfull lifestyle. Suitable for all ages.

Ingredients:
(Percentage %/weight): Rhizoma Polygonati Odorati (37%/38 g), Rhizoma Dioscoreae (22%/23 g), Fructus Lycii (19%/19 g), Radix Panacis Quinquefolii (3%/3 g), Arilus Longan (19%/19 g).

Instruction:
Ingredients Required: One packet of Soup ingredients with 300 g to 500 g of meat and 1500 ml of water. May add more water if desired. Conventional Cooker: Place soup ingredients and meat into a pot. Add water and bring to boil. Continue to simmer over low heat for 1.5 hours. Pressure Cooker > Empty soup ingredients into pot. Add meat and water to boil for 5 minutes on high heat. Reduce heat and simmer for another 15 minutes. Follow precautionary procedure when using pressure cooker. Slow Cooker: Place soup ingredients and meat into pot. Add water and cook for 2 hours on HIGH heat. Add salt to taste.

Price: 102 g — $10.00

Packed & Distributed by:
EU YAN SANG (Singapore) Pte Ltd (Company Reg. No 195500108C) 269A South Bridge Road, Singapore 058818;

14. **American Ginseng with Cordyceps & Radix Notoginseng Capsules (Mei Hua Brand)**

Actions:
Replenish deficiency of vital energy and nourish blood, strengthen the heat and mental ability and eliminate fatigue.

Ingredients:
Each capsule contains 300 mg: *Radix Panacis Quinquefolii* (American Ginseng) 90 mg, *Cordyceps Sinensis* (Fermented) 90 mg, *Radix et Notoginseng* 120 mg

Dosage:
For maintaining good health: Take 2 capsules daily before breakfast. For curative purposes: Take 2 capsules three times a day before food.

Price: 60 capsules — $50.00 (sealed)

Manufacturer:
Science Arts Co. Pte Ltd 150 MacPherson Road, Science Arts Building, Singapore 348525.

15. **American Ginseng with Cordyceps Capsule (Mei Hua Brand)**

Actions:
It is effective for tranquilizing the mind and combating fatigue.

Ingredients:
Each capsule contains 300 mg: American Ginseng 120 mg, *Cordyceps* 180 mg.

Dosage:
For health- 2 times daily, 2 capsules at a time. For treament- 3 times daily, 3 capsules at a time. Take with warm water.
60 capsules: $50.00 (sealed) 300 capsules: $210.00 (sealed)

Manufacturer:
Science Arts Co. Pte Ltd. 150 MacPherson Rd, Science Arts Building Singapore 348524.

16. **American Wisconsin Ginseng Root Tea (Prince of Peace®)**

Instruction:
Prince of Peace® American Ginseng Root Tea (*Panax quinquefolius*) has been selected, processed and packaged for your enjoyment from what is prizcd as one of the highest valued Ginsengs in the world. This ancient but still sought after natural gift to mankind has long been treasured and safely consumed by millions throughout the world for its exclusive properties — the Rb ginsenosides, for example, are double the potency compared to Korean ginseng. Prince of Peace® offers a complete line of teas. Please try our American Ginseng Root Tea, American Ginseng Root Tea with Honey, American Ginseng Green Tea, American Ginseng Root Tea with Jasmine, American Ginseng Root Tea with Chrysanthemum and American Ginseng Tea with Rose Hips.

Ingredients:
American Wisconsin Ginseng (*Panax Quinquefolius*) Root.

Instruction:
Brewing Instructions: To make tea, pour about 4 fl. oz. Boiling water over the ginseng teabag in the cup. Cover the cup and let the tea steep for 3–5 minutes before drinking.

Price: 20 Teabags (1.8 g each sachet); Net Wt. 13 oz/36 g — $16.00

Exclusively Distributed By:
Prince of Peace Enterprises, Inc.®, 3536 Arden Road, Hayward, CA 94545-3908, U.S.A.; Consumer Service Number: 1 (510) 887-1899; Please Visit: www.popus.com; www.popsfoundation.org; www.princeofpeace.hk; Distributor (China, Hong Kong & Macau): Prince of Peace (Hong Kong) Ltd., Unit 1 5/F., Block B, hatin Industrial Centre, 5-7 Yuen Shun Circuit, Shatin, N.T., Hong Kong; Tel: (852) 2314-8919; Website: www.princeofpeace.hk; made in U.S.A.

17. **Ant Joint Care Capsules (Nature's Green)**

Actions and indications:
Invigorates vital energy, relieves swelling and arrests joint pain. It helps relieve the symptoms of joint swelling, stiffness and pain, and difficulty in extension and flexion of limbs caused by rheumatoid arthritis.

Ingredients:
Each 450 mg capsule contains extracts equivalent to raw herbs: *Formica Fusca* (Ant) 120 mg, *Radix Notoginseng* 75 mg, *Rhizoma Paridis* 120 mg, *Herba Erodii Seu Geranii* 75 mg, *Rhizoma Homalomenae* 75 mg, *Herba Lycopodii* 120 mg, *Radix Dipsaci* 120 mg, *Radix Angelicae Pubescentis* 120 mg, *Radix Clematidis* 120 mg, *Herba Epimedii* 75 mg, *Rhizoma Drynariae* 75 mg, *Rhizoma Cibotii* 75 mg, *Radix Saposhnikoviae* 75 mg, *Flos Carthami* 50 mg, *Radix Paeoniae Alba* 75 mg, *Radix Rehmanniae* 75 mg, *Radix Rehmanniae Preparata* 50 mg, *Rhizoma Anemarrhenae* 50 mg, *Spina Gleditsiae* 50 mg.

Dosage:
For oral administration, take 4 capsules, 3 times daily. The recommended course of treatment is 1 month.

Price: 60 capsules — $25 (sealed)

Manufacturer:
Tong Jum Chew Pte Ltd 21 Kaki Bukit View Tech Park II Singapore 415957 Tel: 62781134 Fax: 62781246 Singapore Manufacturer Licence No. MLCP 0400040 Singapore CPM Product Reference No. 115068

18. **Anti-Distention capsule (H & F)**

Actions:
Fortify spleen and harmonize the stomach, Eliminate abdominal distention.

Indications:
Abdominal distention, Eructation with foul odor, acid regurgitation, loose stool, fatigue caused by low Functionality of spleen and stomach.

Ingredients:
Each capsule contains extracts equivalent to raw herbs: *Panax Ginseng* 30 mg, *Rhizoma Atractylodis Macrocephalae* 30 mg, *Cortex Magnoliae Officinalis* 100 mg, *Fructus Aurantii* 100 mg, *Pericarpium Citri Reticulatae* 100 mg, *Poria Cum Radix Pini* 30 mg, *Radix Curcumae* 150 mg, *Herba Hedyotis Diffusae* 20 mg, *Semen Ziziphi Spinosae* 30 mg, *Flos Albiziae* 30 mg.

Dosage:
2 capsules, twice a day. To be taken before breakfast and after dinner.

Safety considerations:
No known side effects. No known contraindication.

Price: 60 capsules — $48 (sealed bottle)

Manufacturer:
Kim Sin Manufactory Pte Ltd. Blk 1022, Tai Seng Ave, #07-3530 Tai Seng Industrial Estate Singapore 534415.

Sole agent:
Herb & Fashion Pte Ltd. 1, Jurong East St 32 #14-04 Singapore 609477.

19. **Anti-constipation capsules (AL)**

Actions and indications:
Moisturise intestines and active bowel movement, promote the vital energy and strengthen your body. It is effective for all types of constipation, suitable for the aged, youth, children, women who just give birth and habitual constipation. Always keeping intestine unblocked and smooth can contribute to strengthen physical body and promote health and long life.

Ingredients:
Each 0.3 g capsule contains extract equivalent to raw herbs: *Radix Polygoni Multiflori* 500 mg, *Radix Rehmanniae* 400 mg, *Radix Ginseng* 200 mg, *Radix Angelicae Sinensis* 400 mg, *Rhizoma Alismatis* 100 mg, *Flos Sophorae* 200 mg.

Dosage:
Adult: 3–4 capsules each time, twice a day, morning and evening. For severe cases, take the prescription regularly for a full course of one month.

Safety considerations:
Side effects and contraindications not known.

Price: 30 capsules — $6.80 Package is sealed.

Manufacturer and sole distributor in singapore:
ALL Link Medical & health products pte ltd. 10 Kaki Bukit Road 1, #03-27 K B Industrial Building, Singapore 416175. Tel: 68460337. Fax: 68460336.

20. **Antihyperlipidemic Capsules (AL)**

Actions:
Removing indigestion, reducing blood fat, benefiting qi and blood.

Indications:
It is effective for hyperlipidemia, improving blood viscosity and plasma viscosity, and protecting against arteriosclerosis and coronary heart diseases. It is suitable for symptoms of palpitation, dyspnea, feeling of oppression in the chest, dizziness, headache, amnesia, tinnitus, sweating and fatigue.

Ingredients:
Each capsule (340 mg) contains extract equivalent to raw herbs: *Radix Notoginseng* 250 mg, *Radix Polygoni Multiflori* 180 mg, *Ganoderma Lucidum* 60 mg, *Auricularia* 35 mg, *Radix Salviae Miltiorrhizae* 200 mg, *Fructus Crataegi* 400 mg, *Spica Prunellae* 200 mg, *Herba Plantaginis* 200 mg, *Semen Cassiae* 350 mg, *Rhizoma Chuanxiong* 200 mg, *Folium Nelumbinis* 200 mg.

Dosage:
2 capsules each time, 2 times a day. Minor cases require continuous medication for 30–60 days; serious cases require continuous medication for 60–90 days.

Safety considerations:
Side effects not known. Not recommended for pregnant women.

Price: 30 capsules — $10.30. Package is sealed.

Manufacturer and sole distributor in singapore:
ALL Link Medical & health products pte ltd. 10 Kaki Bukit Road 1, #03-27 K B Industrial Building, Singapore 416175. Tel: 68460337. Fax: 68460336.

21. **Anti-Hyperosteogeny Capsules (AL)**

Actions and indications:

Anti-Hyperosteogeny works specially for hyperosteogeny of abdominal vertebra. It is effective to nourish loins and kidny and strengthen the tendons and bones, activate blood circulation and to relieve pain. Used for hyperplastic spndulitis, cervical syndrome and spur.

Ingredients:

Each capsule (0.4 g) contains extract equivalent to raw herbs: *Radix Notoginseng* 100 mg, *Radix Rehmanniae Preparata* 200 mg, *Fructus Ligustri Lucidi* 100 mg, *Rhizoma Drynariae* 100 mg, *Rhizoma Dioscoreae Nipponicae* 300 mg, *Caulis Spantholobi* 200 mg, *Radix Cyathulae* 100 mg, *Radix Salviae Miltiorrhizae* 200 mg, *Flos Carthami* 100 mg, *Semen Persicae* 100 mg, *Rhizoma Chuanxiong* 100 mg, *Cortex Eucommiae* 100 mg, *Fructus Psoraleae* 100 mg, *Herba Epimedii* 100 mg.

Dosage:

3 capsules each time, twice a day. Each course of medication lasts 2 months.

Safety considerations:

Side effects not known. Not recommended for pregnant women.

Price: 48 capsules — $10.40 (sealed)

Manufacturer and sole distributor in Singapore:

All Link Medical and Health Products Pte Ltd 10 Kaki Bukit Road 1, #03-27 KB Industrial building, Singapore 416175. tel: 68460337 fax: 68460336.

22. **Authentic Bak Kut Teh (Chwee Song)**

Description:

Renowned for its tender pork ribs and aromatic herbal soup, Bak Kut Teh is a traditional dish well-loved by generations. Keeping to our zealously guarded recipe of specially selected herbs and spices. Authentic Bak Kut Teh brings you the robust flavours and rich aftertastes that have made this dish a perennial favourite. A unique combination of herbs and spices are grounded and packed in sachets for convenient cooking. To prepare a sumptuous meal of Authentic Bak Kut Teh, simply add spare ribs and a pre-packed sachet to boiling water. Chicken, beef or mutton may also be used in place of pork ribs. Apart from being a favourite dish year-round, Authentic Bak Kut Teh is also an ideal gift for all occacions. A savoury present appreciated by both the young and old.

Ingredients:

Membranous Milkvetch Root, Fragrant Solomonseal Rhizome, Chuaxiong Rhizome, Cinnamon, Ginseng, Chinese Angelica Root, Fennel Fruit, Ural Licorice Root.

Dosage:
No information available

Price: 6 × 40 g — $28.00

Packed by:
Chwee Song Supplies Pte Ltd. Blk 5, Ang Mo Kio Ind'l Park 2A Tech II #07-14 to 16 Singapore 567760. Tel: 65-6482 3935; Fax: 65-6778 5028; http://www.chweesong. com.sg; E-Mail: sales@chweesong.com.sg.

23. Ba Zhen He Ji (QianJin)

Actions and indications:
Invigorate qi and nourish blood. Marked by pale or sallow complexion, dizziness, lassitude, shortness of breath etc.

Ingredients:
Each 300 ml of this product contains the following raw herbs: Radix Angelicae Sinensis (2.8 g), Rhizoma Chuanxiong (2.0 g), Radix Paeoniae Alba (2.8 g), Radix Rehmanniae Praeparata (3.8 g), Radix Et Rhizoma Ginseng (2.0 g), Rhizoma Atractylodis macroephalae (2.8 g), Poria (2.0 g), Radix Et Rhizoma Glycyrrhizae Praeparata Cum Melle (1.0 g), Rhizoma Zingiberis Recens (0.2 g), Fructus Jujubae (0.6 g).

Dosage:
30 ml each time, 2 times daily

Safety considerations:
Side effects not known. Not to be taken by pregnant women or patients with diabetes.

Price: 500 ml — $18.00

Manufacturer:
Kiat Ling Health Products & Trading, Blk 3017 Bedok North St. 5 #04-15 Singapore 486121; Tel: 6744 1868 Fax: 6743 5267.

24. Bai Feng Wan [aka "Wu Ji Bai Feng Wan"] (Li Shih Chen)

Actions:
Improve energy and blood circulation, smooth flow of period and decrease discharge.

Indications:
Indicated for general debility, physical tiredness, weakness and irregular period.

Ingredients:
Each 6 g contains to raw herbs: *Pullus Cum Osse Nigro* 1024 mg, *Radix Rehmanniae* 410 mg, *Ootheca Mantidis* 77 mg, *Radix Angelicae Sinensis* 230 mg, *Raidx Ginseng*

205 mg, *Rhizoma Cyperi* 205 mg, *Radix Paeoniae Alba* 205 mg, *Radix Salviae Miltiorrhizae* 211 mg, *Carapax Trionycis* 102 mg, *Concha Ostreae* 77 mg, *Mel* 1741 mg, *Rhizoma Dioscoreae* 205 mg, *Semen Euryales* 102 mg, *Radix Glycyrrhizae* 51 mg, *Radix Asparagi* 102 mg, *Rhizoma Chuanxiong* 102 mg, *Radix Astragali* 211 mg, *Radix Stellariae* 42 mg, *Colla Cornuc Cervi* 211 mg, *Cornu Cervi Pantotrichum* 77 mg, *Radix Rehmanniae Preparata* 410 mg.

Dosage:
One pill each time, twice daily taken with lukewarm boiled water or rice wine.

Safety considerations:
No known side effect. 1. Pregnant individual prohibited from consumption. 2. Avoid taking cold sour food, tea, radish etc. 3. Restrict from taking other medicines while consuming this product.

Price: 10 × 6 g — $13.80 (sealed)

Manufacturer:
Henan ShiZhen Medicines Products Co. Ltd. Henan, China.

Imported by:
Wideway Pte Ltd. 2 Kallang Ave, #06-07 Kallang Bahru Complex S'pore 339407. Tel: 62923618 Fax: 62966956.

25. **Bai Feng Wan Paoshen Chongcao [aka "American Ginseng with Cordyceps pills"] (Mei Hua Brand)**

Indications:
Traditionally used for general weakness, fatigue, improve appetite, headache, backache and to regulate menstruation.

Ingredients:
Each bottle (10 g of pills) contains the following: *Cordyceps Sinensis* 0.2 g, *Radix Panacis Quinquefolii* 0.6 g, *Radix Salviae Miltiorrhizae* 1.8 g, *Rhizoma Ligustici Chuanxiong* 1.0 g, *Herba Leonurus* 2.0 g, *Radix Astragali* 1.0 g, *Radix Rehmannia Preparata* 1.0 g, *Radix Codonopsis Pilosulae* 1.0 g, *Radix Angelicae Sinensis* 1.0 g, *Rhizoma Dioscorea* 0.4 g.

Dosage:
For treatment: One bottle (10 g) each time to be taken with warm water, one time per day. For Health Maintenance: One bottle each time to be taken with warm water, once in every 3 day. If symptoms persist, consult a doctor.

Safety considerations:
Side effects not known. Forbidden to take pill when having cold, diarrhoea or fever. Used with caution in pregnancy.

Price: 6 bottles × 10 g — $46.80 (sealed).

Manufacturer:

S.H. Uniflex Chinese Medical Factory SDN. BHD. No. 21A, Jalan Lambak, Taman Johor Light Ind. Est, 81200 Johor Bahru, Johor, Malaysia.

Imported by:

Science Arts Co. Pte Ltd. 150 MacPherson Rd, Science Arts Building Singapore 348524.

26.　**Bai Feng Wan with Collagen (Ren Xin Tang)**

Description:

Specially formulated with Traditional Chinese Medicinal (TCM) method, Ren Xin Tang's Collagen Bai Feng Wan embraces the benefits of Chinese herbs, which have been used for centuries to enhance women's well-being and immune system. Combined with Marine Fish Collagen Peptides, Ren Xin Tang Bai Feng Wan provides support for a glowing and radiant complexion, as well as nourishes the body to promote skin health.

Indications:

A health and beauty product for women's overall well-being. Supplement diet with quality collagen formula to improve skin health. Regular consumption can help enhance skin health and support the immune system for women's well-being.

Ingredients:

Marine Fish Collagen Peptides, *Radix Et Rhizoma Ginseng (Panax Ginseng)*, *Radix Codonopsis, Radix Rehmanniae Praeparata, Radix Paeoniae Alba, Radix Angelicae Dahuricae, Radix Dipsaci, Rhizoma Cyperi, Herba Leonuri, Herba Taxilli, Radix Angelicae Sinensis, Radix Astragali, Rhizoma Chuanxiong, Semen Trigonellae, Rhizoma Atractylodis Macrocephalae, Fructus Amomi, Radix Scutellariiae, Radix Et Rhizoma Glycyrrhizae Praeparata Cum Melle* (Strength not provided).

Dosage:

2 capsules 2 times daily

Safety considerations:

No known side effects and no known contraindications.

Price: 60 capsules — $49.90 (sealed)

Wholesaler:

LIXR Enterprise #11-15, 9 Penang Road Singapore 238459.

27. **Baifeng Wan (Keyi)**

Actions and Indications:
Invigorates energy and enriches blood. Regulate menstrual cycle. Treat energy and blood deficiency, as well as irregular menstruation due to blood stasis. For symptoms such as watery menses, small in quantity, lack of energy and weak limbs.

Ingredients:
Each capsule (300 mg) contains raw herbs: *Radix Panacis Quinquefolii* (American Ginseng) 100 mg, *Radix Rehmanniae Praeparata* 150 mg, *Rhizoma Atractylodis Macrocephalae* 100 mg, *Poria* 100 mg, *Radix Angelicae Sinensis* 150 mg, *Radix Paeoniae Alba Praeparata* 100 mg, *Radix Et Rhizoma Glycyrrhizae Praeparata* 100 mg, *Rhizoma Chuanxiong* 100 mg, *Herba Leonuri* 300 mg, *Rhizoma Zingiberis Recens* 20 mg, *Fructus Jujubae* 30 mg.

Dosage:
Take 3 times daily after meals, 3 capsules each time or as directed by physician.

Safety considerations:
PIL: side effects not known. Precaution: Avoid raw, cold food and mental aggravations. Not to be suitable for pregnant woman.

Price: 60 capsules — $24.00 (not sealed)

Manufacturer:
Science Arts Co Pte Ltd. 150 MacPherson Rd, Science Arts Building Singapore 348524. Enquires: 67442651

28. **Bakuteh Kau Herb's & Spices Mix (Clay-pot)**

Description:
Improved Recipe! NO ADDED MSG; EASY TO COOK; WITH GINSENG

Ingredients:
Angelica Sinensis, Polygonatum Odoratum, Cinnamon (Kayu Manis), Lycii Fructus, Glycyrrhiza uralensis, White Pepper (Lada Putih), Codonopsis Pilosulae, Astractylodis Macrocephalae, Flavour Enhancer (E635) (Perisa Tambahan), Sugar (Gula), Salt (Gaam), Ligustici Wallichii, Star Anise (Bunga Lawang), Radix Panax Ginseng and Yeast Extract.

Instruction:
Preparation: 1 packet Bakuteh Kau Herb's & Spices Mix (2 filter bags); 1 kg ribs or meat (chicken, mutton or other), cut to preferred size; 1500 ml (6 rice bowls) water; 3 whole garlic bulbs; 1 1/2 tsp dark soy sauce; 1/2 tsp soy sauce; 2 tbsp oyster sauce; COOKING METHOD: 1. In a large pot, boil the 2 filter bags (do not open the bags) in 1500 ml of

water for 30 mins. 2. Add the meat, garlic, dark soya sauce, light soya sauce and oyster sauce to the boiling soup. 3. Simmer for 1 hour. Serves 4–6 persons.

Price: 40 g — $2.65

Manufacturer:
LINACO FOOD INDUSTRIES S/B (117276-K) 12, Lintang Sg. Keramat 2B, Tmn Klang Utama, 42100 Klang, Selangor Darul Ehsan, Malaysia. Tel: 603-3291 4589 Website: www.linaco.com.my.

Imported/Distributed by:
Australia: ORIENTAL MERCHANT PTY LTD 10, Westgate Drive, Laverton North, Vic 3206, Australia. Singapore: ALPHICO MARKETING PTE LTD 48, Toh Guan Road East # 02-131/132, Enterprise Hub, Singapore 608586, Tel: 65-6272 3288; Product of Malaysia.

29. **Bee Pollen Ginseng + Vitamin E (21st Century)**

Description:
21st Century labs has combined Ginseng & Natural Vitamin E-with Bee Pollen, royal jelly and Propolis which are produced by bees to give you a complete natural energizing supplement. Bee Pollen: Contains 18 amino acids, 16 vitamins, 16 minerals and 18 enzymes for youthful zest and vitality. Royal Jelly: The food of the Queen Bee which has a life span 30–40 times of ordinary worker bees. Contains an abundance of vitamins, proteins, and amino acids. Propolis: A sweet-smelling resin produced and used by bees to keep their hives free from infection. Ginseng: The rejuvenating herb highly regarded over the centuries in the East. Natural Vitamin E: The antioxidant that slows the aging process and protects against cell destruction.

Ingredients:
Each tablet contains: Bee Pollen 200 mg, Natural Vitamin E 50 IU, Ginseng 200 mg, Royal Jelly 50 mg, Propolis 100 mg

Dosage:
Take 1 tablet daily in the morning.

Price: 40 tablets — $13.00 (Sealed)

Manufacturer:
21st Century HealthCare Inc., 2119 S. Wilson Street, Tempe, Arizona 85282-2034 USA.

Distributed by:
21st Century HealthCare Pte Ltd. Singapore.

30. **Beijing Baifeng Wan (Tong Ren Tang)**

Actions:
To invigorate the vital energy, nourish the blood, regulate the menstruation and stop leukorrhea.

Indications:
Irregular menstruation, dysmenotthea, cold pain of the lower abdomen, general debility, feeling weak, lassitude of loins and legs, puerperal debility, night sweat due to the deficiency of the refined material in the viscera, these caused by deficiency of both vital energy and blood.

Ingredients:
Each 6 gms contains raw herbs: *Pullus Curn Osse Nigro* (Preparata) 1113.7 mg, *Colla Cornus Cervi* 222.7 mg, *Carapax Trionycis* (Preparata) 111.4 mg, *Concha Ostreae* (Preparata) 83.5 mg, *Ootheca Mantidis* 83.5 mg, *Radix Ginseng* 222.7 mg, *Radix Astragali* 55.7 mg, *Radix Angelicae Sinensis* 250.6 mg, *Radix Paeoniae Alba* 222.7 mg, *Rhizoma Cyperi* (Preparata) 222.7 mg, *Radix Asparagi* 111.4 mg, *Radix Glycyrrhizae* 55.7 mg, *Radix Rehmanniae* 445.5 mg, *Radix Rehmanniae* (Preparata) 445.5 mg, *Rhizoma Chuanxiong* 111.4 mg, *Radix Stellariae* 45.2 mg, *Radix Salviae Miltiorrhizae* 222.7 mg, *Rhizoma Dioscoreae* 222.7 mg, *Semen Euryales* (Preparata) 111.4 mg, *Cornu Cervi Degelatinatum* 83.5 mg ** Same as No. 138

Dosage:
Twice daily, all the water-honeyed pills (6 g) in one wax ball each time.

Instruction:
Take out the wax ball, squeeze the wax ball to open, take out the inner plastic capsule, open the inner plastic capsule and take the pills.

Price: 6 g × 6 balls — $20 (Sealed)

Manufacturer:
Beijing Tongrentang Co. Ltd. Tongrentang Pharmaceu-tical Factory Beijing China.

Imported by:
Science Arts Co. Pte Ltd. 150 MacPherson Rd, Science Arts Building Singapore 348524.

31. **Beijing Dahuoluo dan (Tong Ren Tang)**

Actions:
To dispel wind and remove dampness, to relax muscles and tendons, activate the collaterals.

Indications:
Arthralgia due to wind-cold dampnss, marked by pain of the limbs, numb hands and feet, muscular constriction.

Ingredients:
Each pill weight 3.6 gram contains raw herbs: *Agkistrodon, Benzoinum, Bombyx Bartryticatus, Borneolum Syntheticum, Calculus Bovis Synthetic, Carapac Et Plastrum Testudinis, Colophonium, Cornu Bubali, Cortex Cinnamomi, Flos Caryophylli, Fructus Amomi Rotundus, Herba Ephedrae, Lignum Aquilariae Resinatum, Myrrha, Olibanum, Pericarpium Citri Reticulatae Viride Praeparata, Pheretima, Poria, Radix Aconiti Kusnezoffii Praeparata, Radix Aconiti Lateralis Praeparata, Radix Angelicae Sinensis, Radix Aucklandiae, Radix Clematidis Clematis Chinensis, Radix Et Rhizoma Asari, Radix Et Rhizoma Rhei Praeparata, Radix Et Rhizome Glycyrrhizae, Radix Ginseng, Radix Linderae, Radix Paeoniae Rubra, Radix Polygoni Multiflori Praeparata, Radix Puerariae Lobatae, Radix Rehmanniae Praeparata, Radix Saposhnikoviae, Radix Acrophulariae, Radix Scutellariae, Rhizoma Anemones Raddeanae, Rhizoma Arisaematis Praeparata, Rhizoma Atractylodis Marcocephalae Praeparata, Rhizoma Cyperi, Rhizoma Drynariae, Rhizoma Dryopteris Crassirhizomae, Rhizoma Et Radix Notopterygii, Rhizoma Gastrodiae, Sanguis Dranconis, Scorpio, Zaocys, Honey Mel.*

Dosage:
1–2 pills, twice a day, to be taken with warm yellow rice wine or boiled water.

Safety considerations:
Precaution: Contraindicated in pregnancy

Price: $30.00 (sealed)

Manufacturer:
Beijing TongRenTang Limited Company. Tongrentang Pharmaceutical Factory. Beijing, China.

Imported by:
Science Arts Co. Pte Ltd. 150 MacPherson Rd, Science Arts Building Singapore 348524

32. **Be-Well Capsule (Keyi)**

Actions and Indications:
Calms mind and relaxes nerves. Invigorates energy, improves blood circulation and stops/relieves pain. Treat anxiety, insomnia and chest distension.

Ingredients:
Each capsule (300 mg) contains raw herbs: *Folium Notoginseng* 500 mg, *Rhizoma Gastrodiae* 120 mg.

Dosage:
Take 3 times daily after meals, 2 capsules each time or as directed by physician.

Safety considerations:
Side effects not known.

Price: 60 capsules — $18 (not sealed)

Manufacturer:
Science Arts Co. Pte Ltd. 150 MacPherson Rd, Science Arts Building Singapore 348524. Enquires: 67442651.

33. **Bird's Nest Ginseng with White Fungus & Rock Sugar (Songshan Mountpine)**

Description:
Songshan Brand Bird's Nest, Ginseng with White Fungus and Rock Sugar is made from genuine ingredients to a traditional recipe. Consume within 24 hours after opening as it contains no artificial preservatives.
Rock Sugar Solution (79%), White Fungus (15.0%), Ginseng (5.0%), Permitted Stabilizer (0.8%), Bird's Nest (0.2%).

Dosage:
No information available

Price: 6 × 70 ml — $8.80

Distributor:
Malaysia Adress: Lot 16, Minlon Industrial Park, Jalan Minlon Utama, off jalan Taming 2, Balaakong, 43300 Selangor; Singapore Adress: Blk. 625, Aljunied Industrial Complex, #02-02, Aljunied Road, Singapore 389836.

Manufacturer:
Herculean Food Industries Sdn. Bhd. Lot PT.6913, Kawasan Perindustrian Taman Tasik utama, Ayer Keroh, 75450 Melaka, Malaysia.

34. **Bird's Nest with American Ginseng (Mei Hua)**

Description:
Chinese have treasured Bird's Nest as a valued delicacy and tonic. Mei Hua Brand Bird's Nest with American Ginseng consists of high quality, 100% genuine bird's nest and premium grade American Ginseng. It's all natural, with no preservatives or artificial flavouring.

Ingredients:
No information available

Dosage:
No information available

Price: 75 g × 6 — $50.00

Sole Agent:
Science Arts Co Pte Ltd. 150 MacPherson Road Science Arts Building Singapore 348524.

35. **Bird's Nest with American Ginseng & Rock Sugar (Brand's®)**

Description:
BRAND's® Bird's Nest with American Ginseng & Rock Sugar is prepared using premium grade 100% genuine Indonesian bird's nest and high quality American Ginseng. It is meticulously hand-cleaned and brewed with pure rock sugar solution, which is free from preservatives, flavouring and colouring. This natural product is vacuum sealed to preserve its guaranteed freshness.

Ingredients:
Bird's nest, Rock Sugar, American Ginseng Root and Stabiliser

Instruction:
This product may be consumed straight from the bottle at room temperature, chilled or warmed according to one's preference. Once bottle is opened, contents should be refrigerated and consumed within 24 hours.

Price: 6 bottles × 70 g — $46.80

Manufactured in Thailand under licence from Cerebos Pacific Ltd., Singapore;

Distributed in Singapore by:
DKSH Singapore Pte Ltd 34 Boon Leat Terrace Singapore 119866; Comments? Suggestions? We'd love to hear from you. Call BRAND's® Customer Care Line at 1800-732-4748 or write to us at Cerebos Pacific Ltd., 18 Cross Street #12-01/08, China Square Central; Singapore 048423.

36. **Bird's Nest with American Ginseng, White Fungus & Rock Sugar (Chwee Song)**

Description:
FU GUI Brand Bird's Nest with American Ginseng, White Fungus & Rock Sugar is traditionally prepared from clean Swallow Nest, with selected American Ginseng, White Fungus and Rock Sugar. It is manufactured by latest technology innovations.

The process of manufacturing is completely hygienic, with no addition of artificial colouring, flavouring and preservatives. Bird's nest is a natural nutritional product, suitable to be taken by people of all ages. FUI GUI Bird's Nest with American Ginseng, White Fungus & Rock Sugar can be consumed direct from bottle, chilled or warmed, depending on individual's taste. Consume within 24 hours after opening.

Ingredients:
Bird's Nest (7%), American Ginseng (8.0%), White Fungus (15.0%), Rock Sugar Solution (70.0%).

Dosage:
No information available

Price: 6×70 g — $13.70

Packed by:
Chwee Song Supplies Pte Ltd. Blk 5, Ang Mo Kio Ind'l Park 2A Tech II #07-14 to 16 Singapore 567760. Tel: 65-6482 3935; Fax: 65-6778 5028; http://www.chweesong. com.sg; E-Mail: sales@chweesong.com.sg; Product of Malaysia.

37. **Black-Bone Chicken & White-Phoenix Capsules (Nature's Green)**

Actions and Indications:
Regulating menstruation and arresting leukorrhea. Use for emaciation and general feebleness, aching, weakness and limpness of lions and kness, irregular menstruation with abnormal bleeding and leukorrhea, fatigue, lassitude, and weakness after delivery.

Ingredients:
Each 300 mg capsule contains extracts equivalent to raw herbs: *Pullus cum Osse Nigro* 376 mg, *Cordyceps* 55 mg, *Margarita* 25 mg, *Colla Cornus Cervi* 75 mg, *Cornu Cervi Degelatinatum* 28 mg, *Carapax Trionycis* 38 mg, *Radix Ginseng* 75 mg, *Radix Astragali* 19 mg, *Radix Anglica Sinensis* 84 mg, *Radix Paeoniae Alba* 75 mg, *Rhizoma Cyperi* 75 mg, *Radix Asparagi* 38 mg, *Radix Rehmanniae* 150 mg, *Radix Rehmanniae Preparata* 150 mg, *Rhizoma Chuanxiong* 38 mg, *Radix Stellariae* 15 mg, *Radix Salviae Miltiorrhiae* 75 mg, *Rhizoma Dioscoreae* 75 mg, *Concha Ostreae Preparata* 28 mg, *Ootheca Mantidis* 28 mg, *Semen Eutyales* 38 mg, *Radix Glycyrrhizae* 19 mg.

Dosage:
For treatment, 3 capsules each time, 2 times daily. For health maintenance, 1 capsule each time, 2 times daily.

Price: 30 capsules — $25.00, 2×30 capsules — $44.00 (sealed)

Manufacturer:
Tong Jum Chew Pte Ltd 21 Kaki Bukit View Tech Park II Singapore 415957 Tel: 62781134 Fax: 62781246 Singapore Manufacturer Licence No.: MLCP 0400040 Singapore CPM Product Reference No. 113468.

38. **Blood Circulation Promoting Capsules (Nature's Green)**

Actions and Indications:
Actives blood circulation and resolves stasis. Relieves the symptoms of weak limbs and lassitude, numbness and spasm of hands and feet, stiffness of muscles and joints, difficulty in walking, dizziness and blurred vision caused by blood stasis in brain vessles. Used as auxiliary treatment for the recuperation stage of serious health problems stricken by pathogenic wind.

Ingredients:
Each 480 mg capsule contains extracts equivalent to raw herbs: *Radix Notoginseng* 156 mg, *Rhizoma Chuanxiong* 156 mg, *Flos Carthami* 182 mg, *Radix Puerariae* 522 mg, *Fructus Crataegi* 314 mg.

Dosage:
For oral administration, 3 capsules each time, 3 times daily. The recommended treatment course is one month.

Safety considerations:
Side effects not known (not on packaging of 60 capsules but available in PIL). To be contraindicated for pregnant women (not on packaging of 60 capsules but available in PIL).

Price: 300 capsules — $44; 60 capsules — $10.

Manufacturer:
Tong Jum Chew Pte Ltd. 21 Kaki Bukit View Tech Park II Singapore 415957 Tel: 62781134 Fax: 62781246 Singapore Manufacturer Licence No. MLCP: 04000400 Singapore CPM Product Reference No.: 113698.

39. **Blood Flo-eze capsule (Camellia Brand)**

Actions:
Activates blood circulation, dredging arteries and veins, restrains conglomeration of blood platelets, and increases blood flow to the brain.

Indications:
It helps relieve the symptoms of chest pain and tightness, weak limbs, and lassitude, numbness and spasm of hands and feet stiffness of muscles and joints, difficulty in walking, dizziness and headaches caused by obstruction of Qi in the chest and brain.

Ingredients:

Each capsule of 180 mg ingredients contains 100 mg extracts equivalent to raw *Radix Notoginseng* 1000 mg.

Dosage:

For oral administration, take 1 capsule, 3 times daily.

Safety considerations:

No known side effects. Not to be taken by pregnant lady.

Price: 20 capsules — $11.20; 300 capsules — $110.00 (sealed).

Manufacturer:

Yunnan Weihe Pharmaceutical Co. Ltd. Exporter: Yunnan Camellia Pharmaceutical I/E Co. Ltd. Importer: Hygeian Medical Supplies (Pte) Ltd 203 Henderson Road #07-06 Henderson Industrial Park, Singapore 159546 Tel: 62702993 Fax: 63395034.

40. **Body Cleanser (Yi Shi Yuan)**

Actions:

Clear away blood stasis, promote blood circulation, clear toxic materials, relieve pain. Promote blood immunity, enhance metabolism, strengthen physique, antibacterial, enrich vital energy.

Indications:

Suitable for Inflammation, blood stasis, enhance "qi" and blood flow, rheumatism, coarse skin, disease, infection and coughing.

Ingredients:

Each capsule contains raw herbs 344 mg as below: *Herba Hedyotis Diffusae* 85.50 mg, *Semen Pruni* 16.60 mg, *Herba Andrographitis* 19.90 mg, *Herba Scutellariae Barbatae* 19.90 mg, *Radix Glehniae* 19.90 mg, *Pseudobulbus Cremastrae seu Pleiones* 13.30 mg, *Folium Isatidis* 19.90 mg, *Massa Medicata Fermentata* 16.60 mg, *Sargassum* 9.80 mg, *Herba Dianthi* 13.30 mg, *Semen Persicae* 13.30 mg, *Rhizoma Sparganii* 19.90 mg, *Fructus Gardeniae* 6.50 mg, *Radix Et Rhizoma Notoginseng* 19.90 mg, *Radix Angelicae Dahuricae* 19.90 mg, *Radix Stemonae* 6.50 mg, *Radix Linderae* 13.30 mg, *Radix Aucklandiae* 8.30 mg, *Camphora* 1.70 mg.

Dosage:

Take 5 capsules, 1–2 times daily.

Safety considerations:

No known side effect. Patient who has bleeding tendency takes cautiously. Avoid use in pregnant women.

Price: 60 vegetarian capsules — $48.00 (sealed)

GMP Manufatcurer:
Yi Shi Yuan Pte Ltd 20, Bukit Batok Crescent #13-11/12/13 Enterprise Centre Singapore 658080 Tel: 65670900 (5 lines) Fax: 65672256 Website: www.ysy.com.sg Email: enquiry@ysy.com.sg.

41. **Body Elements Balance Tablets (Nature's Green)**

Actions and Indications:
This product helps adjust metabolic function and relieves the "wasting and thirsting" syndrome characterized by excessive eating, unusual thirst, frequent and profuse urination, fatigue, feeble limbs, and loss of weight.

Ingredients:
Each 420 mg tablet contains extracts equivalent to raw herbs: Radix Ginseng 32 mg, Radix Astragali 52 mg, Radix Salviae Miltiorrhiae 52 mg, Radix Trichosanthis 209 mg, Rhizoma Dioscoreae 209 mg, Radix Rehmanniae 52 mg, Fructus Lycii 32 mg, Rhizoma Anemarrhenae 32 mg, Radix Asparagi 16 mg, Poria 21 mg, Fructus Corni 21 mg, Fructus Schisandrae 16 mg, Hirudo 16 mg, Radix Puerariae 21 mg, Endothelium Corneum Gigeriae Galli 21 mg.

Dosage:
For oral administration, take 4 capsules, 3 times daily before meals. The recommended forst treatment course is twenty days.

Safety considerations:
Side effects not known. Avoid alcohol, cigarette, and any food containing sugar. Not to be taken by pregnant women.

Price: 500 tablets — $59 (sealed bottle)

Manufacturer:
Tong Jum Chew Pte Ltd. 21 Kaki Bukit View Tech Park II Singapore 415957. Tel: 62781134 Fax: 62781246. Singapore Manufacturer Licence No. MLCP 0400040, Singapore CPM Product Reference No. 112879

42. **Body Fluid & Vital Energy Enhancing Capsule [60 vegecaps] (Borsch Med)**

Description:
Genuine Dendrobium Stem (*Herba Dendrobii*), Tian Qi (*Pseudo-Ginseng*) and high-quality American Ginseng (*Radix Panacis Quinquefolii*) are combined to formulate Borsch Med Body Fluid & Vital Energy Enhancing Capsule. American Ginseng is prominent for strengthening vital energy which is essential for blood and it also has the abilities to boost the body fluid-promoting effect of Dendrobiumstem. TianQi

promotes blood circulation. Each ingredient complements each other to achieve optimum efficacy of this product. This product is especially suitable for post illness recuperation and for those lacking in body fluid.

Actions:

This product reinforces the vital energy and promotes body fluids production, improves blood circulation and eases pain and discomfort. Overall, it also strengthens the immune system.

Ingredients:

Ingredients per capsule of 450 mg: *Radix Panacis Quinquefolii* 225.00 mg, *Radix Notoginseng* 112.50 mg, *Herba Dendrobii* 112.50 mg.

Safety considerations:

Adverse-Reactions: There are no known side effects for Borsch Med Body Fluid & Vital Energy Enhancing capsule. Not to be taken by pregnant women. Children of 12 years old or younger should take with caution.

Dosage:

1 capsule to be taken each time with lukewarm water, twice a day.

Price: 60 vege caps — $59.00

Manufacturer:

Union Chemical & Pharmaceutical Pte Ltd. 113 Eunos Avenue 3 #06-06, Gordon Industrial Building, Singapore 409838. Distributed by: Borsch Med Pte Ltd. 60 Alexandra Terrace #03-28, The Comtech, Singapore 118502. Borsch Med Inc. Suite #300 PMB #1024, 2711 Centreville Road, Wilmington, DE 19808, USA.

43. **Brain Nourishing Capsules (Nature's Green)**

Description:

PIL: Brain Nourishing Capsules are made from 19 beneficial herbs and prepared by modern pharmaceutical technology. This product is the typical formulation that helps nourish brain and relieve uneasiness of the mind. It is suitable for people engaged in heavy brainwork or forgetful elderly persons. It is effective in relieving the symtoms of neurasthenia, forgetfulness, insomnia, palpitations, dizziness, restlessness, fatigue, weakness and lumbago.

Actions:

Nourishes the brain and calms the mind.

Indications:

Suitable for people engaged in heavy brainwork or forgetful elderly persons. Relieves the symptoms of neurasthenia, forgetfulness, insomnia, palpitations, dizziness, restlessness, fatigue, weakness and lumbago.

Ingredients:
Each 300 mg capsule contains: *Fructus Alpiniae Oxyphyllae Preparata* 20 mg, *Concretio Silicea Bambusae* 13.3 mg, *Herba Cistanches Preparata* 26.7 mg, *Dens Draconis Preparata* 13.3 mg, *Succinum* 13.3 mg, *Fructus Schisandrae Preparata* 20 mg, *Rhizoma Gastrodiae* 6.7 mg, *Semen Platycladi Preparata* 5.3 mg, *Radix Polygalae Preparata* 6.7 mg, *Radix Salviae Miltiorrhiae* 6.7 mg, *Radix Ginseng* 6.7 mg, *Radix Angelicae Sinensis* 33.3 mg, *Rhizoma Dioscoreae* 26.7 mg, *Flos Chrysanthemi* 6.7 mg, *Rhizoma Anemones Altaicae* 13.3 mg, *Haematitum* 10 mg, *Arisaema Cum Bile* 13.3 mg, *Semen Ziziphi Spinosae Preparata* 53.3 mg, *Fructus Lycii* 26.7 mg.

Dosage:
For oral administration, take 2 capsules, 3 times daily.

Safety considerations:
Side effects not known (on the PIL of 60 capsules and on the packaging of 300 capsules).

Price: 60 capsules — $10.50 (not sealed); 300 capsules — $45.00 (sealed bottle).

Manufacturer:
Tong Jum Chew Pte Ltd. 21 Kaki Bukit View Tech Park II Singapore 415957 Tel: 62781134, Fax: 62781246. Singapore Manufacturer Licence No. MLCP 0400040. Singapore CPM Product Refernece No. 114070.

44. **Brain Tonic Tablets (Nature's Green)**

Actions:
Nourishes brain and clams the mind.

Indications:
Relieves the symptoms of neurasthenia, forgetfulness, insomnia, palpitations, dizziness, fatigue, spontaneous sweating, weakness and emission.

Ingredients:
Each 320 mg tablet contains extracts equivalent to raw herbs: *Rhizoma Polygonati Preparata* 99 mg, *Ganoderma Lucidum* 99 mg, *Herba Epimedii* 82 mg, *Radix Panacis Quinquefolii* 3.3 mg, *Carapax et Plastrum Testudinis Preparata* 8 mg, *Colla Cornus Cervi* 3.3 mg, *Radix Polygalae Preparata* 33 mg, *Semen Ziziphi Spinosae Preparata* 16 mg, *Fructus Schisandrae* 66 mg, *Fructus Lycii* 33 mg, *Radix Ophiopogonis* 16 mg, *Poria* 16 mg, *Radix Rehmanniae Preparata* 17 mg, *Fructus Jujubae* 33 mg, *Fructus Xanthii* 66 mg.

Dosage:
For oral administration, take 2–3 tablets, 2–3 times daily.

Safety considerations:
Side effects not known. Not to be taken by the patients suffering from hypertension, or with poor liver or kidney functions.

Price: 500 tabs — $46.00 (sealed bottle)

Manufacturer:
Tong Jum Chew Pte Ltd. 21 Kaki Bukit View Tech Park II Singapore 415957 Tel: 62781134, Fax: 62781246. Singapore Manufacturer Licence No. MLCP 0400040. Singapore CPM Product Refernece No. 114112

45. **Buyao Jing with Duzhong Cordyceps Baji (Mei Hua)**

Actions and Indications:
Promoting health, keeping body fit, increasing vigour, mourishing the loin, relaxing tendons and ligaments. It is effecive for debility and depletion of physical energy and physical work.

Ingredients:
Each 85 ml of liquid contain extracts of the following: Cordyceps (300 mg), Cortex Eucommiae (500 mg), Radix Morindae officinalis (500 mg), Fructus Psoraleae (500 mg), Radix Notoginseng (500 mg), Radix Astragali Seu Hedysari (500 mg), Fructus Lycii (500 mg).

Instruction:
The product is from natural extracts and does not contain any preservatives. When administering, add a little bit of salt, as desired to enhance taste; and take it orally either hot or cold. After opening the bottle, finish the content within the same day.

Dosage:
Adult: Take one bottle; Children: Take half bottle either hot or cold.

Price: $20.00

Manufacturer:
S.H. UNIFLEX CHINESE MEDICAL FACTORY SDN. BHD., No 21A, Jalan Lambak, Taman Johor Light Ind Est. 82100, Johor Bahru, Malaysia.

Imported by:
Science Arts Co. Pte Ltd., 150 MacPherson Rd, Science Arts Building Singapore 348524;

46. **Campuran Herba untuk Sup Ginseng-Ginseng Herbal Soup Mix (Claypot)**

Instruction:

Ginseng Herbal Soup Mix highlights the delicate aroma and flavours of a blend of natural herbs. No Added MSG. Soup is ready to serve in as little as 1 hour. Enjoy traditional goodness the modern way.

Ingredients:

Polygonatum Odoratum, Codonopsis Pilosulae, Radix Panax Ginseng (10%), Angelica Sinensis, Lycii Fructus, Ziziphi Jujubae Fructus, Glycyrrhiazae Preparata and Rehmanniae Glutinosa.

Instruction:

Preparation: 1 packet Ginseng Herbal Soup Mix (comprising 2 filter bags); 800 g — 1 kg chicken (duck or others), cut to preferred size; 1500 ml (6 rice bowls) water; Salt to taste; COOKING METHOD: Put in the 2 filter bags (do not open filter bags) and chicken into boiling water. Simmer for at least 1 hour. Serve 4–6 persons.

Price: 40 g — $2.65

Manufacturer:

LINACO FOOD INDUSTRIES S/B (117276-K) 12, Lintang Sungai Keramat 2B, Taman Klang Utama, 42100 Klang, Selangor, Malaysia. Tel: 603-3291 4589 Fax: 603-3291 4588 Website: www.linaco.com.my.

Imported/Distributed by:

Australia: ORIENTAL MERCHANT PTY LTD 10, Westgate Drive, Laverton North, Vic 3206, Australia. Singapore: ALPHICO MARKETING PTE LTD 48, Toh Guan Road East # 02-131/132, Enterprise Hub, Singapore 608586, Tel: 65-6272 3288; Product of Malaysia.

47. **Chan Yat Hing Tin Chi Green Bamboo Medicated Oil (Chan Yat Hing Medicine Factory)**

Description on PIL:

Chan Yat Hing Tin Chi Green Bamboo Medicated Oil is a safe and reliable remedy for the treatment of all skin diseases. It is a clear non-greasy liquid, which has the power of penetrating rapidly through the epidermis to the lower layers of the skin. The soothing ingredients quickly put on and to itching and irritation, giving the patient heat, and stopping him from scratching, thus preventing him from further irritating the skin. The antiseptic components of "Chan Yat Hing Tin Chi Green Bamboo Medicated Oil" distroy the germs which cause the disease, and promote rapid and natural healing.

Indications:
PIL: Athlete's foot, Sealies, Tinea crecris, Eczema, Tinea trichophyina, Phthiriasis capitis, Phthiriasis inguinalis, impetigo conlagiosa, insect bites, Seborrhea capitis.

Ingredients:
Formula: Menthol 20%, Camphor Oil (White) 20%, Eucalyptus Oil 2%, Clove Oil 3%, Turpentine Oil 25%, Methyl Salicylate Oil 20%, *Notoginseng* 2%, *Flos Carthami* 2%, *Notopterygium* 2%, *Angelical Pubescentis* 2%, *Notopterygium* 2%.

Instruction on PIL:
Clean and dry the affected area. Freely apply "Chan Yat Hing Tin Chi Green Bamboo Medicated Oil: thinly over the area with some cottons and rub in. Being three or four times daily the best result will be consist in continued application.

Safety considerations:
Warnings (PIL): For external use only. Avoid contact with the eyes, mouth and other mucous membranes. If condition worsens, or if symptoms persist for more than 7 days or clear up and occur within a few days, discontinue use of this product and consult a physician. Do not apply to wounds or damaged skin. Do not bandage tightly. Do not use otherwise than as directed. If you are pregnant or nursing a baby, seek the advice of a health professional before using this product. Keep out of reach of children to avoid accidental poisioning. In case of accidental ingestion, contact a doctor or poison control center immediately.

Price: 30 ml — $4.80 (PIL available)

Manufacturer:
Chan Yat Hing Medicine Factory. Made in H.K. Flat 3, 9/F., Fuk Keung Ind. Bldg., 66-68 Tong Mi Rd., Mong Kok, Kowloon. Tel: 23952966.

48. **Climacterium Support Capsules (AL)**

Actions:
Nourishing the kidney-essence, enriching blood and tranquilizing.

Indications:
It is a concentrated herbal medicine effective to relieve the symptoms of climacterium or neurovegetative imbalance, manifested as irregular menstrual cycle, dizziness, irritability, unstable emotion, enxiety, bad temper, insomnia, tiredness, dreaminess and amnesia, osteoporosis with symptoms of sour pains at lumbar and back, skin dry or itchy.

Ingredients:
Each capsule (400 mg) contains extract equivalent to raw herbs: *Margarita* 50 mg, *Ganoderma Lucidum* 50 mg, *Radix Ginseng* 100 mg, *Radix Polygoni Multiflori*

150 mg, *Radix Rehmanniae Preparatae* 180 mg, *Radix Salvia Miltiorrhizae* 150 mg, *Colla Corii Asini* 50 mg, *Fructus Schisandrae* 150 mg, *Radix Angelicae Sinensis* 200 mg, *Radix Paeoniae Alba* 200 mg, *Rhizoma Chuanxiong* 100 mg, *Radix Bupleuri* 150 mg.

Dosage:
3 capsules each time, 2–3 times a day. Each course of medication lasts 1 month. It is a natural herbal preparation, can be taken combined with western medicine, no contraindication found. Do not eat fried, spicy and oily food.

Price: 60 capsules — $18.90 (sealed)

Manufacturer and Sole Distributor in Singapore:
All Link Medical & Health Products Pte Ltd. 10 Kaki Bukit Road 1, #03-27 K B Industrial Building, Singapore 416175. Tel: 68460337, Fax: 68460336.

49. **CO. Danshen Tablets (Jin Pai Trademark)**

Description on PIL:
Coronary arteriosclerosis is abbreviated as coronarism, which is a kind of heart illnesses commonly found in the middle-aged and elderly people. The illness causes the inner side of the coronary artery to become narrow, and results in cardiac muscles at farther end suffering from oxygen deficiency and will finally lead to angina pectoris. (PIL: In the worse case, coupled with the acute myocardial infarction, the angio-vascular track can be completely clogged, and physical health can be critically damaged. Among 400 coronary cases, the clinical observation of COMPOSITE DANSHEN TABLETS was conducted in 19 clinical units covering one city and three provinces, namely, Shanghai, Jiangsu, Anhui and Zhejiang. In angina pectoris cases, the obvious efficacy was 34.7% and total effectiveness 85.6%. In electrocardiogram cases, the obvious efficacy was 20.1%, and total effectiveness 58.1%. The clinical treatments proved that Composite Danshen Tablets was able to relieve angina pectoris faster, to recover from blood and oxygen deficiency, and to improve metabolism in myocardium more effectively. For dosing, it is rather convenient.

Actions:
Activating blood, relieving clog; Expanding blood vessels; Pungently easing the circulatory system; Regulating 'Qi' and relieving pain.

Indications:
The product is suitable for coronary illnesses, chest uneasiness, and angina pectoris.

Ingredients:
Radix Salviae Miltiorrhizae 80.9%, *Radix Notoginseng* 18.1%, *Borneolum Syntheticum* 1%

Dosage:
Take 3 tables each time, and 3 times daily.

Price: 100 tablets — $6 (not sealed); 500 tablets — $20 (sealed)

Manufacturer:
Li Wah Pharmaceutical Co. Ltd. Ningbo Zhejiang, China.

Assembler & Importer:
Kinhong Pte. Ltd. 297 Kaki Bukit Avenue 1. Shun Li Industrial Park Singapore 416083. Tel: (65) 67415561 Fax: (65) 67413705.

50. **Collaterals Activating Capsules [New Formula] (Nature's Green)**

Description on PIL:
Collaterals Activating capsules are made from highly concentrated, selected Chinese herbs and produced in accordance to a traditional Chinese formula. It helps activate blood circulation, relax tendons and activate energy flow in the meridians and collaterals, dispersing stagnant blood and phlegm, dispelling wind and cold in the joints, and strengthening the kidney. This product is used for joint and back pain, stiff muscles, and difficulty in walking caused by stagnation of blood and rheumatic disease.

Actions and Indications:
Pain in the limbs and trunk, numbness of hands and feet, stiffness of muscles and joints and difficulty in walking caused by stagnation of blood and rheumatic disease.

Ingredients:
Each 460 mg capsule contains extracts equivalent to raw herbs: *Agkistrodon* 20 mg, *Zaocys* 20 mg, *Radix Clematidis* 20 mg, *Rhizoma Ahemones Daddeanae* 20 mg, *Rhizoma Dryopteris Crassirhizomae* 20 mg, *Radix Glycyrrhizae* 20 mg, *Rhizoma et Radix Notopterygii* 20 mg, *Cortex Cinnamomi* 20 mg, *Herba Pogostemonis* 20 mg, *Radix Linderae* 20 mg, *Radix Rehmannaiae Praeparata* 20 mg, *Radix et Rhizoma Rhei* 20 mg, *Radix Aucklandiae* 20 mg, *Lignum Aquilariae Resinatum* 20 mg, *Radix Asari* 10 mg, *Radix Paeoniae Rubra* 10 mg, *Myrrha* 10 mg, *Flos Caryophylli* 10 mg, *Olibanum* 10 mg, *Bombyx Batryticatus* 10 mg, *Rhizoma Arisaematis Praeparata* 10 mg, *Pericarpium Citri Reticulatae Viride* 10 mg, *Rhizoma Drynariae* 10 mg, *Fructus Amomi Rotundus* 10 mg, *Benzoinum* 10 mg, *Radix Scutellariae* 10 mg, *Rhizoma Cyperi Praeparata* 10 mg, *Radix Scrophulariae* 10 mg, *Rhizoma Atractylodis Macrocephalae* 10 mg, *Radix Saposhnikobiae* 25 mg, *Radix Puerariae* 15 mg, *Radix Angelicae Sinensis* 15 mg, *Resina Draconis* 7 mg, *Pheretima* 5 mg, *Colophonium* 5 mg, *Calculus Bovis* 2 mg, *Borneolum Syntheticum* 2 mg, *Radix Ginseng* 30 mg, *Rhizoma Gastrodiae* 20 mg, *Scorpio* 20 mg, *Radix Polygoni Multiflori* 20 mg.

Dosage:
for oral administration, take 4 capsules, 1-2 times daily.

Safety considerations:
Side effects not known (on PIL). Not to be taken by pregnant women (PIL).

Price: 50 capsules — $20 (not sealed)

Manufacturer:
Tong Jum Chew Pte Ltd 21 Kaki Bukit View Tech Park II Singapore 415957 Tel: 62781134 Fax: 62781246 Singapore Manufacturer Licence No. MLCP 0400040 Singapore CPM Product Reference No. 113324

51. **Compound E-Jiao Syrup (DEEJ)**

Actions:
Invigorate vital energy and nourish blood stream.

Indication:
Effective for the relief of dizziness, palpitation, lack of appetite, anemia and for combating deficiency of vital energy and blood.

Ingredients:
Each 20 ml contains extract equivalent to raw herbs: *Asini Gelatinum* 0.870 g, Red Ginseng 0.434 g, *Rhizome Rehmanniae Preparata* 3.044 g, *Radix Codonopsis Lanceolatae* 3.044 g, *Fructus Crataegi* 1.304 g.

Dosage:
Take 20 ml three times a day.

Safety considerations:
Side effects not known. 1. Not to be used during flu. 2. Used before food. 3. Children, pregnant women and patient with hypertension and diabetics should seek doctor advice.

Price: 20 ml × 12 vials — $15.00 (sealed)

Manufacturer:
Shandong Dong-E E-Jiao Company Limited. Shandong China. Imported by: Science Arts Co. Pte Ltd. 150 MacPherson Rd, Science Arts Building Singapore 348524.

52. **Compound HongJingTian Capsule (Mei Hua Brand)**

Actions and Indications:
Replenish the essence of vital organs, invigorate energy and blood circulation, promote the function of metabolism and delay senility.

Ingredients:
320 mg per capsule contains extracts equivalent to raw herbs: *Herba Saussureae* 440 mg, *Radix Rhodiolae* 480 mg, *Cordyceps* 528 mg, *Radix Notoginseng* 32 mg, *Fructus Lycii* 400 mg.

Dosage:
Take 1 capsule two times daily with warm water.

Safety considerations:
Side effects not known. Do not use while you are having cold/flu or during pregnancy.

Price: 60 capsules — $33.00 (Sealed)

Manufacturer:
Science Arts Co Pte Ltd. 150 MacPherson Rd, Science Arts Building Singapore 348524.

53. **Compound Salvia Granules (Nature's Green)**

Actions and Indications: Promotes blood circulation and alleviates chest pain. Relieves the symptoms of oppressed feeling and pain in the chest.

Ingredients:
Each dosage (5 g) contains extracts equivalent to raw herbs: *Radix et Rhizoma Salviae Miltiorrhiae* 1350 mg, *Radix et Rhizoma Notoginseng* 425 mg, *Broneolum Syntheticum* 24 mg.

Dosage:
For oral administration, take 5 g with warm water, 3 times daily.

Safety considerations:
Side effects not known. To be contraindicated in pregnant women.

Price: 100 g — $11.50 (sealed bottle)

Manufacturer:
Tong Jum Chew Pte Ltd. 21 Kaki Bukit View Tech Park II Singapore 415957. Tel: 62781134 Fax: 62781246. Singapore Manufacturer Licence No. MLCP 0400040 Singapore CPM Product Reference No.: 117648.

54. **Cool Man (90 tablets) (Q & N)**

Description:
Male hormone is the key substance that dictates men's youth, vitality and libido; maintains strong bones and muscles; supports optimal health and energy as well as immune

function. It brings out men's confidence and charm internally and externally. But when age increases, energy, vitality, kidney function, libido, bone and muscle are dramatically affected because of male hormone decrease. COOL MAN is scientifically formulated with several plants which help to maintain the well-being of male hormone, thus enhancing the localized and general men's health. It is the natural ideal supplement for adult men to stay young, strong, energetic and healthy. Cool Man has been scientifically proven to ensure optimal: Vitality and Energy — Enhances vitality and energy. Sexual Health. Bone & Muscle Health — Increases bone mass density, strengthens bones, strengthens muscles. General well-being — Delays the aging process, maintains optimal immune function, maintains good blood circulation.

Ingredients:
Epimedium 250 mg, *Morindae Officinalis Radix* 100 mg, American Ginseng 50 mg, Lycium Barbarum 50 mg, Calcium L-aspartate 50 mg

Dosage:
Suggested use: Oral. Take 1 tablet 2–3 times daily.

Safety considerations:
Side effects not known.

Price: 90 tabs — $69.55

Formulated and marketed by:
Q&N Pte Ltd. 178 Paya Lebar Road #06-08 Singapore 409030. Website: www.qn-nutrition.com. Email: enquiry@qn-nutrition.com.

Manufacturer:
He Zhi Pharmaceutical Co. Ltd, Tianjin (China) under license and supervision by Q&N Pte Ltd (Singapore).

55.   Cordyceps & American Ginseng Capsules (AL)

Actions:
Tonifying the heart and transquilizing. Supplement the vital energy, invigorating the spleen and stomach.

Indications:
It is effective for conditions related to insomnia, palpitation, amnesia, tiredness, shortness of breath, dizziness, feeling of suppression in the chest, arrhythmia, loss of appetite, pale complexion, relieving cough and removing phlegm. The product also helps to reduce oxygen consumption in myocardium. Regular taking can strengthen physical conditions.

Ingredients:
Each capsule (0.35 g) contains: Cordyceps 210 mg, *Radix Panacis Quinquefolii* 140 mg.

Dosage:
2 to 3 capsules each time, twice a day. For health maintenance: Take 2 capsules each time, once a day.

Safety considerations:
Side effects not known.

Price: 80 capsules — $39.90 (sealed)

Manufacturer and Sole Distributor in Singapore:
All Link Medical & Health Products Pte Ltd. 10 Kaki Bukit Road 1, #03-27 K B Industrial Building, Singapore 416175. Tel: 68460337 Fax: 68460336.

56. **Cordyceps Essence with American Ginseng (Mei Hua)**

Description:
This product is most suitable for cases of weakness with mental sluggishness, low appetite, mental exhaustion, disorder in diggestive function and convalescent feebleness.

Ingredients:
Every 85 ml of liquid contain extracts of the following: Cordyceps (300 mg), Radix Astragali (700 mg); Radix Panacis Quinquefolii (1200 mg).

Instruction:
When administering, add a little bit of salt, as desired to enhance taste; and take it orally either hot or cold. After opening the bottle, finish the content within the same day.

Dosage:
For adults: 1 bottle each time; For children: Half bottle each time, once or twice daily.

Price: 85 ml × 6 — $20.00

Manufacturer:
S.H. UNIFLEX CHINESE MEDICAL FACTORY SDN. BHD., No 21A, Jalan Lambak, Taman Johor Light Ind Est. 82100, Johor Bahru, Malaysia.

Imported by:
Science Arts Co. Pte Ltd., 150 MacPherson Rd, Science Arts Building Singapore 348524.

57. **Cordyceps Tonic & Strengthener Capsules (Gold Floral)**

Indications:
Invigorate vital energy and promote blood circulation. It is effective for congenitally poor constitution and poor memory of teenagers, and for adult weakness of lumber region and knee joints, aging before one's time, insomnia, osteoporosis, poor appetite, frequent nocturnal urination, dripping of urine, palpitation and shortness of breath.

Ingredients:
Each 0.35 g capsule contains extract equivalent to raw herbs: *Cordyceps* 20 mg, *Hippocampus* 50 mg, *Radix Ginseng* 60 mg, *Fructus Lycii* 60 mg, *Os Draconis* 50 mg, *Geoko* 50 mg, *Cornu Cervi Pantotrichum* 50 mg, *Fructus Psoraleae* 50 mg, *Fructus Corni* 20 mg, *Herba Cistanches* 15 mg, *Cortex Eucommiae* 30 mg, *Radix Morindae Officinalis* 30 mg.

Dosage:
2 capsules each time, twice a day.

Safety considerations:
Side effects and contraindications not known.

Price: 48 capsules — $27.30 (sealed)

Manufacturer and Sole Distributor in Singapore:
All Link Medical & Health Products Pte Ltd. 10 Kaki Bukit Road 1, #03-27 K B Industrial Building, Singapore 416175. Tel: 68460337, Fax: 68460336.

58. **Cordyceps Vigour Capsules (Nature's Green)**

Description:
PIL: Nature's Green Cordyceps Vigour Capsule is made from 32 precious herbs and prepared by modern pharmaceutical technology in accordance with a traditional Chinese medicine formula. It can strengthen the body, regulate the body's internal functions and promote metabolism. It is useful for relieving symptoms of weakness and soreness in the waist and knees, vertigo, tinniyus, night sweat and emission.

Actions:
Strengthens organic functions, vitalizes spirit and stamina.

Indications:
Relieves symptoms such as weakness and soreness of the waist and knees, vertigo, tinnitus, fatigue, palpitation, amnesia and hypofunction.

Ingredients:
Each 300 mg capsule contains extracts equivalent to raw herbs: *Cordyceps* 40 mg, *Cortex Eucommiae* 40 mg, *Radix Morindae Officinalis* 40 mg, *Testis et Penis Equus*

18 mg, *Testis et Penis Canis* 30 mg, *Testis et Penis Bovis* 30 mg, *Os Draconis* 48 mg, *Radix Ginseng* 60 mg, *Radix Codonopsis* 31 mg, *Gecko* 16 mg, Dried Shrimps 16 mg, *Radix Angelicae Sinensis* 10 mg, *Cortex Cinnamomi* 10 mg, *Radix Astragali* 10 mg, *Fructus Corni* 10 mg, *Fructus Psoraleae* 20 mg, *Rhizoma Cibotii* 60 mg, *Fructus Lycii* 20 mg, *Semen Juplandis* 10 mg, *Semen Cuscutae* 31 mg, *Herba Cistanches* 31 mg, *Semen Astragali complanati* 31 mg, *Herba Epimedii* 31 mg, *Rhizoma Dioscoreae* 31 mg, *Poria* 10 mg, *Radix Rehmanniae Preparata* 31 mg, *Fructus Rubi* 20 mg, *Fructus Caryophylli* 20 mg, *Fructus Foeniculi* 20 mg, *Radix Achyranthis Bidentatae* 20 mg, *Fructus Schisandrae* 10 mg, *Radix Glycyrrhizae* 10 mg.

Dosage:
For oral adminis-tration, take 4 capsules, 3 times daily.

Safety considerations:
PIL: Side effects not known. Contraindications/Cautions: Contraindicated for patients with cold and pyrexia.

Price: 60 capsules — $20.00 (not sealed. PIL available)

Manufacturer:
Tong Jum Chew Pte Ltd. 21 Kaki Bukit View Tech Park II Singapore 415957. Tel: 62781134 Fax: 62781246. Singapore Manufacturer Licence No. MLCP: 0400040 Singapore CPM Product Reference No. 113325.

59. **Dieda Zhuang Gu Shui (QianJin)**

Description:
Activates blood and dispels stasis. Relieves swells. For injuries from falls and knocks.

Actions:
Dieda Zhuang Gu Shui is effective in promoting blood circulation, removing blood stasis, relieving pain and swell, easing rheumatism, curing numbness, and strengthening tendon and bone.

Indications:
It is indicated for all injuries from falls and contusions, blood stasis, swells, pains, aching body and limbs resulting from rheumatism, numbness and pain because of stiff joints etc.

Ingredients:
Menthol Crystals (5 mg), Camphor Powder (5 mg), Menthol Salicylate (10 mg), Turpentine Oil (10 mg), Citronella Oil (10 mg), Menthae Oleum (8 mg), Radix et Rhizoma Rhei (4 mg), Flos Carthami (4 mg), Radix Notoginseng (4 mg).

Instruction:
Apply to the affected area 2 or 3 times daily, using much as desired.

Price: 60 ml — $3.50

Sole Agent:
Kiat Ling Health Products and Trading, Blk 3017 #04-16 Bedok North Street 5, Singapore 486121; Tel: 6744 1868; Fax: 6743 5267.

60. **Dietary Supplement with Ginseng (Neovita)**

Description:
For health and vitality. PIL: Neovita Fortified Capsules are a food supplement incorporating controlled doses of important vitamins and minerals with Ginseng suiting the daily requirements of the human body. Neovita Fortified Capsules are suitable for both men and women and help overcome stress and weariness. Certain groups of people have a special need for Neovita: Business men and office workers, the elderly, people who have lost their appetite, people who tire easily, people on a diet, anyone making an increased mental and physical effort such as athletes and sportsmen.

Ingredients:
Vitamin A 2400 IU, Vitamin B1 2.5 mg, Vitamin B2 2.5 mg, Vitamin B6 1 mg, Vitamin B12 4.9 mcg, Vitamin C 40 mg, Vitamin D 240 IU, Vitamin E 2 mg, Nicotinamide 20 mg, Calcium Pantothenate 10 mg. Calcium Phosphate (dibasic) 100 mg, Ginseng Extract equivalent to Root 100 mg, Magnesium Oxide 10 mg, Copper Sulphate 2 mg, Zinc Oxide 5 mg, Manganese Sulphate 2 mg, Ferrous Sulphate (dried) (iron content 10 mg) 33 mg, lecithin 9.5 mg.

PIL:
Vitamin A — essential for health and especially the skin. Vitamin B1 — essential for carbohydrate metabolism, Vitamin B2 — important for cell-respiration and body energy, Nicotinamide works with the other members of the B-complex family of vitamins to convert carbohydrates into energy, Vitamin B12 — essential for the nerve metabolism, blood formation and the sound development of body cells, vitamin D — important for strong bones and teeth; helps the body to utilise calcium and phosphorus, Vitamin E-necessary for normal muscular function, Vitamin C — increases efficiency and energy; essential for the health of gums and tissues, Vitamin B6 — necessary for the health of the nervous system and the skin; good for the teeth and gums, Calcium Pantothenate- supplies further B-complex vitamin which is also essential for the health of the nervous system. In addition each capsule contains: Iron — the body's most important mineral requirement, essential to the formation of red blood cells. Together with five other minerals to help maintain health and vitality and Ginseng

(*Eleutherococcus senticosus*)-Referred to in medical texts dating from the Han Dynasty in China (206BC to AD24). It contains a unique blend of nutrients which help combat fatigue and relieves symptoms of stress. Eleutherococcus has also been demonstrated to have improved anti-oxidant activity compared to other forms of ginseng.

Dosage:
One Neovita Capsule a day makes good any deficiency in a normal diet. Remember your body cannot store all these vitamins so you need one per day. PIL: Adults should take one capsule daily, preferably taken during meals.

Price: 20 capsules — $22.80 (not sealed)

Manufacturer:
Savoy Laboratories (International) Limited. 52 Queen Anne Street, London WIM 9LA. An Alinter Company.

61. **Dragon Herbal Tonic 170 ml (nil)**

Description:
Made from natural Ingredients; Dragon Herbal Tonis is specifically formulated to restore vitality.

Ingredients:
Cortex Eucommiae (20%), Cordyceps (20%), Hippocampus (15%), Radix Ginseng (10%), Radix Morindae Officinalis (10%), Rhizoma Cibotium Borometz (5%); Radix Achranthes Bidentata (5%); Radix Dipsacus Asperoides (5%), Radix Polygonum Multiflorum (5%), Freuctus Lycii (5%)

Dosage:
Consumed 20 ml every night before bedtime for best result.

Price: 170 ml — $11.21

Imported by:
Ang Leong Huat Pte Ltd, 16 Tagore Lane Singapore 787476

62. **Dragon's blood capsules (Nature's Green)**

Actions and Indications:
Promotes blood circulation to remove stasis. Used for traumatic injuries, distension and pain in the costal region and back, flaccidity and weakness of the limbs.

Ingredients:
Each 460 mg capsule contains extracts equivalent to raw herbs: *Resina Draconis* 42 mg, *Radix et Rhizoma Notoginseng* 42 mg, *Radix Aucklandiae* 42 mg, *Radix Angelicae*

Sinensis 42 mg, *Rhizoma Cyperi Praeparata* 42 mg, *Radix et Rhizoma Salviae Miltiorrhizae* 21 mg, *Eupolyphaga Seu Steleophaga* 21 mg, *Radix Paeoniae Rubra* 21 mg, *Olibanum Praeparata* 42 mg, *Myrrha Praeparata* 42 mg, *Flos Carthami* 11 mg, *Catechu* 6.5 mg, *Radix Angelicae Dahuricae* 21 mg, *Rhizoma Kaempferiae* 21 mg, *Radix et Rhizoma Nardostachyos* 21 mg, *Radix et Rhizoma Asari* 10 mg, *Rhizoma Cibotii* 10 mg, *Rhizoma Drynariae* 10 mg, *Herba Lycopodii* 21 mg, *Caulis Spatholobi* 10 mg, *Pericarpium Citri Reticulatae* 21 mg, *Herba Centellae* 42 mg, *Pyritum Praeparata* 6.5 mg, *Borneolum Syntheticum* 1 mg.

Dosage:
For oral administration, take 3–6 capsules, 1–2 times daily. Reduce the dosage for children.

Safety considerations:
Side effects not known. To be contraindicated for pregnant women.

Price: 60 capsules — $12.50 (No PIL)

Manufacturer:
Tong Jum Chew Pte Ltd 21 Kaki Bukit View Tech Park II Singapore 415957 Tel: 62781134 Fax: 62781246. Singapore Manufacturer Licence No: MLCP 0400040 Singapore CPM product reference number: 119539.

63. **Elderly Health Capsules (Nature's Green)**

Description:
PIL: Elderly Health Capsules are made from 10 beneficial herbs and prepared by modern pharmaceutical technology. This product is the typical formulation that helps strengthen the immune system and restore and maintain vitality in middle-aged and elderly persons. It is effective in relieving the symptoms of insomnia, tinnitus, aching pains of the loins, fatigue, chest oppression, and frequent night urination.

Actions:
Nourishes the kidney, adjusts the immune system in middle-aged and elderly persons, and restores the vital energy and builds up health.

Indications:
Relieves the symptoms of insomnia, tinnitus, aching pains of the loins, fatigue, chest oppression, and frequent night urination.

Ingredients:
Each 300 mg capsule contains extracts equivalent to raw herbs: *Radix Panacis Quinquefolii* 150 mg, *Ganoderma Lucidum* 330 mg, *Cordyceps Hypha* 300 mg, *Margarita* 40 mg, *Herba Epimedii* 200 mg, *Radix Polygoni Multiflori Preparata*

150 mg, *Rhizoma Polygonati Preparata* 150 mg, *Fructus Lycii* 150 mg, *Radix Salviae Miltiorrhiae* 150 mg, *Radix Glycyrrhizae* 60 mg.

Dosage:
For oral administration, take 1–2 capsules, 3 times daily.

Safety considerations:
Side effects not known (PIL for 60 capsules and on the packaging of 300 capsules). Use with caution for pregnant women. Not suitable for the patients suffering from flu. Avoid greasy or spicy foods. (PIL for 60 capsules and on packaging of 300 capsules).

Price: 60 capsules — $10.00 (not sealed). 300 capsules — $44.00 (sealed bottle)

Manufacturer:
Tong Jum Chew Pte Ltd. New Address: 21 Kaki Bukit View Tech Park II Singapore 415957 Tel: 62781134. Fax: 62781246

64. ELEGin (Cotton Plant)

Description:
ELEGIN has remarkable effects in promoting health. It can be taken as a long term health tonic, which builds up body immunity and resistance to illnesses. It can help the body to excrete unwanted substances, enhance body organs function, stimulate absoprtion of nourishment, promotes blood circulation, and control body cells from being abnormal. Thus enhancing a healthy body.

Ingredients:
500 ml of this preparation contains the extract as below: *Radix Polygoni Multiflori* 15.20 g, *Fructus Ziziphi Jujubae* 15.20 g, *Radix Salviae Miltiorrhizae* 13.70 g, *Radix Aucklandiae* 6.22 g, *Radix Notoginseng* 13.70 g, *Fructus Lycii* 15.20 g, *Radix Glehniae* 13.70 g, *Cortex Eucommiae* 13.70 g, *Radix Rehmanniae* 6.22 g, *Radix Puerariae* 6.22 g, *Radix Stemonae* 0.92 g, *Rhizoma Polygonati Odorati* 1.51 g, *Rhizoma Ligustici Chuanxiong* 1.51 g, *Radix Glycyrrhizae* 3.02 g, *Ramulus Mori* 1.51 g, *Radix Ginseng* 24.40 g.

Dosage:
Each time 20 ml, 1–2 times daily with warm water.

Safety considerations:
No known side effect. No known contraindication.

Price: 500 ml — $49.90 (sealed)

Manufacturer:
Yi Shi Yuan Pte Ltd (GMP Manufacturer) No. 20, Bukit batok Crescent #13-11/12/13 Enterprise Centre Singapore 658080 Tel: 65670900 Fax: 65672256 Email: enquiry@ ysy.com.sg. Singapore Manufacturer's Licence No.: CPMM0001.

65. **Emperor Genuine Herbs Chicken Spices (Star-flower)**

Details:

No information available

Ingredients:

Ginseng, Wolfberry Fruit, Tangkuei, Dandshan, Ligusticum, Yuzhu, Beiqi, Pepper, Red Date and Flavouring

Instruction:

Preparation: One Chicken (approx. 1 kg); One packet of Emperor Genuine Herbs Chicken Spices. Aluminium foil and HDPE wrapper. Method of Cooking: (1) First boil 500 ml of water (about 2 rice bowl) than add the sachet of herbs into the boiling water and boil for another 15 minutes; (2) Clean the chicken and remove its head and feet then place it on the HDPE wrapper. Apply Emperor Genuine Herbs Chicken Spices onto the skin and inside the body. Next, apply the herbs and Herb water for Step 1 onto and inside the chicken (if some Shao Hsing Chiew is added, it is more tasty). Wrap chicken with HDPE wrapper followed by Aluminium foil. Steam for about 2 hours under slow fire and ready to serve. Can also be cooking with pork or mutton. *This ingredients also can be use for cooking chicken soup.

Price: 70 gm — $4.20

Packed By:

Packed in Singapore; Hong Seah Food Industries Pte. Ltd. 10, TUAS BAY WALK, #03-18, Singapore 637780 Tel 626 59728: Fax: 62681143: Website: http://www.hongseah.com.sg; E-mail: hongseah@cyberway.com.sg.

Distributor:

HUP HUAT NODDLES Pte. Ltd., No. 8, Wan Lee Rd, Singapore 627940; Tel: 62688335; 62688011, 62614044; Fax: 62661215.

66. **Energins American Ginseng Essence (Avalon)**

Description:

American ginseng (*Panax quinquefolius*) belongs to the same species of Panax ginseng. The Ginsenosides of American ginseng is similar to that of Panax ginseng. American ginseng is probably the best known supplement for keeping energy up. As a nutritional support for energy, it is well known to enhance endurance adn support healthy immune system. Energins American Ginseng Essence contains HB802 standard American Ginseng Extract. With the advanced technology, the true essence of American ginseng is extracted and standardised to 4% Ginsenosides and 5% Ginseng Polysaccharides. The standard extract ensures the consistency of dosage and free of heavy metal and pesticide residues. Vitamin D3 helps to properly utilize calcium necessary for strong bones and teeth as well as enhance immunity. Specially formulated together, American ginseng can synergized with vitamin D3 in keeping energy.

Indications:
Amercian ginseng is traditionally used as a prophylactic and restorative agent for enhancement of mental and physcial capacities and general health.

Ingredients:
Standard American Ginseng Extract HB802 (4% Ginsenosides and 5% Ginseng Polysaccharides) 200 mg, Micocrystalline cellulose, MCC 150 mg, Vitamin D3 150 IU.

Dosage:
For general healthcare, take one capsule daily after breakfast or lunch. Adult: the recommended daily dosage is 1 capsule after breakfast or lunch. The capsule is best taken with some liquid. Children: Not recommended for use in children under 12 years.

Safety considerations:
So far no side effect has been found. Precaution on PIL: At the recommended doses, no special precautions are necessary. This product is not intended to diagnose, treat, cure or prevent any disease. If the symptoms persists, please consult a doctor. Energins American Ginseng Essence should not be taken in known hypersensitivity to any of the ingredients of the compound.

Price: 60 vegecaps — $63.20 (PIL available)

Developed and distributed by:
Hi-beau international Pte Ltd, 18 Boon Lay Way, #07-102, Tradehub 21, Singapore 609966.

67. **Energins Ginseng Essence (Avalon)**

Description:
Panax ginseng is probably the best known supplement for keeping energy up. It has been used for thousands of years in Asian countries. As a nutritional support for energy, Panax ginseng is well known to enhance endurance and support healthy immune system. Energins Ginseng Essence contains HB801 standard Panax Ginseng Extract. With the advanced technology, the true essence of Panax ginseng is extracted and standardised to 4% Ginsenosides and 5% Ginseng Polysaccharides. The standard extract ensures the consistency of dosage and free of heavy metal and pesticide residues. Vitamin D3 helps to properly utilize calcium necessary for strong bones and

teeth as well as enhance immunity. Specially formulated together, Panax ginseng can synergize with vitamin D3 in keeping energy up. PIL: Energins Ginseng Essence is indicated for both men and women at every stage of life. It is particularly useful for those who need to boost the energy.

Indications:
PIL: Panax ginseng is traditionally used as a prophylactic and restorative agent for enhancement of mental and physical capacities and general health.

Ingredients:
Standard Panax Ginseng Extract HB802 (4% Ginsenosides and 5% Ginseng Polysaccharides) 200 mg, Microcrystalline cellulose, MCC 150 mg, Vitamin D3 150 IU

Dosage:
For general healthcare, take one capsule daily after breakfast or lunch. PIL: Adults: The recommended daily dosage is 1 capsule after breakfast or lunch. The capsule is best taken with some liquid. Children: not recommended for use in children under 12 years.

Safety considerations:
PIL: So far no side effect has been found. At the recommended doses, no special precautions are necessary. This product is not intended to diagnose, treat, cure or prevent any disease. If the symptoms persist, please consult a doctor. Pregnancy and lactation: controlled studies with pregnant women are so far not available. As with any dietary suppplement, you should consult your healthcare practitioner prior to using this product if you are nursing, pregnant or considering pregnancy. Effects on the ability to drive and use machines: No effects on the ability to drive and use machines are known with the intake of the product. Energins Panax Ginseng Essence should not be taken in known hypersensitivity to any of the ingredients of the compound.

Price: 60 vege-caps — $49.00

Manufacturer:
Hi-Beau International Pte Ltd. Enquiries: 65159818. http://www.hibeau.com.

68. **Enervon with Ginseng and Vitamin E (Enervon)**

Description:
Enervon with Ginseng and vitamin E series 1: Guaranteed Endurance Staying up late again for whatever reason. Travelling long haul. Non-stop hectic activities. Even marathon babysitting or shopping. It's one of those times when you need more than just a burst of energy. You need energy that endures. Sustained stamina that will see

you through a longer period of time. You can't afford to take chances. Your energy has to stay up as long as you want it to. So what are you going to do about it? What is energy that endures? This is a much desired condition whereby your body is able to maintain energy longer than usual. The sustained length of time varies from one individual to another, depending on certain factors like state of health or well being, age, mental/psychological disposition, etc. External factors like weather conditions also affect one's energy. Vitamins as a solution Because life is one continuous struggle with daily tasks and stress, vitamins like the B complex group and E are rapidly depleted. Hence you need a daily vitamin supplement that will help augment this loss. For more information, ask your doctor about Enervon with Ginseng and Vitamin E.

Ingredients:
Composition per caplet: Ginseng Extract 100 mg, Vitamin E (d-Alpha Tocopheryl Acetate 100 IU, Vitamin B1 (Thiamine Mononitrate) 50 mg, Vitamin B2 (Riboflavin) 25 mg, Vitamin B6 (Pyridoxine HCl) 10 mg, Vitamin B12 5 mcg, Niacinamide 50 mg, Calcium Panthothenate 20 mg.

Dosage:
Take 1 caplet once a day. May be taken with or without food.

Price: 30 caplets — $15.30. 100 caplets — $45.00

Manufacturer:
Medifarma Laboratories under the authority of United American Pharmaceutical. Distributed by: Zuellig Pharma Pte Ltd. 15 Changi North Way #01-01 Singapore 498770 Tel No: 65468188

69. Essence of Bird's Nest Ginseng & Cordyceps (Ferragold)

Description:
This essence Birdnest ginseng with cordyceps uses traditional recipe togehter with advance technology, to extract a high and pure concentration of herbal content. It is effective against bodily weakness caused by late night study or heavy workload, weakness due to sickness, poor appetite & fatigue. Taken regularly it will energize the body and prolong life, really invaluable remedy as well as nourishment.

Ingredients:
Cordyceps (400 mg); Brid Nest (400 mg); Radix Panax Quinnefolium (800 mg); Rhizoma Polygonati (600 mg); Radix Panax Rehmanniae (600 mg).

Dosage:
Adult — 1 bottle each time, 2 times a day. Children — 1/2 bottle each time, 2 times a day.

Safety considerations:
Side effects and contraindication not known.

Price: 6 bottles × 75 g — $22.80.

Sole Agent:
Ferragold (S) Pte Ltd. Blk 32 Defu Lane #04-08 Singapoore 537923; Tel: (65) 6744 6656; Fax: (65) 6742 4968; Email: ferragold@hotmail.com.

70. **Essence of Chicken with American Ginseng (Brand's®)**

Description:
BRAND's® Essence of chicken with American Ginseng is an extract of fine quality chicken in an easily digestible form combined with the goodness of choice quality American Ginseng. It is hygienically processed under high temperature to give it its unique flavour and vacuum sealed to preserve its freshness. Take it regularly anytime, anywhere as part of a balanced diet. Brand's® Essence of Chicken with American Ginseng does not contain any preservatives. Only fine quality chicken and choice American Ginseng are used in every bottle of BRAND's® Essence of Chicken with American Ginseng. This product may be consumed straight from the bottle at room temperature, chilled or warmed according to one's preference. Once bottle is opened, contents should be refrigerated and consumed within 24 hours.

Ingredients:
Essence of Chicken, Panax quinquefolium (American Ginseng Root), Caramel (Natural Source), Glycyrrhiza uralensis.

Dosage:
No information available
Price: 6 bottles × 70 g — $17.50

Manufacturer:
Manufactured in Malaysia under license from Cerebos Pacific Ltd., Singapore.

Distributor:
Distributed in Singapore by: DKSH Singapore Pte Ltd, 34 Boon Leat Terrace Singapore 119866; Comments? Suggestions? We'd love to hear from you. Call BRAND's® Customer Care Line at 1800-732-4748 or write to us at Cerebos Pacific Ltd., 18 Cross Street #12-01/08, China Square Central; Singapore 048423.

71. **Essence of Chicken with American Ginseng & Cordyceps (Fu Gui)**

Description:
FU GUI Essence of chicken with American ginseng and cordyceps is prepared by using fresh chicken with selected American Ginseng and Cordyceps. It is

manufactured by vacuum seal filling machine which is under completely hygienic environment. It does not contain fats cholesterol, preservatives and artificial colouring. It can be consumed direct from the bottle, chilled or warmed, depending on individual's taste. Consume within 24 hours afer opening.

Ingredients:
Essence of Chicken (80%); American Ginseng (10%), Cordyceps (5%); Caramel (5%)

Dosage:
No information available

Price: 6 × 70 ml — $14.70

Packed by:
Chwee Song supplies Pte Ltd., Blk 5, Ang Mo Kio Ind'l Park 2A Tech II; #07-14 to 16 Singapore 567760; Tel: 65-6482 3935; Fax: 65-6778 5028; http://www.chweesong.com.sg; E-Mail: sales@chweesong.com.sg.

72. **Essence of Chicken with Ginseng and Cordyceps (E-Health)**

Indications:
This essence is effective against bodily weakness caused by late night study or heavy workload, before and after pregnancy or weakness due to sickness, poor appetite & fatigue. Taken regularly it will energize the body and prolong life, really invaluable remedy as well as nourishment.

Ingredients:
Wild Ginseng (15%), Cordyceps (20%); Essence of Chicken (65%)

Dosage:
Adult — 1 bottle each time, 2 times a day; Childen — 1/2 bottle each time, 2 times a day.

Price: 6 bottles × 75 g — $20.00

Sole Agent:
Ferragold (S) Pte Ltd. Blk 87 Circuit Road #01-975 Singapore 370087; Tel: (65) 6744 6656; Fax: (65) 6742 4968.

73. **Essence of Cordyceps Cortex Eucommiae Ginseng Waist Tonic (QianJin)**

Description:
QianJin Tonic Essence is made through refining and extracting a fine selection of cordyceps and other traditional herbs. This health product is suitable for men and women. It promotes health and vitality; strengthens and nourishes the body while improving one metabolism.

Actions and Indications:
Relieves backaches and sores in the knees; Strengthens the body and waist; Relieves rigidity of the muscles and tendons and activates the flow of qi and blood in the channels and collaterals; Restores energy and relieves tiredness; Strengthens the spleen and gastric; Nourishes the hair; Nourishes the body after delivery.

Ingredients:
Each 100 ml of this product contains extracts equivalent to: Cordyceps (700 mg), Cortex Eucommiae (6000 mg), Radix Ginseng (2000 mg); Radix Morindae Officinalis (9000 mg); Radix Polygoni Multiflori Preparata (5000 mg), Radix Astragali (4000 mg), Radix Codonopsis (5000 mg); Fructus Lycii (12000 mg).

Dosage:
2 or 3 times daily 25 ml (small cup enclosed) each time.

Safety considerations:
No known side-effects. No known contraindication.

Price: 750 ml — $40.00

Quality Assured by:
Kiat Ling Health Products & Trading; Blk 3017 Bedok North St 5; #044-15 Singapore 486121; Tel: 6744 1868; Fax: 6743 5267.

74. **Essence of Fish with American Ginseng & Cordyceps (Fu Gui)**

Description:
Fu Gui Essence of Fish with American ginseng and cordyceps is prepared by using high quality freshwater fish with selected american ginseng and cordyceps. It is manufactured by latest technology innovations. The process of manufacturing is completely hygienic, with no addition of artificial colouring, flavouring and preservatives. This nutritious essence of fish is suitable to be taken by people of all ages. With its rich content of essence of fish and natural nutritions, it can be easily absorbed into the body system. It can be consumed direct from the bottle, chilled or warmed, depending on individual's taste. Consume within 24 hours after opening.

Ingredients:
Essence of Fish (90%), American Ginseng (5.0%), Cordyceps (5%)

Dosage:
No information available

Price: 6 × 70 ml — $14.70

Packed by:
Chwee Song supplies Pte Ltd., Blk 5, Ang Mo Kio Ind'l Park 2A Tech II; #07-14 to 16 Singapore 567760; Tel: 65-6482 3935; Fax: 65-6778 5028; http://www.chweesong. com.sg; E-Mail: sales@chweesong.com.sg.

75. **Essence of Ginseng & Cordyceps (nil)**

Description:
This product may be consumed straight from the bootle at room temperature, chilled or warmed according to one's preference. Once bottle is openend, contents should be refrigerated and consumed withing 24 hours. Ginseng and Cordyceps is an easily digestible form combined with the goodness of quality Cordyceps. It is hygienically processed under high temperature to give it its unique flavour and vacuum sealed to preserve its freshness. Take it regularly, anytime, anywhere as part of balanced diet.

Ingredients:
Each 70 ml contains following ingredients: Cordyceps 3.5 gm, American Ginseng Root 3.5 gm, Polygonatum Cyrtonema 3 gm, Rehmannia Glutinosa 3 gm; Essence up to 70 ml

Dosage:
No information available

Price: 6 bottles × 70 ml — $22.80

Sole Agent:
Ferragold (S) Pte. Ltd., Blk 3015A#05-07, Ubi Road 1 Singapore 408705; Tel: (65) 6744 6656.

76. **Essence of Tienchi Flowers (Camellia)**

Description:
This product is manufactured by a scientific process of extraction from the flowers of Tienchi, a precious and well-known herbal medicine indigenous to Yunnan. Retaining the rich fragrance of the original flowers and possessing various therapeutic effects, it constitutes an excellent refreshing beverage.

Actions and Indications:
Relieves heat and cools blood. Indicated for sores and carbuncles due to pathogenic heat, as well as frustration, palpitation, headache and lack of sleep due to liver heat.

Ingredients:
Each sachet of 15 gm contains: *Flos Notoginseng* 0.112 g, Folium Notoginseng 2.24 g.

Dosage:
No information available

Price: 10 sachet × 15 g — $2.80 (sealed)

Manufacturer:
Yunnan Weihe Pharmacueticals Co. Ltd, Add: Yuxi, Yunnan, China;

Imported by:
Tong Jum Chew Pte. Ltd. 21 Kaki Bukit View Tech Park II Singapore 415957, Tel: 62781134; Fax: 62781246.

77. **Essence of Tienchi Flowers (Shen Bao Trade Mark)**

Description:
This product is manufactured by a scientific process of extraction from the flowers of Tienchi, a precious and well-known herbal medicine indigenous to Guang Xi. Retaining the rich fragrance of the original flowers and possessing various therapeutic effects, it constitutes an excellent refreshing beverage which, if drunk frequently, can prevent, alleviate or cure the following diseases: 1. Facial pimples of puberty, boils, blisters around the mouth, etc; 2. Dizziness, nausea, vomiting, head-ache, insomnia, emotional inquietude, etc; 3. Heat on the palms, temperamental, grinding of the teeth during sleep etc., which are caused by biliousness of the liver.

Ingredients:
Each sachet of 15 g contains extract equivalent to raw herbs: *Flos Notoginseng* 0.75 g, Cane Sugar 14.25 g.

Dosage:
1 sachet twice daily.

Price: 10 sachet × 15 g — $1.70 (sealed)

Manufacturer:
Guangxi Guixi Pharmaceutical Corporation Ltd. (China). Importer: Winter Honey Trading Company. 32 Kallang Pudding Road #05-01, Elite Industrial Building 1, Singapore 349313. Tel: 68416976. Fax: 68416096

78. **External Injury Relief Tablets (AL)**

Actions and Indications:
Promoting blood circulation to remove blood stasis and relieve swelling and pain as traumatic injury, sprain, lumbar sprain.

Ingredients:
Each tablet (400 mg) contains extract equivalent to raw herbs: *Radix Notoginseng* 120 mg, *Rhizoma Drynariae* 100 mg, *Herba Lycopodii* 80 mg, *Radix Et Rhizoma Rhei* 100 mg, *Rhizoma Cyperi* 150 mg, *Radix Bupleuri* 100 mg, *Radix Angelicae Sinensis* 100 mg, *Semen Persicae* 120 mg, *Flos Carthami* 150 mg, *Olibanum* 60 mg, *Myrrha* 60 mg, *Radix Glycyrrhizae* 60 mg.

Dosage:
For oral administration, take 4 tablets, 2 times daily.

Safety considerations:
Long-term intake could result in impair yin and blood as the recipe has many ingredients that can promote the flow of blood circulation. It is contraindicated in pregnancy.

Price: 60 tablets — $6 (sealed)

Manufacturer and sole distributor in singapore:
All Link medical and health products pte ltd. 10 kaki bukit road 1, #03-27. KB Industrial building, Singapore 416175 tel: 68460337 fax: 68460336.

79. Extract of Sheep Placenta (Jin Pai Trademark)

Description:
Placenta- Life's Cradle→ In human, the placenta forms during conception. The human embryo and fetus absorbs oxygen, nutrients and other substances from the mother and excretes carbon dioxide and other wastes through the placenta. Without the placenta, the fetus cannot develop hence it is aptly named as Life's Cradle. Extract of Sheep Placenta → Placenta essence is made from extracts of sheep placenta containing abundance nutrients that are beneficial and delay the aging of the human skin. A Swiss Professor, discovered the extraction process. This was formulated as a treatment and skin beautification product. The launching of this product created history in the cosmetic industry; Internationally known and very popular among film stars, singers, models. In USA, Japan and Switzerland intensive research has confirmed the miraculous properties of this extract. It contains abundance nutrients and active ingredients. Besides it's noted rejuvenating effect on the human skin, it's immunogenic and nourishment effects are well recognized. For Rejuvenating, well being and antiaging.

Actions and Indications:
Prevent skin from aging, loosening, eliminate wrinkles, freckles and pigmentation; brighten dull skin; rejuvenate aging skin. Promote blood-making functions and

regulate the endocrine system. Delay the aging process. Promote the balancing of the body's ying and yang.

Ingredients:

Each 200 mg contains: Extract of Sheep Placenta 145 mg, *Ftuctus Lycii* 25 mg, *Herba Cistanches* 20 mg, *Radix Panacis Quinquefolii* 10 mg, Vitamin E 200 iu

Dosage:

To be taken twice a day on an empty stomach. 2 capsules each time. The recommended treatment period is 30 days. Prolong use is safe.

Price: 200 mg × 60 capsules — $60.00 (sealed)

Manufacturer:

Qinghai Jinghui Bio-Tech Co., Ltd. Xining, Qinghai, China. Assembler and importer: Kinhong Pte Ltd 297 Kaki Bukit Avenue 1 Shun Li Industrial Park Singapore 416083 Tel: (65) 67415561 Fax: (65) 67413705.

80. **Eyes Nourishing Tablets (Nature's Green)**

Description:

PIL (60 tablets) — Eyes Nourishing Tablet is a well-known and effective product for maintaining the health of eyes. It is suitable for symptoms of congestive and fatigued eyes as well as dizziness.

Actions and Indications:

Brightens eyes, maintains vision, nourishes the liver, strengthens the kidneys, relieves dizziness and fatigue.

Ingredients

Each 410 mg tablet contains extracts equivalent to raw herbs: *Herba Dendrobii* 25 mg, *Semen Celosiae* 25 mg, *Semen Cassiae* 25 mg, *Radix Rehmanniae* 50 mg, *Radix Rehmanniae Preparata* 50 mg, *Fructus Lycii* 25 mg, *Semen Cuscutae* 25 mg, *Herba Cistanches* 25 mg, *Radix Ginseng* 100 mg, *Rhizoma Dioscoreae* 25 mg, *Poria* 100 mg, *Radix Asparagi* 100 mg, *Radix Ophiopogonis* 50 mg, *Fructus Schisandrae* 25 mg, *Radix Glycyrrhizae* 25 mg, *Fructus Aurantii* 25 mg, *Flos Chrysanthemi* 25 mg, *Radix Saposhnikoviae* 25 mg, *Radix Achyranthis Bidentatae* 25 mg, *Rhizoma Chuanxiong* 25 mg, *Semen Armeniacae Amarum* 25 mg, *Gypsum Fibrosum* 25 mg, *Magnetitum* 20 mg, *Fructus Tribuli* 25 mg, *Pulvis Cornus Bubali Concentratus* 45 mg.

Dosage:

For oral administration, take 4 tablets each time, 3 times daily.

Safety considerations:
PIL (60 tabs) & packaging of 500 tabs — side effects not known. Contraindications/ cautions: Pregnant women should take the medicine under the guidance of TCM practitioner (PIL plus packaging of 500 tabs).

Price: 60 tablets — $7.00 (package not sealed); 500 tablets — $48.00 (sealed bottle)

Manufacturer:
Tong Jum Chew Pte Ltd. 21 Kaki Bukit View Tech Park II Singapore 415957. Tel: 62781134 Fax: 62781246. Singapore Manufacturer Licence No. MLCP 0400040, Singapore CPM Product Reference No. 113335.

81. **Fatigue Relief Capsule [20 vegecaps] (Borsch Med)**

Description:
Radix Rhodiolae is good for regulating vital energy and blood condition. Given its reliability and comprehensive nutritional value, the traditional herb was given an imperial name of 'Xian Ci Cao'. Ginseng, a first-class tonic medicine serves to replenish the vital energy, nourish the lung, generate fluid and promote metabolism. Among numerous types of Ginseng, Changbaishan wild Ginseng is particularly precious and incomparably superior to ordinary Ginseng due to its medicinal effects. Borsch Med Fatigue Relief Capsule is formulated from Tibetan Radix Rhodiolae and Changbaishan wild Ginseng. Perfectly blending the essence of these two herbs, this product is a brillant choice for health nourishment and body strengthening.

Indications:
This product is especially good for treating conditions such as fatigue, poor immunity, poor sleeping quality, forgetfulness, palpitation, deficiency in vital energy and premature aging. It is most suitable for metropolitan people who need mind enhancement due to busy and tired lifestyle.

Ingredients:
Ingredients per capsule of 300 mg: *Radix Rhodiolae* 270 mg, *Radix Ginseng* 30 mg.

Safety considerations:
Adverse-Reactions: There are no known side effects for Borsch Med Fatigue Relief Capsule. This product is not suitable for children and those suffering from cold and fever. For pregnant women, please consult a physician before use.

Dosage:
2 capsules to be taken each time with lukewarm water, 1–2 times a day. Do not take more than 6 capsules per day.

Price: No information available

Manufacturer:

Union Chemical & Pharmaceutical Pte Ltd. 113 Eunos Avenue 3 #06-06, Gordon Industrial Building, Singapore 409838. Distributed by: Borsch Med Pte Ltd. 60 Alexandra Terrace #03-28, The Comtech, Singapore 118502. Borsch Med Inc. Suite #300 PMB #1024, 2711 Centreville Road, Wilmington, DE 19808, USA.

82. **Fu Fang Dan Shen Pian (Nature's Green)**

Description on PIL:

Fu Fang Dan Shen Pian is a natural botanical medicine manufactured through the modern pharmaceutical technology. It is a well-known herbal prescription in China, and can help maintain a healthy heart function. The product will relieve the discomfort symptoms of chest pain or distress and stabbing pain in the anterior pectorial region, and so is an effective natural supplement for coronary heart disease and angina pectoris.

Actions and Indications:

Activates blood circulation and alleviates chest pain. Relieves the symptoms of chest pain or distress, and stabbing pain in the anterior pectorial region caused by coronary heart disease and angina pectoris.

Ingredients:

Each 250 mg tablet contains extracts equivalent to raw herbs: *Radix Salviae Miltiorrhiae* 450 mg, *Radix Notoginseng* 141 mg, *Borneolum Syntheticum.* *This product contains tartrazine.

Dosage:

For oral administration, take 3 tablets, 3 times daily.

Safety considerations:

Side effects not known (not on packaging for 100 tablets but on PIL). Use with caution for pregnant women (not on packaging for 100 tablets but on PIL).

Price: 100 tablets — $5; 1000 tablets — $37 (sealed bottle)

Manufacturer:

Tong Jum Chew Pte Ltd 21 Kaki Bukit View Tech Park II Singapore 415957 Tel: 2781134 Fax: 6278 1246.

83. **Fu Long Wan (SeaGull)**

Actions:

Invigorating vital energy & tonifying blood, benefiting essence of the marrows, strengthening tendons & loins, nourishing the liver & kidney.

Indications:
All kinds of injury or impairment due to deficiency, mental tiredness, dizziness & tinnitus, sallow complexion, body weakness & aversion to cold, soreness of loins & knees, numbness of hands & feet.

Ingredients:
Each bottle weight 60 g (360 pills ±) contains *Fructus Foeniculi* 0.91 g, *Halitum* 0.91 g, *Radix Ginseng* 1.81 g, *Rhizoma Chuanxiong* 1.81 g, *Radix Morindae Officinalis* 1.81 g, *Radix Asparagi* 1.81 g, *Rhizoma Atractylodis Macrocephalae* 1.81 g, *Herba Cistanches* 1.81 g, *Cortex Eucommiae* 1.81 g, *Semen Euryales* 1.81 g, *Fructus Lycii* 1.81 g, *Semen Trigonellae* 1.81 g, *Radix Astragali* 1.81 g, *Colla Cornus Cervi* 1.81 g, *Herba Cynomorii* 1.81 g, *Radix Rehmanniae Preparata* 1.81 g, *Pericarpium Zanthoxyli* 0.91 g, *Lignum Aquilariae Resinatum* 0.91 g, *Rhizoma Dioscoreae* 1.81 g, *Radix Achyranthis Bidentatae* 1.81 g, *Fructus Schisandrae* 1.81 g, *Radix Glycyrrhizae* 1.81 g, *Radix Rehmanniae* 1.81 g, *Radix Angelicae Sinensis* 1.81 g, *Radix Ophiopogonis* 1.81 g, *Pericarpium Citri Reticulatae* 1.81 g, *Poria* 1.81 g, *Fructus Psoraleae* 1.81 g, *Radix Dipsaci* 1.81 g, *Semen Cuscutae* 1.81 g, *Fructus Broussonetiae* 1.81 g, *Fructus Rubi* 1.81 g.

Dosage:
For treatment course, take twice daily, each time 15 pills. For healthcare, take twice daily, each time 10 pills. To be taken with lukewarm water before breakfast and prior to bed time.

Safety considerations:
Side effects not known. Raw & cold foods should be restrained. Not recommended for pregnant women.

Price: 360 pills — $28.00 (sealed)

Manufacturer:
Kang Sheng Chinese Medicine Manufacturer Blk 3015 Bedok North St.5, #06-22 Shimei East Kitchen, Singapore 486350.

Sole Agent:
Sea Gull Trading Pte Ltd. Blk 217 Henderson Industrial Park, #03-05 Henderson Road Singapore 159555. Tel: 62741033, Fax: 62724997 Email: sea_gull@pacific.net.sg.

84. **Gan Bao Capsules (Yulin)**

PIL in package:
Abnormally functioning liver and dark urine caused by damp-heat; the yellowness on the skin will fade very quickly.

Actions and Indications:

To remove toxic heat in the body and to relieve the depressed liver and alleviate pain, relieve from jaundice and other inflammation diseases.

Ingredients:

Each capsule (500 mg) contains extract equivalent to raw herbs: *Herba Abri* 714 mg, *Radix Notoginseng* 380 mg, *Herba Origani Vulgaris* 309 mg, *Herba Artemisiae Scopariae* 286 mg, *Radix Paeoniae Alba* 238 mg, *Fructus Lycii* 190 mg, *Fructus Gardeniae* 143 mg, *Fructus Jujubae* 135 mg, *Calculus Bovis* (Synthetic) 119 mg, *Fel Suillus* 76 mg, *Tartrazine* (Lemon Yellow) 0.295 mg.

Dosage:

3 times a day; for adults 4 pills a time and for children reduce half the dosage. Take with boiled water.

Safety considerations:

Side effects not known. Do not use during pregnancy.

Price: 50 capsules — $6.50 (not sealed)

Assembler & importer:

Kinhong (Pte) Ltd 297 Kaki Bukit Ave 1, Shun Li Industrial Park, Singapore 416083.

Manufacturer:

Guangxi Yulin Pharmaceutical Co., Ltd. Yulin, Guangxi, China.

85. **GinGold (Ginkgo leaf extract formula 60 mg) (Red Sun)**

Description:

Red Sun — GinGold is produced in Japan and specially formulated with ginkgo leaf extract, ginseng, black sesame, vit B1 & vit B6. Ginkgo leaf extract helps to promote blood circulation, increase the mobility of the both arms and legs. It also aids in the transportation of sufficient oxygen to the brain, thus it improves concentration and prevents fatigue. The active properties of ginseng- ginsenosides stimulates brain cells, enhances the power of memory. Consume ginkgo leaf extract with ginseng regularly help to sharpen your memory and slow down the process of aging, particularly in older people. Red Sun — GinGold also contains Vit B1, Vit B6 and black sesame, which is rich in Vit E, providing all the important nutrients to prevent memory loss and enhance the effective functioning of the nervous systems.

Ingredients:

Active ingredients: Ginkgo leaf Extract 60 mg, Ginseng 100 mg, Black Sesame 50 mg, Vitamin B1 2 mg, Vitamin B16 2 mg.

Dosage:
2 capsules per day in the morning after food.

Safety considerations:
Do not take before surgery.

Price: 90 vegecapsules — $69.00 (sealed). Made in Japan.

Manufactured for:
Redsun Singapore Pte Ltd. 43 Kaki Bukit Place EUNOS TECHPACK Singapore 416221. Tel: (65) — 63377133 Fax: (65)-68421810. Website: www.redsunproducts.com

86. **Ginsagel Gold Capsule Korean Ginseng Extract Powder (Il Hwa Co. Ltd)**

Description:
Il Hwa Ginsagel Gold Capsule, soft capsule type of ginseng extract powder, is made of raw materials of ginseng, lecithin, natural tocopherol, etc. Ginseng Extract Powder concentrated from Korean ginseng roots with a unique and special method being processed at low temperature and pressure and then dried, has plentiful ginsenosides over 10 types and a most flavourful taste of fresh roots.

Ingredients:
Ginseng Extract Powder (30.04%), Natural Tocopherol (1.66%), Corn Oil, Palm Oil, Lecithin, Beeswax

Dosage:
Take two capsules three times a day.

Price: 50 × 600 mg — $53.50 (sealed)

Manufacturer:
Ilwah Co., Ltd. 437 Sutaek-Dong, Guri- Si, Gyeonggi-Do, Korea.

Imported by:
Tongil Singapore Pte Ltd. 14 Arumugam Road #03-01F Lion Building C Singapore 409959. http://www.buyginseng.com.sg. Tel: (65) 67422151, Fax: (65) 67422935

87. **Ginseng Beard (Chwee Song)**

Actions and Indications:
Effective relieve Heat, Refreshment

Ingredients:
Ginseng

Instruction:
Put the ginseng beard in a cupful of boiling water for few minutes strain and drink
Price: 37 gm — $4.30

Packed by:
Chwee Song Supplies Pte. Ltd. Blk 5, Ang Mo Kio Industrial Park 2A Tech II, #07-14 to 16 Singapore 567760; e-mail: ccsup@singnet.com; Internet: www.chweesong.com.sg; Tel: (65) 6482 3935, 6482 3386 Fax: (65) 6778 5028 Product of China;

88. **Ginseng chrysanthemum cooling tea (Min Feng)**

Details:
No information available

Ingredients:
Ginseng Root (15%), Chrysanthemum (55%), Licorice (3%), Folium Mori (27%)

Instruction:
Place tea bag in cup. Pour in boiling water and then drink is ready. If desired, suitable amount of sugar or salt may be added; Cold Drink: Place tea bag in cup. Pour in boiling water and add in suitable amount of sugar. After the drink has been cooled, add some ice and a tasty drink is ready.

Dosage:
Each time 1 sachet, twice daily

Safety considerations:
Side effects and contraindication not known.

Price: 5 g — $1.04

Manufacturer:
No information available

89. **Ginseng Green Tea (Gold Kili)**

Description:
Instant Ginseng Green tea, blended with premium American Ginseng and refreshing green tea, giving the authenticity of pure ginseng yet provides the soothing effect from the natural green tea. Together with the benefits of glucose, ginseng and green tea, it is an ideal drink for all. No Preservative, Not Artificial Colouring.

Ingredients:
Glucose, Sucrose, Ginseng, Green Tea.

Instruction:
For Hot Serving: Pour contents, add hot water (250 ml) stir and serve instantly. For Cold Serving: Pour Contents, add Hot Water (100 ml) to dissolve content, add ice, stir and serve.

Price: 18 g × 10 g (6.3 oz/180 g) — $4.80

Manufacturer:
Gold Kili Trading Enterprise (Singapore) Pte Ltd. 9, Woodlands Link, Singp. 738 723; Website: www.goldkili.com; Email: query@goldkili.com; Products of Singapore.

Imported by:
10 Importers around the world (Addresses not indicated)

90. **Ginseng Juice Wine (Hsiang Yang Brand)**

Details:
No information available

Ingredients:
No information available

Dosage:
No information available
Price: 200 ml — $13.25

Produced by:
Liaoning Medicines & Health Products Import & Export Corporation;

Imported by:
Wah Thong co. P/L No. 346/346A King George's Ave Singapore 208577; Tel: 2993722.

91. **Ginseng Nutrition Tablets (Nature's Green)**

Actions and Indications:
Used for mental fatigue and tiredness, sallow complexion, poor appetite, loose stool, and weakness during convalescence due to deficiency of heart and spleen.

Ingredients:
Each 460 mg tablet contains extracts equivalent to raw herbs: *Radix Gingseng* 120 mg, *Rhizoma Atractylodis Macrocephalae* 120 mg, *Radix Astragali* 120 mg, *Radix Paeoniae Alba* 120 mg, *Pericarpium Citri Reticulatae* 120 mg, *Radix Angelicae Sinensis* 120 mg, *Radix Glycyrrhizae* 120 mg, *Cortex Cinnamomi* 120 mg, *Radix Rehmanniae Preparata* 90 mg, *Fructus Schisandrae* 90 mg, *Poria* 90 mg, *Radix Polygalae* 60 mg.

Dosage:
For oral administration, take 4 tablets, 2 times daily.

Safety considerations:
Side effects not known. Not suitable for pregnant women and patients who are sturdy.

Price: 500 tablets — $33.00 (sealed)

Manufacturer:
Tong Jum Chew Pte Ltd. Alexandra Distripark Blk.1 #08-15/17 Pasir Panjang Road Singapore 118478 Tel: 63781134 (3 lines) Fax: 62781246. Singapore Manufacturer Licence No. MLCP 0400040 Singapore CPM Product Reference No. 113721.

92. **Ginseng Pearl Pollen Pai Fong Wan (Chan Kang Brand)**

Indications:
Traditionally used for general weakness, to relieve fatigue, tiredness, backache, giddiness and to regulate menstruation.

Ingredients:
Formulation not given on packaging.

Dosage and instruction:
One bottle to be taken each time with warm water before sleep at night daily. The pills can be taken by steaming together with chicken or other meat. If symptoms persist, please consult the doctor. For health maintenance, one bottle to be taken each time, once in every three days.

Safety considerations:
The pills should not be taken when having cold, diarrhoea or fever.

Price: 10 g — $6.80 (sealed)

Manufacturer:
Kim Sin Medication Supply Blk 625 Aljunied Road #06-06 Aljunied Industrial Complex Singapore 389836.

Packed and distributed by:
China Tangshan Chinese Pharmaceutical Co. Blk 32 Defu Lane 10 #04-06 Singapore 539213.

93. **Ginseng Qing Bu Tang (Chwee Song)**

Description:
Improve General Health

Actions and Indications:
Improve immunity and body resistence, improve blood circulation. Especially good for those who have just recovered from illness.

Ingredients:
Ginseng (25 g), Dioasorea Opposita (25 g), Boxthorn fruit (25 g), Polygonatum Odoratum (35 g).

Dosage:
No information available

Price: 100 gm — $6.40

Packed by:
Chwee Song Supplies Pte. Ltd. Blk 5, Ang Mo Kio Industrial Park 2A Tech II, #07-14 to 16 Singapore 567760; e-mail: sales@chweesong.com.sg; Internet: www.chweesong.com.sg; Tel: (65) 6482 3935, 6482 3386 Fax: (65) 6778 5028 Product of China.

94. **Ginseng Red Date (Allswell)**

Description:
Double boiled for extra goodness!

Ingredients:
Water, Sugar, Ginseng, Red Dates, Honey Dates.

Instruction:
Best served chilled; Keep refrigerated once opened; Shake well before use as product may contain natural sediments.

Price: 250 ml — $2.10

Manufacturer:
Allswell Trading Pte Ltd., 41 Sunset Way # 02-05 Clementi Arcade Singapore 597071; Tel: (65) 6778 8218; Email: service@allswelltrading.com.sg

95. **Ginseng Royal Jelly (Huay Feng Hang)**

Description:
Ren shen feng wang jiang (Ginseng Royal Jelly) is a health remedy for drinking purpose. Ginseng is long reputed by Oriental-for-thousand of years. As a superior and specialty herb. It has been enjoyed by people all over the world for decades. Royal Jelly is a milk-like secretion from worker bee. It is solely for the Queen Bee to consume. By using the Royal Jelly, the Queen Bee is able to survive 20 times longer than

the other bees. This "original and ancient" recipe of Ginseng Royal Jelly is being sold all over the world.

Ingredients:
Each ampule contains 200 mg of Ginseng.and 300 mg of Royal Jally.

Dosage:
One ampule daily before breakfast. and/or another one before supper.

Safety considerations:
Warning: Not recommended for asthmatics or allergy sufferers as it can cause-severe allergic reactions

Price: 10 ampules — $3.90 (sealed)

Import by:
Huay Feng Hang Pte Ltd. Blk 623 Aljunied Road, #06-08, Aljunied Industrial Complex, Singapore 389835, Tel: 67482911, Fax: 67440283. Email: sales@huiji. com.sg. Product of China

96. **Ginseng Saponins capsules (Mei Hua Brand)**

Actions:
Invigorate vital energy, replenish the lungs and spleen, anti-anxiety, promote brain function and increase body resistance.

Indications:
Effective for energy deficiency, weakness in lungs and palpitation and low blood pressure. Help to reinforce the functions of the stomach, relieve dizziness and vertigo, combat fatigue and delay aging. (30 capsules)

Ingredients:
Each capsule (300 mg) contains extract equivalent to raw herb *Radix Ginseng* 3800 mg. 300 caps: 380 mg per capsule contains extract equivalent to raw herbs: *Radix Ginseng* 3800 mg.

Dosage:
For curative purpose: Take 2 capsules twice daily. As health supplement, take 1 capsule once daily with warm water, best taken half an hour before meal.

Safety considerations:
(Side effects and contraindications not on packaging of 30 capsules. Package is sealed)

Price: 30 capsules — $15; 300 capsules — $130 (sealed)

Manufacturer:
Science Arts Co Pte Ltd 150 MacPherson Rd, Science Arts Building Singapore 348524

97. Gold Label Bak Foong Pill (Eu Yan Sang)

Description:
Gold Label Bak Foong Pill is made of precious Chinese herbs, based on an ancient formula. Traditionally used for health, stomachache, malnutrition after childbirth and regulating menstrual ailments.

Indications:
Traditionally used for health, stomachache, malnutrition after childbirth and regulating menstrual ailments.

Ingredients:
Composition per 19 grams pill: *Radix Angelicae Sinensis* 542.59 mg, *Cortex Eucommiae* 542.59 mg, *Cortex Cinnamomi* 161.83 mg, *Folium Artemisiae Argyi* 609.22 mg, *Rhizoma Corydalis* 809.12 mg, *Radix Astragali* 1085.17 mg, *Radix Ginseng* 266.54 mg, *Radix Paeoniae Alba* 656.82 mg, *Radix Polygalae* 542.59 mg, *Semen Sesami Nigrum* 409.31 mg, *Fructus Amomi* 428.36 mg, *Faeces Trogopterori* 809.12 mg, *Cornu Cervi Pantotrichum* 266.54 mg, *Rhizoma Ligustici Chuanxiong* 409.31 mg, *Rhizoma Atractylodis Macrocephalae* 266.54 mg, *Poria* 542.59 mg, *Rhizoma Cyperi* 542.59 mg, *Herba Leonuri* 609.22 mg, *Mel* 9499.95 mg.

Safety considerations:
Avoid consumption when suffering from fever or influenza or during menstruation period.

Recommended Dosage:
For promoting youth and health: 1 pill taken once weekly. For general weakness: 1 pill taken at every two days interval. For malnutrition after childbirth: 1 pill taken daily repeating for several days. It should be taken after clearing labour discharge (normally about 10 days). For regulating menstrual ailments: 1 pill taken daily. If symptoms persist, consult your physician.

Price: 6 pills × 19 g — $45.30 (Sealed)

Manufacturer:
Weng Li Sdn. Bhd. (053874-D) (Wholly owned by Eu Yan Sang Int. Ltd.) 4 Persiaran 1/118C, Fasa II Desa Tun Razak Industrial Park, 56000 Kuala Lumpur, Malaysia. Reg. No.: MAL19988046T.

Distributed by:
Eu Yan Sang (1959) Sdn Bhd (3544-P) L2-01 & L2-12, 2nd Floor, Shaw Parade, Changkat Thambi Dollah, 55100 Kuala Lumpur, Malaysia. Eu Yan Sang (Singapore) Pte Ltd 151 Lorong Chuan, #05-05/06 New Tech Park, Singapore 556741.

98.   Health Maintenance Capsules (Nature's Green)

Description:
Health Maintenance Capsules are made from highly concentrated, 60 precious Chinese herbs and produced in accordance to the well-known Chinese herbal formula. It helps activate blood circulation, relax tendons and activate energy flow in the meridians and channels, disperse stagnant blood and phlegm, dispel wind and cold in the joints, and tonify kidney. This product helps relieve the symptoms of weak limbs and lassitude, numbness and spasm of hands and feet, stiffness of muscles and joints, difficulty in walking, dizziness and headache. It is used as a powerful health supplement that reduces the risk of blood stasis and benefits the recuperation stage of serious health problem stricken by pathogenic wind.

Actions:
Promotes blood circulation, resolves stasis and activates channels.

Indications:
Relieves the symptoms of weak limbs and lassitude, numbness and spasm of hands and feet, stiffness of muiscles and joints, difficulty in walking, dizziness and headache. Used as a health supplement at the recuperation stage of serious health problem stricken by pathogenic wind.

Ingredients:
Each 480 mg capsules contains extracts equivalent to raw herbs: *Benzoinum* 10 mg, *Lignum Aquilariae Resinatrm* 10 mg, *Lignum Santali Albi* 10 mg, *Radix Aucklandiae* 20 mg, *Flos Caryophylli* 10 mg, *Herba Pogostemonis* 20 mg, *Olibanum* 10 mg, *Myrrha* 10 mg, *Resina Draconis* 3 mg, *Succinum* 5 mg, *Calculus Bovis* 5 mg, *Concretio Silicea Bambusae* 10 mg, *Agkistrodon* 20 mg, *Zaocys* 20 mg, *Scorpio* 15 mg, *Hirudo* 20 mg, *Bombyx Batryticatus* 10 mg, *Lumbricus* 5 mg, *Eupolyphaga Seu Steleophaga* 40 mg, *Cornus Bubali* 30 mg, *Carapax et Plastrum Testudinis* 10 mg, *Radix Notoginseng* 5 mg, *Radix Ginseng* 20 mg, *Radix Astragali* 20 mg, *Radix Polygoni Multiflori Praeparata* 20 mg, *Raidix Scrophulariae* 20 mg, *Radix Angelicae Sinensis* 10 mg, *Radix Rehmanniae preparata* 20 mg, *Rhizoma Gastrodiae* 20 mg, *Herba Taxilli* 20 mg, *Rhizoma Drynariae* 10 mg, *Radix Clematidis* 15 mg, *Rhizoma Dioscoreae Nipponicae* 80 mg, *Radix Salviae Miltiorrhiae* 120 mg, *Flos Carthami* 40 mg, *Semen Persicae* 40 mg, *Radix Paeoniae Rubra* 20 mg, *Rhizoma Chuanxiong*

20 mg, *Radix Puerariae* 15 mg, *Broneolum Syntheticum* 3 mg, *Rhizoma Atractylodis Macrocephalae* 10 mg, *Poria* 10 mg, *Rhizoma Vyperi* 10 mg, *Radix et Rhizoma Rhei* 20 mg, *Rhizoma Dioscoreae Hypoglaucae* 20 mg, *Cortex Cinnamomi* 20 mg, *Pericarpium Citri Reticulatae Viride* 10 mg, *Fructrs Amomi Rotundus* 10 mg, *Rhizoma Wenyujin Concisum* 2.5 mg, *Semen Alpiniae Katsumadai* 20 mg, *Radix Linderae* 10 mg, *Exocarpium Citri Rubrum* 40 mg, *Massa Fermentata Medicinalis* 40 mg, *Arisaema Cum Bile* 10 mg, *Radix Angelicae Dahuricae* 20 mg, *Radix Saposhnikoviae* 20 mg, *Rhizoma Seu Radix Notopterygii* 20 mg, *Radix Asari* 10 mg, *Radix Glycyrrhizae* 20 mg.

Dosage:
For oral administration, take 4 capsules, 2 times daily. The recommended treatment course is one month.

Price: 50 capsules — $25.00 (sealed)

Manufacturer:
Tong Jum Chew Pte Ltd. 21 Kaki Bukit View Teck Park II Singapore 415957. Tel: 62781134. Fax: 62781246. Singapore CPM Product Reference No. 113827.

99. **Healthy Heart Capsules (Nature's Green)**

Description on PIL:
Chest pain that is caused by a heart disease may be a sign of a serious health problem. Heartonic Tablets are made from 17 special selected herbs based on the classical Chinese herbal prescription and prepared by modern pharmaceutical technology. This product can effectively relieve heart disease with the symptoms of a feeling of tightness or pressure on the chest, heart pain, palpitation, shortness of breath, mental fatigue, dizziness and insomnia. It is a natural herbal medicine designed to maintain a healthy heart function for middle-aged and elderly person.

Actions and Indications:
Promotes blood circulation and alleviates heart pain. Relieves heart disease with the symptoms of chest distension, heart pain, palpitation, shortness of breath, mental fatigue, dizziness and insomnia.

Ingredients:
Each 480 mg tablet contains extracts equivalent to raw herbs: *Radix Salviae Miltiorrhiae* 107 mg, *Radix Notoginseng* 80 mg, *Cor Cervi* 80 mg, *Folium Ginkgo* standardized Extract (equivalent to dry Ginkgo biloba leaf 1300 mg) 26 mg, *Radix Polygoni Multiflori Preparata* 80 mg, *Radix Puerariae* 80 mg, *Radix Paeoniae Rubra* 80 mg, *Flos Carthami* 53 mg, *Rhizoma Chuanxiong* 80 mg, *Lumbricus* 80 mg, *Radix*

Curcumae 8 mg, *Rhizoma Anemones Altaicae* 80 mg, *Radix Achyranthis Bidentatae* 80 mg, *Fructus Lycii* 80 mg, *Rhizoma Alismatis* 80 mg, *Radix Polygalae Preparata* 80 mg, *Semen Ziziphi Spinosae* 53 mg, *Radix Glycyrrhizae* 53 mg, *Borneolum Syntheticum* 8 mg.

Dosage:
For oral administration, take 3 capsules, 3 times daily.

Safety considerations:
Side effects not known (Not on packaging for 60 capsules but in PIL). Not to be taken by pregnant women (not on packaging for 60 capsules).

Price: 60 capsules — $11.50
      300 capsules — $50

Manufacturer:
Tong Jum Chew Pte Ltd. 21 Kaki Bukit View Tech Park II Singapore 415957 tel: 62781134 Fax: 6278 1246.

100. **Healthy Life Capsules (Nature's Green)**

Actions and Indications:
Used in coordination with radiotherapy or chemotherapy. Helps relieve patient's symptoms, support healthy energy, and promotes the recovery of normal functions after disease. Promotes blood circulation, counteracts toxicity, disperses accumulation and alleviates pain.

Ingredients:
Each 500 mg capsule contains extracts equivalent to raw herbs: *Moschus* (Synthetic) 5 mg, *Calculus Bovis* (Synthetic) 20 mg, *Margarita* 20 mg, *Radix Panacis Quinquefolii* 60 mg, *Ganoderma Lucidum* 80 mg, *Cordyceps Hypha* 80 mg, *Radix Astragali* 300 mg, *Fructus Ligustri Lucidi* 120 mg, *Radix Salviae Miltiorrhiae* 100 mg, *Flos Carthami* 40 mg, *Radix Ranunculi Ternati* 200 mg, *Herba Hedyotidis Diffusae* 150 mg, *Rhizoma Sparganii* 100 mg, *Rhizoma Curcumae* 100 mg, *Herba Scutellariae Barbatae* 200 mg, *Radix Sophorae Flavescentis* 120 mg, *Radix Trichosanthis* 80 mg, *Radix Clematidis* 80 mg, *Arisaema Cum Bile* 80 mg, *Polyporus* 100 mg, *Semen Impatientis* 80 mg, *Periostracum Serpentis* 40 mg, *Scolopendra* 10 mg, *Olibanum* 10 mg, *Myrrha* 10 mg, *Broneolum Syntheticum* 10 mg.

Dosage:
For oral administration, take 2–3 capsules half an hour after meal with honey water or warm water, 3 times daily. The recommended treatment course is one month. Stop taking this medicine 3–7 days before the start of next period.

Safety considerations:
Side effects not known. Not to be taken by pregnant women. Contraindicated for patients with poor liver or kidney functions. Avoid cold, hard, pungent or offensive smell food.

Price: 300 capsules — $105.00 (Sealed)

Manufacturer:
Tong Jum Chew Pte Ltd. 21 Alexandra Distripark Blk. 1. #08-15/17 Pasir Panjang Road Singapore 118478. Tel: 62781134 (3 lines) Fax: 62781246 Manufacturer Licence No. MLCP: 0400040 Singapore CPM Product Reference No. 114069.

101. **Heart Caring Capsule (Keyi)**

Actions:
To reinforce Qi and promote blood circulation, activates meridians and collaterals to relieve pain.

Indications:
Used for discomfort and pains in chest caused by obstruction of collaterals by blood stasis, which manifested as tiredness, dizziness, poor breathing, palpitation, chest distress and pains.

Ingredients:
Each capsule (300 mg) contains extracts equivalent to raw herbs: *Folium Ginkgo* 960 mg, *Radix et Rhizoma Salviae Miltiorrhizae* 900 mg, *Radix et Rhizoma Notoginseng* 252 mg, *Radix et Rhizoma Ginseng* 290 mg.

Dosage:
Oral administration: For health supplement: 2 times a day, 1 or 2 capsules each time. For curative purpose: 2 times a day, 3 capsules each time.
Price: 60 capsules — $48 (sealed)

Manufacturer:
Science Arts Co Pte Ltd 150 MacPherson Road, Science Arts Building Singapore 348524.

102. **Heartonic Tablets (Nature's Green)**

Description on PIL:
Chest pain that is caused by a heart disease may be a sign of a serious health problem. Heartonic Tablets are made from 17 special selected herbs based on the classical Chinese herbal prescription and prepared by modern pharmaceutical technology. This product can effectively relieve heart disease with the symptoms

of a feeling of tightness or pressure on the chest, heart pain, palpitation, shortness of breath, mental fatigue, dizziness and headache. It is a natural herbal medicine designed to maintain a healthy heart function for middle-aged and elderly person.

Actions and Indications:
Promotes blood circulation and alleviates heart pain. Relieves heart disease with the symptoms of chest distension, heart pain, palpitation, shortness of breath, mental fatigue, dizziness and headache.

Ingredients:
Each 420 mg tablet contains extracts equivalent to raw herbs: *Radix Salviae Miltiorrhiae* 107 mg, *Radix Notoginseng* 80 mg, *Radix Polygoni Multiflori Preparata* 80 mg, *Radix Puerariae* 80 mg, *Radix Paeoniae Rubra* 80 mg, *Flos Carthami* 53 mg, *Rhizoma Chuanxiong* 80 mg, *Lumbricus* 80 mg, *Radix Curcumae* 8 mg, *Rhizoma Anemones Altaicae* 80 mg, *Radix Achyranthis Bidentatae* 80 mg, *Fructus Lycii* 80 mg, *Rhizoma Alismatis* 80 mg, *Radix Polygalae* 80 mg, *Semen Ziziphi Spinosae* 53 mg, *Radix Glycyrrhizae* 53 mg, *Borneolum Syntheticum* 8 mg

Dosage:
For oral administration, take 3 tablets, 3 times daily.

Safety considerations:
PIL: Side effects not known. Not to be taken by pregnant women (Not stated on packaging of the 60 tablets)

Price: 60 tablets — $8.50; 500 tablets — $52 (sealed)

Manufacturer:
Tong Jum Chew Pte Ltd 21 Kaki Bukit View Tech Park II Singapore 415957 Tel: 62781134 Fax: 62781046 Singappre Manufacturer Licence No. MLCP 0400040 Singapore CPM Product Reference No. 114415

103.   **Heel Pain Relief Capsules (Nature's Green)**

Description on PIL:
Gout typically affects the joint at the base of the big toe. Almost any other joint can be affected, but the joints of the lower limbs are more commonly than those of the ipper limbs. The pain is so fiery and the foot so sensitive that you cannot bear to be touched by anything. Nature's Green Heel Pain Relief Capsules is made into capsules from 8 natural herbs and prepared by modern pharmaceutical technology. It helps to remove turbidity and to reduce pain and inflammation in the foot.

Actions and Indications:
Helps relieve disabling foot ailments such as heel pain on one or two sides, and difficulty in walking.

Ingredients:
Each 300 mg capsule contains extracts equivalent to raw herbs: *Herba Lycopodii* 300 mg, *Caulis Sargentodoxae* 200 mg, *Radix Notoginseng* 100 mg, *Radix Salviae Miltiorrhiae* 100 mg, *Rhizoma Dioscoreae Septemlobae* 300 mg, *Rhizoma Alismatis* 200 mg, *Semen Coicis* 200 mg, *Rhizoma Smilacis Glabrae* 200 mg.

Dosage:
For oral administration, take 3 capsules, 3 times daily. The recommended treatment course is sixty days.

Safety considerations:
Side effects not known. 1. Avoid alcoholic drink (beer, wine, etc.), which can trigger gout. 2. Avoid seafood with high concentrations of purines. 3. Avoid high protein foods such as red meat and organ meats. 4. Avoid peanut, soybean and its products. 5. Stay away from coffee and tea. 6. Reduce eating certain vegetables such as mushroom, laver, spinach, kelp and hyacinth bean. 7. Not suitable for pregnant women.

Price: 30 capsules — $7.50 (not sealed)

Manufacturer:
Tong Jum Chew Pte Ltd 21 Kaki Bukit View Tech Park II Singapore 415957 Tel: 62781134 Fax: 62781246

104. **Heel Pain Relief Tablets (Nature's Green)**

Actions and Indications:
Helps relieve disabling foot ailments such as heel pain on one or two sides, and difficulty in working caused by gout.

Ingredients:
Each 420 mg tablet contains extracts equivalent to raw herbs: *Herba Lycopodii* 225 mg, *Caulis Sargentodoxae* 150 mg, *Radix Notoginseng* 75 mg, *Radix Salviae Miltiorrhiae* 75 mg, *Rhizoma Dioscoreae Hypoglaucae* 225 mg, *Rhizoma Alismatis* 150 mg, *Semen Coicis* 150 mg, *Rhizoma Smilacis Glabrae* 150 mg, *Radix Achyranthis Bidentatae* 75 mg, *Radix Angelicae Pubescentis* 75 mg.

Dosage:
For oral administration, take 4 tablets, 3 times daily. The recommended treatment course is thirty days.

Price: 500 tablets — $46

Manufacturer:

Tong Jum Chew Pte Ltd. 21 Kaki Bukit View Tech Park II Singapore 415957 Tel: 62781134 Fax:62781246 Singapore Manufacturer Licence No. MLCP: 04000400 Singapore CPM Product Reference No.: 113840.

105.   **Hengzhi Cough Capsules (Heng Chun Brand)**

Actions:

Reinforces and warms the vital energy and nourishes blood and fluid; dispels fluid retention; arresting cough and relieves asthma.

Indications:

For deficiency in vital energy and blood and fluid; resolves phlegm, cough and breathlessness induced by deficiency of yang, stagnation of fluid or phlegm in the chest, fatigue.

Ingredients:

Each capsule (0.25 g) contains extract equivalent to: *Radix Ginseng Rubra* 28.8 mg, *Radix Panacis Quinquefolii* 28.8 mg, *Cortex Cinnamomi* 28.8 mg, *Rhizoma Pinelliae Praeparata* 480.8 mg, *Pericarpium Citri Reticulatae* 14.4 mg, *Flos Caryophylli* 14.4 mg, *Folium Perillae* 28.8 mg, *Herba Menthae* 14.4 mg, *Lignum Aquilariae Resinatum* 28.8 mg, *Fructus Amomi* (Amomum Villosum) 14.4 mg, *Rhizoma Zingiberis Recens* 120.2 mg, *Radix et Rhizoma Glycyrrhizae* 14.4 mg, *Flos Carthami* 14.4 mg, *R*hizoma Bletillae* 50.4 mg, *Fructus Citri Sarcodactylis* 14.4 mg, *Fructus Citri* 14.4 mg, *Fructus Amomi Rotundus* 14.4 mg, *Haematitum* 4.2 mg. Capsule material contains food coloring tartrazine.

Dosage:

Oral, 2–4 capsules each time, twice daily.

Safety considerations:

Side effects not known. Not for pregnant women. Women should exercise discretion in taking this product during menstruation.

Price: 24 capsules — $7.2 (sealed)

Manufacturer:

Wuhu Zhanghengchun Medicine Co Ltd. Anhui, China.

Importer:

Ban San Tong Koong Kee 2 Alexandra Road #06-05 Singapore 159919.

106. **Herba Dendrobii Capsules (Mei Hua Brand)**

Actions:
Replenish vital energy, nourish the stomach and promote the secretion of body's fluid.

Indications:
Effective for all febrile diseases showing symptoms of blurred vision, dry mouth, fatigue, irritability, anxiety and feeling feverish. It is benefical for those undergone treatment of chemotherapy or radiotherapy.

Ingredients:
Each Capsule (250 mg) contains raw herbs: *Herba Dendrobii* 175 mg, American Ginseng 75 mg.

Dosage:
Take 4 capsules three times a day with warm water. For health supplement: Take 2 capsules twitch a day.

Safety considerations:
Side effects and contraindications not known.

Price: 60 capsules — $33 (sealed)

Manufacturer:
Science Arts Co. Pte Ltd. 150 MacPherson Rd, Science Arts Builidng Singapore 348524

107. **Herbal Braised Duck Spices Sachet (nil)**

Details:
No information available

Ingredients:
Cinnamon, Star Anise, Pepper, Ginseng Root, Radix

Instruction:
Preparation: 1. use 3 litres of water. Bring to boil. Add in 1 packet of Braised Duck Sachet. (1 packet for 1 whole duck) 2. Add in 4 spoonful of Dark Sooy Sauce, 3 spoonful of Light Soy Sauce, 2 spoonful of Oyster Saue, 1 tea spoonful of Salt, 1 spoonful of Sugar, 1 slice of galangal(Ginger). 3 heat at low temperature for 2 hours until the duck has the fragrance taste smell. *This ingredients also suitable for boiled egg, bean curd and others type of meat. This is a tasty local Teochew treat! It is your best choice!

Price: 32 gm — $2.50

Packed by: Unita Enterprise No.9 Jalan Saga 3, Taman Desa Cemerlang, 81800 Ulu Tiram, Johor, Malaysia. H/P: 016-730 6256, 019-752 0501; Fax: 07-861 0288;

Singapore Distributor:

Hua Bao Agency Pte Ltd. 105, Sims Avenue #06-10, Chancelodge Complex Singapore 387429; Tel: 6749 0809, Fax: 6749 3662.

108.   **Herbal Chicken Soup Spices (Seah's Spices)**

Details:

No information available

Ingredients:

Chinese Angelica, Frucuts Fig, Coastal Glehnia Root, Fragrant Solomonseal Rhizome, Szechuan Lovage Rhizome, Ginseng, Salt, Sugar, Permitted Food Enhances [E631, E627]

Instruction:

Preparation: 1 sachet of spices, 500 g skinless chicken meat (Bite sizes), 1 canned button mushrooms (425 g), 10 g snow fungus (soak bite sizes in hot water until soft), 6 bowls water (1500 ml/50 oz); Method: 1. Boil 500 ml water, 2. Place sachet and all ingredients in boiling water, 3. Slimmer for 45 mins on low heat, 4. Turn off fire and gamish with spring onion. Serve hot.

Price: 32 gm — $2.30

Manufacturer:

Seah's Spices Food Industries, Pte. Ltd, No. 18 Senoko Crescent, Senoko Food Connection, Singapore 758284 Tel (65) 6759 9551, Fax (65) 67599552; E-mail: spices@singnet.com.sg, www.seahspices.com.

109.   **Herbal Essence Health Tonic (Harvest)**

Actions:

Promote blood and Qi energy circulation, strengthen kidneys and back, nourish blood, calm nerves and promote quality sleep, improving skin complexion and promote growth of black hair.

Indications:

Tiredness from working, illness, hectic lifestyle resulting in weak health and blood. Individuals with good health my use it to improve skin condition and for beautifying purpose.

Ingredients:
Each 750 ml contains: Cordyceps (2.2 g), Cortex Eucommiae (6.6 g), Radix Ginseng (52 g), Radix Polygoni Multiflori Preparata (35 g), Radix Angelicae Sinensis (108 g), Radix Rehmanniae Praeparatae (22 g), Fructus Ziziphi Jujubae (66 g), Fructus Lycii (35 g), Radix Glycyrrhizae (66 g), Rhizoma Chuanxiong (46 g)

Instruction:
Consume one cup as given (20 ml) orally once in morning and once in night. May consume before of after meal.

Safety considerations:
No known side-effects. No known contraindication.

Price: 750 ml — $36.00

Proudly Made in Singapore by GMP certified factory:
Union Chemical & Pharmaceutical Pte Ltd., No. 113, Eunos Ave 3, Gordon Industrial Building, #06--06/10, Singapore 409838; Website: www.union.com.sg; GMP Licence: GMP00020H; Manufacturer Licence: CPMM0010; Consumer Hotline: 6747 7242.

110. **Herbal Slimming Tea (Honey Lemon, Natural, Orange Spice) (21st Century)**

Description:
21st Century's Herbal Slimming Tea is a blend of 100% natural herbs which provides a light, delicious caffeine free beverage that helps achiece results in aiding digestion and contributing to weight loss. This all natural herbal tea offers a rich, satisfying taste in hot or iced tea and provides slimming and digestive benefits that may be enjoyed after every meal. 21st Century's Herbal Slimming Tea combines herbs to promote a "thermogenic" reaction which increases metabolic activity. The result is that excess calories and toxins will be eliminated.

Ingredients:
Senna leaves, Malva leaves, Licorice root, Panax ginseng root, Orange Oil.

Instruction:
Steep one tea bag in a cup of boiling water for 2–5 minutes to desired strength and taste. Drink 15 minutes before or during meals. If desired, add sugar or sweetener to taste. Begin drinking at half strength by diluting with water and reducing the steeping time. Gradually increase the tea strength as your digestive system adjusts.

Price: Herbal — $15.50 (24's); Natural — $25.85 (2 × 24's)

Herbal: Made in USA.
21st Century Laboratories Inc. 2119, South Wilson Street, Tempe, Arizona 85282-2034 USA. www.21stcenturyvitamins.com, www.21stcentury.sg.

Honey Lemon: Made in USA.

21st Century Laboratories Inc. 2119, South Wilson Street, Tempe, Arizona 85282-2034 USA. www.21stcenturyvitamins.com, www.21stcentury.sg.

Distributed by:

21st Century HealthCare Pte Ltd. No.40, Jalan Pemimpin, #03-07 Tat Ann Building, Singapore 577185.

Orange Spice: Made in USA.

21st Century Laboratories Inc. 2119, South Wilson Street, Tempe, Arizona 85282-2034 USA. www.21stcenturyvitamins.com, www.21stcentury.sg.

Distributed by:

21st Century HealthCare Pte Ltd. No.40, Jalan Pemimpin, #03-07 Tat Ann Building, Singapore 577185.

111. **High Strength Men's Tonic Capsules (Nature's Green)**

Actions:

Strengthens organic functions, energizes spirit and stamina.

Indications:

Relieves symptoms such as weakness and soreness of waist and kness, vertigo, tinnitus, emission, mental fatigue and poor appetite.

Ingredients:

Each 300 mg capsule contains extracts equivalent to raw herbs: *Cortex Eucommiae* 17.04 mg, *Radix Morindae Officinalis* 17.04 mg, *Testis et Penis Equus* 37.47 mg, *Testis et Penis Canis* 8.52 mg, *Colla Corii Asini* 17.04 mg, *Hippocampus* 8.52 mg, *Radix Ginseng* 34.05 mg, *Radix Astragali* 34.05 mg, *Herba Cistanches* 34.05 mg, *Radix Angelicae Sinensis* 34.05 mg, *Fructus Lycii* 34.05 mg, *Fructus Corni* 34.05 mg, *Herba Cynomorii* 34.05 mg, *Semen Trigonellae* 34.05 mg, *Fructus Psoraleae* 345.08 mg, *Cornu Cervi Pantotrichum* 17.04 mg, *Semen Cuscutae* 17.04 mg, *Radix Rehmanniae Preparata* 17.04 mg, *Fructus Rubi* 17.04 mg, *Cortex Moutan* 17.04 mg, *Raidix Scrophulariae* 17.04 mg, *Raidix Ophiopogonis* 16.56 mg, *Rhizoma Curculiginis* 16.56 mg, *Cortex Cinnamomi* 13.62 mg, *Herba Epimedii* 8.52 mg, *Radix Achyranthis Bidentatae* 8.52 mg, *Radix Dipsaci* 8.52 mg, *Poria* 8.52 mg, *Rhizoma Atractylodis Macrocephalae* 8.52 mg, *Radix Glycyrrhizae* 17.04 mg.

Dosage:

For oral administration, take 2–3 capsules 2 times daily, morning and night.

Price: 30 capsules — $38.00 (sealed); 2 × 30capsules — $66.80 (sealed)

Manufacturer:
Tong Jum Chew Pte Ltd. 21 Kaki Bukit View Tech Park II Singapore 415957. Tel: 62781134 Fax: 62781246.

112. **High Strength Zheng Gu Plaster (Jin Pai Trademark)**

Description:
The plaster is of high medicinal potency, strong penetration and fragrant smell. It is effective for falls, blows, injuries, rheumatic bone aching, muscular pain, sprain, trauma and fatigue in exercises.

Actions:
This plaster is prepared according to the dialectic therapeutics of traditional Chinese medicine. The elements of the various drug and herbs it contains, when applied to the skin, will penetrate into the subcutaneous tissues so as to stimulate circulation and producing a local analgesic effect. It helps to cure inflammation of muscles and to promote the healing of bonetractures.

Indications:
Falls, blows injuries rheumatic bone aching, muscular pain, sprain, trauma and fatigue in exercises.

Ingredients:
Radix Pseudoginseng 18%, *Croton Tiglium* 14%, *Cinnanmomum Camphora Nees Et Eberm* 14%, *Radix Angelicae* 12%, *Moghania Macrophylla* 12%, *Inula Cappa* 12%, *Boswellia Carterii Birdw* 6%, *Commiphora Myrrha Engl* 7%, *Menthol* 3%, *Camphora* 2%.

Instruction:
Method of Usage: Firstly, wash and clean the surface of the skin till dry, then paste the plaster on the affected portion. In case of pregnancy, cautiously apply.

Price: 1 box (4 pieces) — $2.50

Manufacturer:
Made in China.

113. **Honeyed Korean Red Ginseng Slices (Korean Ginseng Corp.)**

Details:
No information available

Ingredients:
6-Year-Old Korean Red Ginseng Slices, Honey, Isomaltooligosaccharides, Fish Collagen

Dosage:
No information available

Price:
Net Wt. 37.05 OZ (Each pack 20 g)x10packs/Box — $138.00

Manufacturer:
Korea Ginseng Corp. (www.kgc.or.kr) 926, Dunsan-dong, Seo-gu, Daejeon, Korea;
Sole Authorized Distributor: Wing Joo Loong Ginseng Hong (S) Co Pte. Ltd, 30&31
North Canal Road, Singapore 059286 Tel: 6538-3838; Fax: 6534-2800.

114.   **Hong Sam Won (Korea Ginseng Corp.)**

Details:
No information available

Ingredients:
Water, Fructose syrup, Mixed herbal extract (Jujube extract, Dried ginger extract,
Cinnamon bark extract, Lycium Fruit extract), Caramel sugar syrup, Korean Red
ginseng Extract, Cola flavor, Citric acid. Oringin: South Korea.

Dosage:
Adult: Take 1 bottle one or two times daily. Children under 15: Take on half of the
adult serving.

Safety considerations:
Caution: Edges at opening may be sharp.

Price: $11

Manufacturer:
Korea Ginseng Corporation 926 Dunsan-dong, Seo-gu, Daejeon, Korea. Imported
by: Wing Joo Loong Ginseng Hong (S) Co Pte Ltd. 31 North Canal Road (S) 059287

115.   **Hua Qu Shen Soup (Yew Chian Haw)**

Details:
No information available

Ingredients:
American Ginseng, Rhizoma polygonati odorati, Fructus lycii, Rhizoma dioscoreae
batatuo, Euphoria longan, Fructus Ziziphi jujube.

Instruction:
Method: After boiling 2 litres of water, add in Yew Chian Haw Hua Qu Shen Soup
ingredients and boil vigorously. Then add in 500 gm of meat (any kind) and simmer.
Lastly add in one tea spoon of salt and serve.

Price: 105 gm — $5.86

Made & Distributed by:
YEW CHIAN HAW (MALAYSIA) SDN. BHD., (Company No. 218632-A) 2, Lingiang Beringin 2, Jalan Permatang Damar Laut, 11960 Batu Maung, Penang, Malaysia. Tel: 604-626 2020: Fax: 604-626 1010: Email: ych@e-ych.com; Product of Malaysia: GMP Standard with 100% Genuine Ingredients; Serves 4–6 people; Life Span: 18 months.

Distributed by:
YEW CHIAN HAW (Singapore) Pte. Ltd (Company No. 199200237-N) 7 Fan Yoong Road Singapore 629 785: E-mail: ych.sg@e-ych.com.

116. **"Hua Tuo" Anti-Contusion Rheumatism Plaster (Kong Fong)**

Description:
This plaster are elaborated with scientific methods selecting super Chinese medicinal herb, according to popular traditional prescriptions; so that it has the effective of invigorating the circulation of blood, subsidence of a swelling, analgesic and curing rheumatism. The plaster has good curing effect to treatment of injuries from falls, sprain and rheumatalgia. This plaster is a good one in common use for family and travelling.

Actions:
Anti-contusion, antiphlogistic, antioncotic, analgetic, anti-rheumatism, promoter blood circulation.

Indications:
Bruise & Sprain, Muscular Aching, Rheumatic Pains, Lumbago Backache, Arthritis Pains, Neuralgia and Sciatica etc.

Ingredients:
Moschus 0.03%, Mastix 2%, Myrrha 2%, Radix Pseudoginseng 2%, Flos Carthami 2%, Radix Sileris 5%, Herba Schizonepetae 5%, Radix Angelicae 5%, Rhizoma Kaempferiae 5%, Cortex Acant Radicis 5%, Rhizoma Drynariae 5%, Glechoma Hederacea 5%, Radix Angelicae Tuhuo 2%, Rhizoma Zingiberis 5%, Borneolum 2%, Oleum Caryophylli 0.5%, Oleum Cinnamomi 1%, Oleum Menthae 3%, Excipient add to 100%.

Instruction:
Remove the plaster from the sheet and stick it to the affected parts. Each sheet will be effective for 24 hrs.

Safety considerations:
Notice: Not recommended for pregnant women due to its strong effects.

Price: 1 pack (5 plaster sheets) — $1.90

Manufacturer:
Not indicated, but is Product of China.

Imported by:
Winlykah Trading Block 8, Lorong Bakar Batu #06-09 Singapore 348743.

117.   **Hua Tuo Rheutatism (Medicking)**

Description:
According to the secret prescriptions from Chan San Feng of "Wu Tam", Tien-Chi Feng-Shi Die-Da Jing is mainly used for the treatment of muscles Bruise and Sprain, Rheumatism Pains, Lumbago Backache, Arthritis Pain, Infeammation of the shoulder.

Indications:
Rheumatism, ostalgia, muscular pain, lumbago, shoulder and neck stiffness, rheumatic neuralgia, arthritis, sprain and contusion, muscular tension and sprain due to over-exercise.

Ingredients:
Ingredients: desorbed in 70 ml per bottle. *Herba Adenosma Glutinosum Druce* 2.33 gm, *Caulis Trachelospermi* 2.92 gm, *Cortex Acanthopanacis* 3.15 gm, *Rhizoma Homalomenae* 2.57 gm, *Caulis Piperis Kadsurae* 2.57 gm, *Oleum Menthae* 0.93 gm, *Radix Notoginseng* 8.12 gm, *Pamulis Mori* 2.92 gm, *Flos Caryopyii* 0.35 gm, *Semen Dryobalanops Aromatica* 2.33 gm, *Cinnamomum Camphora* 0.93 gm, *Oleum Eucalyoli* 0.58 gm, *Oleum Gaultheriae* 0.58 gm, *Ramulus Zanthoxylum* 2.33 gm, Alcohol 49 gm, Distilled Water 35 gm.

Application: Sprays sufficient quantity evenly on the affected part 2–3 times daily, or more when needed.

Price: 70 c.c Spray Action — $8.40

Manufacturer:
Wuzhou Yunshan Pharm. Fty. Guangxi, CHINA.

Singapore Importer:
Winlykah Trading. Blk 1 Alexandra Distripark #06-03 Singapore 118478

118.   **Hua Tuo Zhen Tong Ding Pain Relieving Tincture (Medicking)**

Indications:
Anti-contusion, Bruise & Sprain, Muscular Pain, Stiff Neck and Shoulder, Backache, Arthritic Pains, Rheumatism.

Ingredients:

Composition: (Formula in 30 ML)- *Panax Notoginseng* 10 gm, *Radix Salviae Miltiorrhizae* 16 gm, *Myrrha* 10 gm, *Olibunum Boswellia Carterii* 12 gm, *Oleum Methyl Salicylate* 5 ml, *Oenothera Erythrosepala Borb.* 10 gm, *Flos Rosae Rugosae* 10 gm, *Pericarpium Citri Reticulatae* 8 gm, *Mentholum* 5 gm, *Herba Siegesbeckiae* 14 gm, Alcohol 22 ml.

Instruction:

To apply and rub the affected area, 2–3 times a day. Applying after hot compress will be more effective.

Safety considerations:

Not recommended for pregnant women. Keeps out of reach of children. Do not apply to irritated skin.eyes, mucous membranes or wounds.

Price: 30 ml — $3.20 (sealed)

Manufacturer:

Changshu City Hyginic Chemical Fty. Jiangsu, China.

Imported by:

Winlykah Trading Blk 8 Lorong Bakar Batu #06-09 Singapore 348743

119. **Huiji® Fish Essence with American Ginseng, Cordyceps & Radix Astragali (Huiji)**

Description:

This product is made from fresh Black Fish and high quality American Ginseng, Cordyceps, Radix Astragali, etc using advanced technology. It contains the natural goodness of protein, amino acid and minerals which are easily absorbed by the body. It is suitable for consumption after an illness, an operation, pre/post-pregnancy, working adults and students during exam period. It boasts of excellent health benefits for people of all ages.

Ingredients:

Essence of Black Fish (54.88 ml), Caramel (0.14 ml), Extract of herbs (14.98 ml) (which includes: American Ginseng (7.5 g), Cordyceps (3.5 g), Radix Astragali (5 g), Dried Longan Pulp (4 g), Radix Codonopsitis (5 g)

Dosage:

Adults — 1 bottle; Children — half bottle; 70 ml × 6

Price: $18.00

Manufacturer:
Huay Feng Hang Pte Ltd. Blk 623, Aljunied Road #06-08, Aljunied Industrial Complex Singapore 389835; Tel: 6748; Fax: 6744 0283; Email: sales@huiji.com.sg; Product of China

120. **Huiji® Waist Tonic; Chongcao, Shouwu, Duzhong Bu Yao Jing (Cordycep, Polygonum Multiflorum and Eucommia Ulmoides Waist Tonic) (Huiji Brand)**

Description:
The Huiji Cordycep, Polygonum Multiflorum and Eucommia Ulmoides Waist Tonic is made according to ancient prescriptions improved through repeated research by modern physicians. It consists of selected precious Chinese herbs such as Cordyceps, Eucommia Ulmoides, Polygonum Multiflorum, Dates etc. extracted through one of the most meticulous refining methods. Mild in nature and fragrant in scent, this product has excellent effects. If taken regularly, it can strengthen the body and the waist, invigorate vital energy and blood. It is pure herbal preparations, and has no known side-effects and no known contraindication.

Actions and Indications:
Nourishes vital energy and "zhongjiao" nourishes the blood and promotes the production of the body fluid. Suitable for physical weakness, palpitation and dizziness caused by weakness in "qi" and blood.

Safety considerations:
No known side effects and contraindications.

Ingredients:
Each 100 ml of this product contains extracts equivalent to: Cordyceps Sinensis (500 mg), Radix Polygoni Multiflor Preparata (5000 mg), Cortex Eucommiae (1000 mg), Radix Angelicae Sinensis (14 gm), Radix Ginseng (6 gm), Fructus Jujubae (30 gm)

Dosage:
Taken orally, 10–20 ml each time, 2–3 times a day.
Price: 250 ml — $18.90

Manufacturer:
AnHui FuKang Pharamceutical Co Ltd. An Hui, China; Email: sales@huiji.com.sg;

Imported and Repacked: Huay Feng Hang Pte Ltd., Blk 623 Aljunied Road 206-08, Aljunied Industrial Complex, Singapore 389835; Tel: 67489211; Fax: 6744 0283.

121. **Hwal Sam 28 D [6 Year Old Korean Red Ginseng] (Korea Ginseng Corp)**

Details:

No information available

Ingredients:

Water, Fructose, Caramel Syrup, Mixed herbal Extract (Ginger extract, Jujube extract, Schizandra fruit extract, Lycium Fruit extract, Astragali extract), Korean Red Ginseng Extract, Taurin, Citric acid, Poly sorbate 80, Flavour 26-4399, Trisodium citrate, Nicotinamide, Flavor 26-4397, Thiamine Hydrochloride, Riboflavin 5'-phosphate Sodium. Origin: South Korea

Dosage:

Adult: Take 1 bottle one or two times daily. Children under 15: Take on half of the adult serving.

Safety considerations:

Caution: Edges at opening may be sharp.

Price: $48

Manufacturer:

Korea Ginseng Corporation 926 Dunsan-dong, Seo-gu, Daejeon, Korea.

Imported by:

Wing Joo Loong Ginseng Hong (S) Co Pte Ltd. 31 North Canal Road (S) 059287

122. **Hwal Sam 28D (Korea Ginseng Corp.)**

Details:

No information available

Ingredients:

Water, Fructose, Caramel Syrup, Mixed herbal Extract (Ginger extract, Jujube extract, Schizandra fruit extract, Lycium Fruit extract, Astragali extract), Korean Red Ginseng Extract, Taurin, Citric acid, Poly sorbate 80, Flavour 26-4399, Trisodium citrate, Nicotinamide, Flavor 26-4397, Thiamine Hydrochloride, Riboflavin 5'-phosphate Sodium. Oringin: South Korea

Dosage:

Suggested use: Adult: Take 1 bottle one or two times daily. Children under 15: Take on half of the adult serving.

Safety considerations:

Caution: Edges at opening may be sharp.

Price: 10 bottles × 100 ml — $21.00 (sealed)

Manufacturer:
Korea Ginseng Corporation 926 Dunsan-dong, Seo-gu, Daejeon, Korea.

Imported by:
Wing Joo Loong Ginseng Hong (S) Co Pte Ltd. 31 North Canal Road (S) 059287

123.   **Hwal-Sam 28 (50 ml × 10) (Korea Ginseng Corp.)**

Details:
No information available

Ingredients:
Korean Red Ginseng Extract, Astragalus Root Extract, Ginger Extract, Schisandra Fruit Extract, Lycium Fruit Extract, Jujubae Extract, Cervil Parvum Tinc, Taurin, Nicotinamide, Pyridoxine Hydrochloride, Fructose, Starch Syrup, Caramel, Acidity Regulator: INS #330, INS #331 (iii), Color: INS #101 (ii), Emulsifier, Stabilizer: Polysorbate 80, Flavor: No.2 26-4397, No. 3 26-4399, Purified water.

Dosage:
No information available

Price: $48

Manufacturer:
Korean Ginseng Corporation. 926 Dunsan-dong, Seo-gu, Daejeon.

Sole Agent:
Wing Joo Loong Ginseng Hong (S) Co Pte Ltd. 30 & 31 North Canal Road, Singapore 059286.

124.   **Il Hwa Korean Ginseng Capsules (Il Hwa Co. Ltd)**

Description:
These capsules offer nutritive value of ginseng in a quick, convenient form. They contain finely ground ginseng powder which is manufactured through careful selection and processing of the best quality Korean ginseng roots, the specialty of the Republic of Korea.

Ingredients:
Net weight: Korean Ginseng Powder (100%) 500 mg.

Dosage:
Take 2 capsules a day.

Price: 50 × 500 mg capsules — $33.00; 100 × 500 mg capsules — $60.00 (Sealed)

Manufacturer:
Ilwah Co., Ltd. 437 Sutaek-Dong, Guri- Si, Gyeonggi-Do, Korea.

Imported by:
Tongil(S) Pte Ltd. 113 Eunos Avenue 3 #05-04 Gordon Industrial Building Singapore 409838 tel:68424344

125. **Il Hwa Korean Ginseng Extract (Il Hwa Co. Ltd)**

Details:
No information available

Ingredients:
Korean Ginseng Extract (solid: more than 60%)

Directions:
Put one spoonful of this Korean ginseng extract into a cup of hot or cold water, and add sugar or honey to taste. Stir well.

Price: 50 g — $99.00; 30 g — $63.00; 100 g — $190.00. (all sealed)

Manufacturer:
Ilwah Co., Ltd. 437 Sutaek-Dong, Guri- Si, Gyeonggi-Do, Korea.

Imported by:
Tongil Singapore Pte Ltd. 14 Arumugam Road #03-01F Lion Building C Singapore 409959. http://www.buyginseng.com.sg. Tel: (65) 67422151, Fax: (65) 67422935. Address for 100 g- Tongil Singapore Pte Ltd 61 Club Street Singapore 069436. Tel: 65-67593020, Fax: 65-67596779

126. **Il Hwa Korean Ginseng Powder (Il Hwa Co. Ltd)**

Description:
Il Hwa Korean Ginseng Powder is a delicious food product which can be enjoyed anytime. The powder form is manufactured from the best quality of raw materials carefully selected among Korean ginseng roots, the speciality of the Republic of Korean.

Actions:
Boost immunity, Combat fatigue.

Ingredients:
Panax Ginseng 100%

Directions:
Put one or two spoonfuls of this Il Hwa Korean Ginseng Powder into one cup of hot or cold water, add sugar or honey to taste and stir well. Mixing with some other beverage is recommended.

Safety considerations:
Side effects and contraindications not known.
Price: 50 g — $60.00 (sealed)

Manufacturer:
Ilwah Co., Ltd. 437 Sutaek-Dong, Guri- Si, Gyeonggi-Do, Korea.

Imported by:
Tongil Singapore Pte Ltd. 14 Arumugam Road #03-01F Lion Building C Singapore 409959. http://www.buyginseng.com.sg. Tel: (65) 67422151, Fax: (65) 67422935.

127.   **Il Hwa Korean Ginseng Tea (Il Hwa Co. Ltd.)**
Details:
No information available

Ingredients:
Ginseng Extract (18%), Anhydrous Dextrose (54%), Lactose (28%)

Instruction:
Put the contents inside one packet into a cup of hot or cold water and add sugar or honey for the better taste. Then stir it well.
Price: 90 g (3 g × 30) — $42.00

Manufacturer:
Il Hwa Co Ltd. 437 sulaek-Dong, Guri-St, Gyeonggi-do, Korea;

Distributed by:
Tongil (S) Pte. Ltd., 14 Arumugam Road #03-01F Lion Building C Singapore 409959; Tel: (65) 6742 2151; Fax: (65) 6742 2935;

128.   **Il Hwa Korean Honeyed Ginseng (Il Hwa Co. Ltd.)**
Description:
This honeyed ginseng is a health food which can appeal to everyone. It is Korean ginseng in its original taste and is one of the special products of Korea. This honeyed ginseng is made of only carefully selected raw ginseng roots which are permeated by pure honey. It is one of the best products, and the harmony of the raw ginseng with honey offers a delicate natural taste. Before eating, you may remove the hard top part

of the root if you prefer. When it was hardened, put into the hot water or microwave oven for a moment with the packaged condition and have it when it is soften.

Ingredients:
(in Korean)

Dosage:
No information available

Price: 300 g — $338.00

Manufacturer:
Not stated

129. **Ilex Pubescens Heart Health Capsules (Nature's Green)**

Description on PIL:
Ilex Pubescens Heart Health Capsules are used for maintaining a healthy heart function based on a herbal remedy reccognized by Chinese health authorities. This product can effectively relieve heart disease with the symptoms of a feeling of extreme pressure on the chest, heart pain, palpitation, shortness of breath, mental fatigue, or asthmatic breathing.

Actions and Indications:
Promotes blood circulation and alleviates heart pain. Relieves heart disease with the symptoms of chest distension, heart pain, palpitation, shortness of breath, mental fatigue, or asthmatic breathing.

Ingredients:
Each 470 mg capsule contains extracts equivalent to raw herbs: *Radix Ilicis Pubescentis* 2380 mg, *Radix Notoginseng* 120 mg, *Radix Salviae Miltiorrhiae* 90 mg, *Flos Carthami* 90 mg, *Herba Siegesbeckiae* 480 mg, *Lignum Dalbergiae Odoriferae* 30 mg, *Borneolum Syntheticum* 6 mg

Dosage:
For oral administration, 3 capsules each time, 3 times daily.

Safety considerations:
Side effects not known. Contraindicated for pregnant women (not on packaging for 60 capsules but on PIL).

Price: 60 capsules — $10; 300 capsules — $44 (sealed bottle)

Manufacturer:
Tong Jum Chew Pte Ltd 21 Kaki Bukit View Tech Park II Singapore 415957 tel: 62781134 Fax: 6278 1246. Singapore Manufacturer Licence No. MLCP 0400040 Singapore CPM Product Reference No. 113601

130. **Indigestion Relief Granules (Nature's Green)**

Actions and Indications:
Regulates the functions of spleen and stomach. Used for dyspepsia, abdominal distention and loose stools.

Ingredients:
Each dosage (5 g) contains extracts equivalent to raw herbs: *Rhizoma Atractylodis Macrocephalae* 400 mg, *Rhizoma Dioscoreae* 400 mg, *Poria* 400 mg, *Semen Nelumbinis* 400 mg, *Massa Fermentata Medicinalis* 320 mg, *Radix Ginseng* 200 mg, *Pericarpium Citri Reticulatae* 200 mg, *Fructus Crataegi Praeparata* 200 mg, *Fructus Hordei Germinatus* 200 mg, *Rhizoma Alismatis* 200 mg, *Radix Glycyrrhizae* 200 mg.

Dosage:
For oral administration, take 5 g with warm water, 2–3 times daily.

Safety considerations:
Side effects not known. Avoid raw, cold and spicy food.

Price: 100 g — $9.50 (Sealed)

Manufacturer:
Tong Jum Chew Pte Ltd. 21 Kaki Bukit View Tech Park II Singapore 415957. Tel: 62781134 Fax: 62781246. Singapore Manufacturer Licence No. MLCP 0400040 Singapore CPM Product Reference No.: 117137.

131. **Indigestion Relief Tablets (Nature's Green)**

Description:
PIL: Indigestion is a common gastrointestinal problem. It may be triggered by particular foods, eating too fast or overeating, especially after a holiday meal or party. Some people may find that spicy, high-fibre, or fatty foods can all aggravate this problem. Indigestion Relief Tablets are based on a classical Chinese herbal prescription and made into concentrated tablets with modern pharmaceutical technology. It provides herbal support for indigestion and symptomatic relief of abdominal fullness, loss of appetite and diarrhea.

Actions and Indications:
Regulates the functions of spleen and stomach. Used for dyspepsia, abdominal distention and loose stools.

Ingredients:
Each 420 mg tablet contains extracts equivalent to raw herbs: *Radix Ginseng* 100 mg, *Rhizoma Atractylodis Macrocephalae* 100 mg, *Rhizoma Dioscoreae*

100 mg, *Poria* 100 mg, *Semen Nelumbinis* 100 mg, *Pericarpium Citri Reticulatae* 50 mg, *Fructus Crataegi Preparate* 50 mg, *Fructus Hordei Germinatus* 50 mg, *Massa Fermentata Medicinalis* 80 mg, *Rhizoma Alismatis* 50 mg, *Radix Glycyrrhizae* 50 mg.

Dosage:
For oral administration, take 4 tablets, 2–3 times daily.

Safety considerations:
Side effects not known (on PIL of 60 tablets). On the packaging of 500 tablets.

Price: 60 tablets — $6.00; 500 tablets — $29.00 (not sealed). Contraindications/ Cautions: Avoid raw, cold and spicy food. (on PIL of 60 tablets); Contraindication: Avoid raw, cold and spicy food. (on package of 500 tablets).

Manufacturer:
Tong Jum Chew Pte Ltd. 21 Kaki Bukit View Tech Park II Singapore 415957. Tel: 62781134 Fax: 62781246. Singapore Manufacturer Licence No. MLCP 0400040, Singapore CPM Product Reference No. 113371

132.   **Ji Gong Musk Plaster plus pseudoginseng (Mei Hua Brand)**

Actions:
On the internal packaging: Relieving rheumatism and activating blood circulation dispersing swelling and bruise, penetrating intraculaneous tissue with high efficacies.

Indications:
Anti-rheumatism, anti-contusion, anti-neuralgia, Relieving pain and swelling, efficacious for back, leg and muscular aching. On internal packaging: Wounds and conlusions, rheumatic pain, arthritis, muscular aching, numbness in limb, sciatica etc.

Ingredients:
Radix Pseudoginseng 25%, Flos *Cartiami* 8%, *Mastic* 7%, *Myrrh* 5%, *Cortex Acanthopanacis* 7%, *Aquilaria Sinensis* 5.5%, *Radix Ledebouriellae* 7.8%, Cinnamomum Oil 12.2%, *Daemonorops Draco* 4.5%, Ilex Oil 18%.

Instruction:
Wash and dry affected part. Remove the transparent paper and apply the Plaster on affected area. It is more effective when applying after bath.

Safety considerations:
1. Do not apply on abdomen during pregnancy. 2. In case of rheumatic pain due to deficiency of blood and energy. Mei Hua Brand Shu Jin Huo Wo Plan can be jointly administered with the Plaster to reinforce efficacies.

Price: 1 box (5 plasters) — $2.20

Manufacturer:
Made in Chongqing, China.

Sole Agent:
Science Arts Co. Pte Ltd.

133.   **Ji Gu Cao Wan (Yulin)**

Description:
PIL in package: Ji Gu Cao Wan is of pleasant taste and mild in nature. The clinical experiments prove that it is good for removing toxic heat, relieving the depressed liver and alleviating pain.

Actions and Indications:
Clearing Liver, beneficial to bile, cantidote and anodyne, inflammation

Ingredients:
Each capsule (500 mg) contains extract equivalent to raw herbs: *Herba Abri* 714 mg, *Radix Notoginseng* 380 mg, *Herba Origani Vulgaris* 309 mg, *Herba Artemisiae Scopariae* 286 mg, *Radix Paeoniae Alba* 238 mg, *Fructus Lycii* 190 mg, *Fructus Gardeniae* 143 mg, *Fructus Jujubae* 135 mg, *Calculus Bovis* (Synthetic) 119 mg, *Fel Suillus* 76 mg, *Tartrazine* (Lemon Yellow) 0.295 mg

Dosage:
3 times a day; for adults 4 capsules each time and for children reduce half the dosage. Take with boiled water

Safety considerations:
Do not use during pregnancy.

Price: 50 capsules — $6.00. Not sealed.

Assembler & importer:
Kinhong (Pte) Ltd 297 Kaki Bukit Ave 1, Shun Li Industrial Park, Singapore 416083.

Manufacturer:
Guangxi Yulin Pharmaceutical Co., Ltd. Yulin, Guangxi, China

134.   **Jin Li Bao Highly concentrated capsule (Win Brand)**

Description:
PIL: The product is based on the guidance of the Chinese medicinal theory. The therapeutic effect of tonifying, invigorating the vital organ, replenishing the vital

energy, building up the physique by using essential invigorating tonics in the traditional medicinal way. The meticulous preparation of extracting from the valuable natural medicinal materials by the modern advance technology. It is mainly for the male consumers and has a tonic action that remarkably enhances and improves the vital energy.

Actions and Indications:
Tonifying, invigorating the vital energy, building up the physique and preserving the body functions. It is a product for the male consumers.

Ingredients:
Each 350 mg capsule contains extract equivalent to raw materials — *Radix Ginseng* 50 mg, *Cornu Cervi Pantotrichum* 2 mg, *Testis Et Penis Bovis* 50 mg, *Testis Et Penis Canis* 50 mg, *Herba Epimedii* 226 mg, *Radix Rehmannie Praeparatae* 65 mg.

Dosage:
2 capsules each time, twice a day, morning and bedtime. May take 2 more if needed.

Safety considerations:
No known side effects (PIL). Not for children, the pregnancy and sthenic heat syndrome.

Price: 0.35 g × 24 capsules — $18.40 (not sealed. PIL available)

Manufacturer:
Wuhu Brain Pharmaceutical Co. Ltd. Anhui, China.

Imported by:
Wideway Pte Ltd. 2 Kallang Ave. #06-07 Kallang Bahru Complex Singapore 339407. Tel: 62923618 Fax: 62966956.

135. **Jing Pei Rou Gu Cha Xiang Liao (Chwee Song)**

Details:
No information available

Ingredients:
Astragalus Menbranaceus, Polygonatum Odoratum, Ligusticum Chuan Xiong, Cinnamomum Cassia, Ginseng, Angelica Sinensis, Foeniculum Vulgare, Glycyrrhiza Uralensis.

Cooking instructions:
Boil ingredients together with 1000 ml of water for 20 minutes. Marinate 500 gm of spare ribs with pepper, top grade dark soya for an hour. Add marinated spare ribs

into soup, add in some cloves of garlic, peppercorns, mushroom and cook under low fire for an hour. Ready to serve.

Price: 30 g — $2.00

Packed by:
Chwee Song supplies Pte Ltd., Blk 5, Ang Mo Kio Ind'l Park 2A Tech II; #07-14 to 16 Singapore 567760; Tel: 65-6482 3935, 6482 3386; Fax: 65-6778 5028; Website: http://www.chweesong.com.sg; E-Mail: sales@chweesong. com.sg.

136.   **Jingu Dieshang Capsule (Science Arts)**

Description:
Science Arts Jingu Dieshang Capsule composed of ingredients which provide the healing properties of strengthening the bones and meridians, dispersing blood stasis and activating blood circulating. There are also herbs that helps to eliminate inflammation, reduce swelling and relieve pain. Science Arts Jingu Dieshang Capsule is commonly used for injuries, sprains and strain of ligaments. It is effective for damaged muscular tissues, swellings and bruises caused by physical injuries. The product also provides remedial actions against arthritis.

Actions:
Activating blood circulation to remove blood stasis, expelling swelling and relieving pain.

Indications:
Effective for all types of injuries, sprain, strain and damaged muscular tissues. Disperse bruises, relieve pain and stiffness and to promote mobility. Also beneficial to sufferers of arthritis.

Ingredients:
Each 0.3 g capsule contains raw herbs. *Radix Notoginseng* 23.40 mg, *Sanguis Draxonis* 48.86 mg, *Myrrha* 23.40 mg, *Radix Angelicae Sinensis* 46.76 mg, *Radix Dipsaci* 46.86 mg, *Flos Carthami* 46.86 mg, *Radix Paeoniae Alba* 70.35 mg, *Radix Paeoniae Rubra* 70.35 mg, *Rhizoma Sparganii* 46.86 mg, *Fructus Aurantii Immaturus* 46.86 mg, *Semen Persicae* 46.86 mg, *Herba Artemisiae Anomalae* 46.86 mg, *Lignum Sappan* 46.86 mg, *Radix Saposhnikoviae* 46.86 mg, *Radix Platycodi* 46.86 mg, *Rhizoma CUrcumae Longae* 46.86 mg.

Dosage:
4 capsules each time, three times daily, to be taken with warm water.

Safety considerations:

Side effects not known (not on the packaging for 30 capsules but PIL available). Not recommended for pregnant women (not on the packaging for 30 capsules but PIL available).

Price: 30 capsules — $7.80; 300 capsules — $68 (PIL available).

Manufacturer:

Science Arts Co Pte Ltd. 150 MacPherson Rd, Science Arts Building Singapore 348524

137. **JingZhi WuJi RenShen Bai Feng Wan (Shan Cheng Brand)**

Description:

PIL: Shan Cheng Brand WUJI RENSHEN BAI FENG WAN is a high-value medicine for the treatment of gynecological diseases especially anemia and feebleness. The pills contain Radix Ginseng and prepared Radix Rehmanniae etc. These selected herbs are presented in the form of honeyed bolus preserved in wax shell which are convenient for storage. It is effective in the treatment of general weakness, anaemia, abdominal pains with distention, vague aching in the loins, weak legs, night sweat resulted from deficiency of body-essence, postpastum anaemina and paleness. Administration of the pills over a long term period will enrich the vital energy and blood, build up resistance to diseases and maintain a fresh youthful look. Additionally, it can be an ingredient in soups providing a rich flavour without affecting the curative effect.

Indications:

General weakness, Anaemia, Abdominal pain with distention, Vague aching in the loins, Weak legs, Night sweat result from deficiency of body — essence, Postpastum anaemina and pleness. PIL: General Weakness, Weak Appetite, Insomnia, Amnesia, Weakness in pregnancy to serves illness, Fatigue due to excessive.

Ingredients:

Each pill 6 g contains: *Pullus Cum Osse Nigro* 978 mg, *Radix Salviae Miltiorrhizae* 196 mg, *Radix Ginseng* 196 mg, *Radix Paeoniae Alba* 196 mg, *Rhizoma Cyperi* (processed with vinegar) 196 mg, *Radix Angelicae Sinensis* 220 mg, *Radix Et Rhizome Glycyrrhizae* 49 mg, *Concha Ostreae* (praeparata) 73 mg, *Colla Cornu Cervi* 196 mg, *Ootheca Mantidis* 73 mg, *Radix Rehmanniae Praeparata* 390 mg, *Radix Astragali* 49 mg, *Cornu Cervi Degelatinatum* 73 mg, *Radix Stellariae* 40 mg, *Semen Euryales* (stir-baked) 98 mg, *Rhizoma Dioscoreae* 196 mg, *Radix Rehmanniae* 390 mg, *Carapax Trionycis* (processed) 98 mg, *Radix Asparagi* 98 mg, *Rhizoma Chuanxiong* 98 mg, *Mei* 2097 mg.

Dosage:

6 g each time. 2 times daily. Take with lukewarm water. PIL: Administration: For general health, two or three times weekly, one pill each time. For women suffering from gynecological diseases of anemia and feebleness, two pills daily during morning and evening warm water.

Safety considerations:

No known side effects. PIL: Caution: Avoid taking Raw or Cold food. Not suitable for pregnant ladies.

Price: 6 g — $6 (not sealed)

Manufacturer:

GuangZhou ChenliJi Pharmaceutical Factory.

Imported & Packed by:

Tai Chong Fatt Medical Hall Blk 9005, Tampines Street 93, #04-236 S(528839).

Sole Agent:

Yu Lian Medical Hall Blk 1004, Toa Payoh Industrial Park, #01-1485/1487, S(319076)

138.   **Joint Movement Ease Tablets (Nature's Green)**

Actions:

Promotes blood circulation, to remove blood stasis.

Indications:

Used for traumatic injuries, lumbago, lower back pain or soreness, pain or stiffness of muscles and joints.

Ingredients:

Each 360 mg tablet contains extracts equivalent to raw herbs: *Flos Carthami* 30 mg, *Sanguis Dracanis* 30 mg, *Radix Notoginseng* 100 mg, *Rhizoma Cyperi Praeparata* 100 mg, *Rhizoma Cibotii Praeparata* 140 mg, *Cortex Periplocae* 70 mg, *Caulis Trachelospermi* 100 mg, *Herba Lycopodii* 100 mg, *Herba Lycopi* 100 mg, *Caulis Spatholobi* 100 mg, *Herba Visci* 140 mg, *Pyritum Praeparata* 20 mg.

Dosage:

For oral administration, take 4 tablets, 3 times daily.

Safety considerations:

Side effects not known. Not to be taken by pregnant women.

Price: 500 tablets — $42

Manufacturer:
Tong Jum Chew Pte Ltd. 21 Kaki Bukit View Tech Park II Singapore 415957. Tel: 62781134 Fax: 62781246. Singapore Manufacturer No: MLCP 0400040 Singapore CPM product reference number: 116351.

139. **Joint Pain Relieving Tablets (Nature's Green)**

Description on PIL:
Joint pain is the inflammation of one or more joints and is characterized by pain, swelling, stiffness, and dimished range of motion. Joint Pain Relieving Tablets are made from highly concentrated, selected Chinese herbs and produced in accordance to a traditional Chinese formula. It is the typical prescription that maintains joint health, and helps relieve the symptoms of constant or recurring pain in the joints, swelling in one or more joints, stiffness around the joints, spasm of limbs, and heavy feeling and ache of the body caused by arthritis or rheumatism.

Actions and Indications:
Relieves pain, swelling and stiffness of the joints, spasm of limbs, and heavy feeling and ache of the body caused by arthritis.

Ingredients:
Each 410 mg tablet contains extracts equivalent to raw herbs: *Cortex Eucommiae* 125 mg, *Radix Angelicae Pubescentis* 125 mg, *Radix Dipsaci* 125 mg, *Radix Achyranthis Bidentatae* 125 mg, *Radix Gentianae Macrophyllae* 125 ng, *Radix Saposhnikoviae* 125 mg, *Radix Ginseng* 125 mg, *Radix Astragali* 125 mg, *Radix Angelicae Sinensis* 125 mg, *Rhizoma ChuanXiong* 125 mg, *Radix Paeoniae Alba* 125 mg, *Radix Rehmanniae* 125 mg, *Poria* 125 mg, *Cortex Cinnamomi* 125 mg, *Radix Asari* 125 mg, *Radix Gltcyrrhizae* 125 mg, *Rhizoma Zingiberis Recens* 125 mg, *Fructrs Jujubae* 125 mg

Dosage:
For oral administration, take 4 tablets, 3 times daily.

Safety considerations:
Side effects not known (not on the packaging of 60 tablets but on PIL). Not to be taken by pregnant women (not on packaging of 60 tablets but on PIL).

Price: 60 tablets — $7 (not sealed); 500 tablets — $43 (sealed)

Manufacturer:
Tong Jum Chew Pte Ltd 21 Kaki Bukit View Tech Park II Singapore 415957 Tel: 62781134 Fax:62781246 Singapore Manufacturer Licence No. MLCP: 04000400 Singapore CPM Product Reference No.: 117326

140.   **JointCare Sport Glucosamine Plus Omega-3 Plus Chondroitin, Vitamins, Minerals & Herbs [30 capsules] (Seven Seas)**

Description:

SEVEN SEAS JointCare Sport Glucosamine Plus Omega-3 Fish Oil plus chondroitin, vitamins, minerals and herbs is a multi-nutrient capsule specially developed by Jane Griffin, a leading sports dietician to help maintain a healthy body however you exercise. Choose this if you want... — Extra help to maintain supple and flexible body, however you exercise. — Glucosamine, Omega-3, chondroitin, vitamins, minerals and herbs in one convenient capsule. — A sports supplement formulated by a leading sports dietician. SEVEN SEAS JointCare Sport and Health In nearly every aspect and at nearly every level, taking part in sport and exercise promotes a healthy body and mind. But it is one of life's paradoxes that sport and exercise can make heavy demands on the body, especially the joints. Developed with the knowledge and advice of leading sports dietician, Jane Griffin, and acceptability tested by world class sports players, SEVEN SEAS JointCare Sport capsules contain a unique blend of Glucosamine, Chondroitin, Omega-3, vitamins, minerals and herbs to help you keep supple and flexible before and after exercise. Glucosamine lays down the foundation for the everyday rebuilding of the connective tissues around the joints, including tendons, ligaments and cartilage. Omega-3 are important fatty acids. As well as their important role in keeping joints supple and flexible, they are also proven to maintain heart health and healthy circulation. Chondroitin is present in cartilage and connective tissue and is involved in the attraction of fluid that lubricants the joints. Chondroitin may be obtained from the diet but is present in only a small number of foods. Vitamins, minerals and herbs found in JointCare Sport have been specially selected to help maintain an active body and a healthy immune system.

Ingredients:

Vitamin E 10 mg α-TE, Calcium 270 mg, Iron 14 mg, Zinc 15 mg, Selenium 50 ug, Beta-carotene 4 mg, Omega- 3 nutrients 200 mg, Gamma Linolenic Acid (GLA) 10 mg, Glucosamine Sulphate 2 KCl 540 mg, Chondroitin Sulphate 10 mg, Ginger Extract 4 mg Equivalent to Ginger Root 12 mg, Ginseng Extract 7.4 mg Equivalent to Ginseng Root 20 mg. Ingredients: Capsule Shell (Gelatin, Glycerol, Sorbitol Syrup, Colours, Iron Oxides), Calcium Carbonate, Glucosamine Sulphate 2KCl[1], Cod Liver Oil, Fish Oil, Soya Bean Oil, Vegetable Oil, Chondroitin Sulphate Prep. (Sodium Chondroitin Sulphate, Hydrolyzed Proteins)[2], Emulsifier: Soya Lecithin, Mono-and Diglycerides of Fatty Acids, Beeswax. Starflower (Borage) Oil, Ferrous Fumarate, ZInc Sulphate, Vitamin E, Beta Carotene (Corn Oil, Beta Carotene, DL Alpha Tocopherol), Fish Oil Concentrate (Triomega), Ginseng Extract (Ginseng Extract, Maltodextrin, Colloidal Silica), Ginger Extract prep. (Magnesium

Carbonate, Maize Starch, Dextrin, Ginger Extract, Magnesium Oxide), Sodium Selenite. 1- From Shellfish. 2- From Fish

Dosage:
Recommended Adult Daily Intake: Two capsules with a cold drink each day. Do not exceed the recommended intake.

Safety considerations:
Women who are pregnant or planning a pregnancy should consult their doctor before taking vitamin or mineral supplements. Food supplements are intended to supplement the diet and should not be regarded as a substitute for a varied diet & a healthy lifestyle.

Price: 30 capsules — $29.50

Distributed by:
Zuellig Pharma Pte Ltd. 15 Changi North Way #01-01 Singapore 498770. Tel No.: 65468188.

141. **Joy Tall Capsule (Xian Chau)**

Description:
Nutritional support for growing children.

Ingredients:
Each capsule contains: *Radix Scutellariae* 200 mg, *Fructus Crataegi* 200 mg, *Fructus Alpiniae Oxyphyllae* 100 mg, *Poria* 100 mg, *Fructus Lycii* 100 mg, *Fructus Ziziphi Jujubae* 100 mg, *Radix Notoginseng* 80 mg, *Calcium Lactas* 40 mg, *Zinci Gluconas* 0.6 mg.

Dosage:
8–12 years, 2 pills once, three times a day. 12 years and above, 4 pills once, three times a day, take orally with boiled water or fruit juice.

Safety considerations:
No known side effects or contraindications.

Price: 100 capsules — $41.20 (Sealed)

Manufacturer:
Hainan Phoenix International Pharmaceutical Co. Ltd. Hainan Phoenix Pharmaceutical Factory, China.

Importer:
Chung Kuo Refined Chinese Medicine Dealers Ltd. 554, Haveolck Road, Ganges Centre, #09-00, Singapore 169639.

142. **900 Kang Yan Bao Jia Wei Wan (Cotton Plant)**

Actions:

Clear away blood stasis, promote blood circulation, clear toxic materials, relieve pain. Promote blood immunity, enhance metabolism, strengthen physique, antibacterial, enrich vital energy.

Indications:

Suitable for Inflammation, blood stasis, enhance "qi" and blood flow, rheumatism. coarse skin, skin disease, infection and coughing.

Ingredients:

Each capsule contains raw herbs 344 mg as below: *Herba Hedyotis Diffusae* 85.50 mg, *Semen Pruni* 16.60 mg, *Herba Andrographitis* 19.90 mg, *Herba Scutellariae Barbatae* 19.90 mg, *Radix Glehniae* 19.90 mg, *Pseudobulbus Cremastrae Seu Pleiones* 13.30 mg, *Folium Isatidis* 19.90 mg, *Massa Medicata Fermentata* 16.60 mg, *Sargassum* 9.80 mg, *Herba Dianthi* 13.30 mg, *Semen Persicae* 13.30 mg, *Rhizoma Sparganii* 19.90 mg, *Fructus Gardeniae* 6.50 mg, *Radix Notoginseng* 19.90 mg, *Radix Angelicae Dahuricae* 19.90 mg, *Radix Stemonae* 6.50 mg, *Radix Linderae* 13.30 mg, *Radix Aucklandiae* 8.30 mg, *Camphora* 1.70 mg.

Dosage

Take 5 capsules, 1–2 times daily.

Safety considerations:

No known side effect. Avoid use in pregnant women.

Price: 160 capsules — $80.00 (sealed)

Manufacturer:

Yi Shi Yuan Pte Ltd (GMP Manufacturer) No. 20, Bukit Batok Crescent #13-11/12/13 Enterprise Centre Singapore 658080 Tel: 65670900 Fax: 65672256.

143. **Kidney Health Tablets (Nature's Green)**

Description:

PIL: According to traditional Chinese medicine, deficiency of the kidney can cause fluid to accumulate in the tissues, leading to edema in the face, arms, legs, and feet. Kidney Health Tablets are made from 13 highly concentrated, selected Chinese herbs based on the classical Chinese herbal prescription and prepared by modern pharmaceutical technology. This product is the typical formulation that has satisfactory effect in relieving the symptoms of pitting edema in the limbs and face, soreness and pain in the lower back and loins, lassitude of extremities, sensation of heaviness in the knees, dizziness, vertigo, tinnitus, and abnormal urination due to deficiency of the kidney. As a herbal supplement, it is used as a special tonic for weakened kidneys, reduces water retention and alleviates edema, therefore making it beneficial for maintaining healthy kidney function.

Actions and Indications:
Nourishes kidney and alleviates edema. Helps relieve the symptoms of pitting edema in the limbs and face, soreness and pain in the lower back and loins, lassitude of extremities, sensation of heaviness in the knees, dizziness, vertigo, tinnitus, and abnormal urination due to deficiency of the kidney.

Ingredients:
Each 460 mg tablet contains extracts equivalent to raw herbs: *Radix Panacis Quinquefolii* 80 mg, *Radix Ginseng* 60 mg, *Cortex Eucommiae* 150 mg, *Radix Rehmanniae Preparata* 150 mg, *Radix Astragali* 150 mg, *Rhizoma Dioscoreae* 100 mg, *Radix Salviae Miltiorrhiae* 100 mg, *Herba Hedyotidis Diffusae* 150 mg, *Rhizoma Smilacis Glabrae* 150 mg, *Herba Leonuri* 150 mg, *Rhizoma Alismatis* 200 mg, *Rhizoma Imperatae* 200 mg, *Radix Platycodi* 60 mg.

Dosage:
For oral administration, take 5 tablets, 3 times daily. The recommended treatment course is one month.

Safety considerations:
Side effects not known (on packaging of 500 tabs and on PIL of 60 tabs). 1.Limit salt (sodium) intake. 2. Avoid greasy, fatty, pungent or spicy food. 3. Avoid peanut, soybean and its products. 4. Used with caution for pregnant women.

Price: 60 tablets — $ 8.50 (not sealed-PIL available); 500 tablets — $ 50.00 (sealed bottle)

Manufacturer:
Tong Jum Chew Pte Ltd. 21 Kaki Bukit View Tech Park II Singapore 415957. Tel: 62781134 Fax: 62781246. Singapore Manufacturer Licence No. MLCP: 0400040 Singapore CPM Product Reference No. 113845

144. **Korean Red Ginseng (Korea Ginseng Corp.)**
Details:
(in Korean)

Ingredients:
(in Korean)

Dosage:
(in Korean)

Price: 37.5 g (1.32 OZ) — $180.00

Manufacturer:
(in Korean)

145. **Korean Red Ginseng Extract (Korea Ginseng Corp.)**

Actions and Indications:
Enhance immune system and strengthen your body.

Ingredients:
6-year-old Korean Red Ginseng (Panax Ginseng) Extract 100 g (Equivalent to 142 g of raw ginseng) Origin: South Korea

Dosage:
Take 1 g per serving three times a day, take with water.

Safety considerations:
Side effects and contraindications not known.

Price: 100 g — $176.00 (Sealed)

Manufacturer:
Korea Ginseng Corporation 926 Dunsan-dong, Seo-gu, Daejeon, Korea.

Imported by:
Wing Joo Loong Ginseng Hong (S) Co Pte Ltd. 31 North Canal Road (S) 059287.

146. **Korean Red Ginseng Extract Capsule- Gold (Korea Ginseng Corp.)**

Details:
No information available

Ingredients:
6-Year-Old Korean Red Ginseng Extract Powder, Wheat germ oil, Grape seed oil, Palm oil, Beeswax, Lecithin, d-alpha-Tocopherol, Gelatine, Glycerine, Ethyl Vanillin, Food Color (Cochineal Extract, Gardenia Blue, Gardenia Yellow). 2 capsules: Korean Red Ginseng Extract Powder 420 mg.

Dosage:
Suggested use: As a dietary supplement, Take 2 capsules per serving 3 times a day. Drink with water. Take half of adult dosage for children under the age of 15.

Price: 100 capsules (60 g): $72 (sealed)

Manufacturer:
Korea Ginseng Corporation 926 Dunsan-dong, Seo-gu, Daejeon, Korea.

Imported by:
Wing Joo Loong Ginseng Hong (S) Co Pte Ltd. 31 North Canal Road (S) 059287

147. **Korean Red Ginseng Extract Pill (Korea Ginseng Corp.)**
Details:
No information available

Ingredients:
Korean Red Ginseng Extract, Rice Powder (as binder), Fructo-oligoaccharide, Microcrystalline, L-Ascorbic acid, dl-alpha-tocopherol. 5 pills → Korean Red Ginseng Extract 417 mg

Dosage:
Suggested use: as a dietary supplement, Take 5 pills per servings 3 times a day. Drink with water. Take half of adult dosage for children under the age of 15.

Price: 168 g — $86.00 (sealed)

Manufacturer:
Korea Ginseng Corp. Daejun, Seo-Ku, Dunsan- Dong 926. Made in Korea.

Sole distributor:
Wing Joo Loong Ginseng Hong (S) Co Pte Ltd. 31 North Canal Road (S) 059287. Tel: 65383838. Fax: 65342800.

148. **Korean Red Ginseng Extract Powder Tea (Korea Ginseng Corp.)**

Details:
No information available

Ingredients:
Lactose, 6-Year-Old Korean Red Ginseng Extract, Jujube Extract

Dosage:
No information available

Price: 3 g × 50 packs (150 g) — $75.00

Manufacturer:
Korea Ginseng Corp. (www.kgc.or.kr) 926, Dunsan-dong, Seo-gu, Daejeon, Korea;

Sole Authorized Distributor:
Wing Joo Loong Ginseng Hong (S) Co Pte Ltd 30 & 31 North Canal Road, Singapore 059286; Tel: 6538-3838; Fax: 6534-2800.

149. **Korean Red Ginseng Kid Tonic (Korean Red Ginseng)**

    Details:
    No information available

    Ingredients:
    Purified water, Cyclodextrin syrup, Crystalline fructose, Korean red ginseng extract, Deer antler extract, Agave syrup, Honey, Angelicae gigantis extract, Sea shell calcium, Pear extract, Casein phosphopeptide, Gamma cyclodextrin, Vitamin C, Yogurt flavor, Citric acid anhydrous, Nicotinamide, Germinated brown rice extract, Inositol, L-carnitine, Gellan gum, Trisodium citrate, Vitamin B2, Vitamin D3.

    Dosage:
    No information available

    Price: 15 ml × 30 packs — $175.00

    Manufacturer:
    Korea Ginseng Corporation 926 Dunsan-dong, Seo-gu, Daejon, Korea.

    Imported by:
    Wing Joo Loong Ginseng Hong (S) Co. Pte Ltd. 31 North Canal Road (S) 059287.

150. **Korean Red Ginseng Powder (Korea Ginseng Corp.)**

    Details:
    No information available

    Ingredients:
    6-year-old Korean Red Ginseng (*Panax Ginseng*) Powder 60 g. Origin: South Korea.

    Dosage:
    Take 1 g per serving three times a day with water.

    Safety considerations:
    Side effects and contraindications not known.

    Price: 60 g — $52.00 (sealed)

    Manufacturer:
    Korea Ginseng Corporation 926 Dunsan-dong, Seo-gu, Daejeon, Korea.

    Imported by:
    Wing Joo Loong Ginseng Hong (S) Co Pte Ltd. 31 North Canal Road (S) 059287.

151. **Korean Red Ginseng Powder Capsule (Korea Ginseng Corp.)**

Details:

No information available

Ingredients:

6-year-old Korean Red Ginseng (*Panax Ginseng*) Powder 42 g. Origin: South Korea.

Dosage:

Take 2 capsules per serving three times a day.

Safety considerations:

Side effects and contraindications not known.

Price: 42 g (84 capsules) — $45 (sealed)

Manufacturer:

Korea Ginseng Corporation 926 Dunsan-dong, Seo-gu, Daejeon, Korea.

Imported by:

Wing Joo Loong Ginseng Hong (S) Co Pte Ltd. 31 North Canal Road (S) 059287.

152. **Korean Red Ginseng Tablet (Korea Ginseng Corp.)**

Details:

No information available

Ingredients:

6-year-old Korean Red Ginseng (*Panax Ginseng*) Powder 60 g. Origin: South Korea.

Dosage:

Take 2 tablets per serving three times a day with water.

Safety considerations:

Side effects and contraindications not known.

Price: 60 g (120 tablets) — $56.00

Manufacturer:

Korea Ginseng Corporation 926 Dunsan-dong, Seo-gu, Daejeon, Korea.

Imported by:

Wing Joo Loong Ginseng Hong (S) Co Pte Ltd. 31 North Canal Road (S) 059287.

153. **Korean Red Ginseng Tea (Il Hwa Co. Ltd.)**

Description:

Korean Red Ginseng Tea is made by extracting the major constituents of Korean Red ginseng roots, special products of Korea. Pure Red ginseng extract is mixed with dextrose anhydrous and dried at a low temperature to make the best Korean Red ginseng tea products, having an original flavor and taste just like the fresh Red ginseng roots themselves.

Ingredients:

(in Korean)

Instruction:

Put the contents inside one packet into a cup of hot or cold water, add sweetener or honey to taste and stir well.

Price: 150 g (3 g × 50) — $54.00

Manufacturer:

Il Hwa Co Ltd. 437 sulaek-Dong, Guri-St, Gyeonggi-do, Korea.

Distributed by:

Tongil (S) Pte. Ltd., 14 Arumugam Road #03-01F Lion Building C Singapore 409959; Tel: (65) 6742 2151.

154. **Korean Red Ginseng Tea (Korea Ginseng Corp.)**

Details:

No information available

Ingredients:

Glucose anhydrous, 6-Year-Old Korean Red Ginseng Extract, Lactose, Jujube extract, Ascorbic acid.

Dosage:

No information available

Price: 3 g × 50 packs (150 g) — $32.00

Manufacturer:

Korea Ginseng Corp. (www.kgc.or.kr) 926, Dunsan-dong, Seo-gu, Daejeon, Korea.

Sole Authorized Distributor:

Wing Joo Loong Ginseng Hong (S) Co Pte Ltd 30 & 31 North Canal Road, Singapore 059286; Tel: 6538-3838; Fax: 6534-2800.

155. **Korean Red Ginseng Tonic (Korean Ginseng Corp.)**

Details:
(in Korean)

Ingredients:
(in Korean)

Dosage:
No information available

Price: 40 ml × 10 — $90.00

Manufacturer:
No information available

156. **Korean Red Ginseng Tonic gold (Korean Ginseng Corp.)**

Details:
(in Korean)
(in Korean)

Dosage:
No information available
40 ml × 30 (1,200 ml) — $230.00

Manufacturer:
No information available

157. **Korean Red Ginseng Women Balance (Korean Red Ginseng)**

Details:
No information available

Ingredients:
Germ oil, Korean Red Ginseng Extract, Palm oil, Korean Angelica Extract, Cnidii Rhizoma Extract, Peony Root Extract, Atractylodes Rhizome Extract, Hoelen Extract, Lophatheri Herbal Extract, Yellow Beeswax, Trucal D-50(milk mineral complex D50), Fujiflavone, d-α-Tocopherol, Cholecalciferol, Gelatin, Glycerin, Titanium Dioxide, Ethyl Vanillin, Food Color (Red 40, Yellow 5, Blue 1).

Dosage:
As a Dietary supplement, Take 2 capsules per serving 3 times a day. Drink with water. Take half of adult dosage for children under the age of 15.

Price: 1.79 OZ (51 g, 60 Capsules)/Box × 3, 3 for $158.40

Manufacturer:
Korea Ginseng Corp., Dacjun. Seo-Ku, Dunsan-Dong 926.

Sole Authorized Distributor:
Wing Joo Loong Ginseng Hong (S) Co Pte Ltd. 3D & 31 North Canal Road, Singapore Q59286; Tel: 6538-3838; Fax: 6534-2800.

158. **Korean White Ginseng Root 500 mg (Ginseng Gold)**

Description:
Product Features: Each capsule contains 500 mg Korean White Ginseng Root Extract standardied to provide 3% Ginsenosides (15 mg). Provides assured intake of Ginsenosides, responsible for Korean White Ginseng's efficacy. Ideal for people who leads active and demanding lifestyle. Suitable for vegetarian. Benefits: Traditionally used to support vitality and overall well-being. As adaptogen, it particularly promotes Yang energy which stimulates functions of the central nervous system, brain and circulatory system. Maintains mental alertness hence enable one to concentrate and maintain a sharp mind. Aids recovery from weakness after illness.

Ingredients:
Supplement Facts: Serving Size 1 capsules. Servings per container 90. Amount per serving (%DV) Korean White Ginseng Root Extract 500.00 mg ** (*Panax Ginseng*) (3% Ginsenosides = 15 mg) ** Daily Value (DV) not established. Other Ingredients: Vegetable Cellulose capsule. No Sugar, No Starch, No Artificial Color, No Artificial Flavors, No Wheat, No Gluten, No Corn, No Soy, No Dairy, Yeast Free.

Safety considerations:
Warning: Consult your physician prior to using this product if you are pregnant, nursing or taking medication, or have a medical condition. Discontinue use two weeks prior to surgery.

Dosage:
As a dietary supplement, take one or two capsules daily.

Price: 90 vcaps — $39.95

Manufacturer:
No information available

159. **7 Leaf Ginseng Natural Health Tea (100% Pure Amachazuru Tea) (nil)**

Description:
7-Leaf Ginseng Herbal Tea is specially selected from high grade plant called *Gynostemma Pentaphyllum* Makino, known in Japan as Amachazuru. It is also

widely known as The 2nd Ginseng due to its similar frame structures and contains Sapponins as found in Korean Ginseng, plus abundance of Amino Acids, Vitamins A, E and B complex, calcium, iron, phosphorus, sodium, potassium, etc. Regular drinking will enhance the body's immunological function and improves blood circulation. 7-Leaf Ginseng Herbal Tea is 100% natural. It does not contain any artificial flavours, colours, sweeteners, caffeine, or any addictives.

Ingredients:
Gynostemma Pentaphyllum — 100%

Dosage:
Daily: 1–3 cups

Instruction:
Put one tea bag in a cup of hot water (500 cc). Steep it for 2–3 minutes. Drink it hot or cold.

Safety considerations:
Regular drinking will not cause any side effects. Containdications not known.

Price: 25 × 2 g — $6.10

Manufacturer:
Fujian Longhai Zhengfa Foodstuffs Co. Ltd., Longhai, China

Assembled by:
Chiah Huat (Int'l) Pte Ltd., 705 Sims Drive 06-16A Shun Li Industrial Complex Singapore 387384; Tel: (65) 6844 0233; Fax: (65) 6844 0323

160. **Lipid Health (QianJin)**

Description:
Balances blood lipid at healthy level. For healthy blood functions

Actions and Indications:
Regulates blood lipid, improves blood circulation. Removes stasis, prevents atherosclerosis.

Ingredients:
Each 300 mg of capsule contains the following: *Folium Gemmae Camelliae Sinensis* 30 mg, *Radix Et Rhizoma Seu Caulis Acanthopanacis Senticosi* 15 mg, *Fructus Crataegi* 30 mg, *Semen Raphani* 25 mg, *Folium Nelumbinis* 20 mg, *Radix Puerariae* 20 mg, *Flos Chrysanthemi* 30 mg, *Radix Astragli* 15 mg, *Rhizoma Polygonati* 15 mg, *Radix Rehmanniae Praeparata* 20 mg, *Cortex Eucommiae* 20 mg, *Radix Salviae Miltiorrhizae* 15 mg, *Radix Et Rhizoma Notoginseng* 15 mg, *Flos Sophorae* 15 mg, *Herba Taxilli* 15 mg.

Dosage:
Oral administration: 3 capsules 3 times daily.

Safety considerations:
No known side effects. Not to be taken by pregnant woman.

Price: 50 capsules — $7.50 (not sealed-No PIL)

Manufacturer:
Kiat Ling Health Products & Trading Blk 3017 Bedok North St 5 #04-15 Singapore 486121. Tel: 67441868, Fax: 67435267.

161. **Lipid Health Capsules (Nature's Green)**

Description:
PIL: High blood lipid levels (elevated blood lipid levels) can increases the risk of developing heart disease for middle aged and elderly persons. Lipid Health capsules are made from 6 precious natural herbs based on the classical Chinese herbal prescription and prepared by modern pharmaceutical technology. This product helps to lower blood lipids and prevent the risk for heart disease. It can be used by the middle aged and elderly as a health-care supplement for adjusting high blood lipid levels and maintain healthy blood function.

Actions and indication: Clears waste and decreases blood-lipid. Relieves the symptoms of dizziness, chest distress and dry stool caused by high blood lipid levels

Ingredients:
Each 500 mg capsule contains extracts equivalent to raw herbs: *Rhizoma Alismatis* 500 mg, *Fructus Crataegi* 500 mg, *Semen Cassiae* 500 mg, *Radix Notoginseng* 60 mg, *Folium Nelumbinis* 100 mg.

Dosage:
For oral administration, take 3 capsules, 3 times daily.

Safety considerations:
Side effects not known (not on the packaging for 60 capsules). Avoid fried and greasy foods. Use with caution for pregnant women. (not on packaging for 60 capsules).

Price: 300 capsules — $43; 60 capsules — $10 (sealed)

Manufacturer:
Tong Jum Chew Pte Ltd 21 Kaki Bukit View Tech Park II Singapore 415957 Tel: 62781134 Fax: 62781246 Singapore Manufacturer Licence No. MLCP 0400040 Singapore CPM Product Reference No. 114202.

162. **Lipid Health Tablets (Nature's Green)**

Description:

PIL: Elevated blood lipid levels can increases the risk of developing heart disease for middle aged and elderly persons. Lipid Health tablets are made form 12 precious herbs based on the classical Chinese herbal prescription and prepared by modern pharmaceutical technology. This product helps to lower blood lipids, promote blood flow, improve microcirculation and prevent the risk for heart disease. It can be used by the middle aged and elderly as a health-care supplement for adjusting high blood lipids levels.

Actions and Indications:

Enhances healthy blood circulation and removes blood stasis. It helps reduce blood lipid levels, improve microcirculation and maintain healthy blood function.

Ingredients:

Each 460 mg tablet contains extracts equivalent to raw herbs: *Radix Polygoni Multiflori Preparata* 150 mg, *Radix Notoginseng* 60 mg, *Rhizoma Polygonati* 100 mg, *Radix Puerariae* 200 mg, *Radix Salviae Miltiorrhiae* 200 mg, *Fructus Crataegi* 200 mg, *Semen Cassiae* 100 mg, *Rhizoma Alismatis* 100 mg, *Radix Angelicae Sinensis* 50 mg, *Rhizoma Chuanxiong* 50 mg, *Herba Epimedii* 50 mg, *Cortex Acanthopanacis* 50 mg.

Dosage:

For oral administration, take 4 tablets, 3 times daily.

Safety considerations:

Side effects not known. Avoid fried and greasy foods. Use with caution for pregnant and nursing women.

Price: 500 tablets — $45; 60 tablets — $8 (SE and CI not on packaging but included in PIL)

Manufacturer:

Tong Jum Chew Pte Ltd 21 Kaki Bukit View Tech Park II Singapore 415957 Tel: 62781134 Fax: 62781246. Singapore Manufacturer No: MLCP 0400040 Singapore CPM product reference number: 113974.

163. **Lu Wie Ba Bai Jiu (Snow Mountain)**

Description:

Cauda Cervi Tonic Wine; Lu Wie Ba Bu Jiu is prepared from the extraction of Cauda Cevi, i.e. the tail of female deer (Cerrus Nippon). a speciality of Hun Chun in Northeastern China. as main material with support of adequate other precious

Chinese medicines. Cornu Cervi Parvum Ligamentium Cervi, Radix Ginseng, Radix Astragali, Poria, Fructus Lycii and Radix Polygalae macerated in pure Kao — liang wine for a long time. (Action: A nutrient and roborant for improving health, strengthening the sinew and bone, increasing vigour, bracing up energy, regulating blood curculation and prolonging life. The thick matter or sediment, if any found in the wine, is the effective elements of drugs and by no means deterioration.

Ingredients:
Cauda Cervi (20%), Cornu Cervi Parvum (15%), Ligamentium Cervi (15%), Radix Ginseng (15%), Radix Astraagali (10%), Poria (10%), Fructus Lycii (10%), Radix Polygaiae (5%).

Dosage:
No information available

Price: 500 ml; Alc. 35% — $24.00

Manufacturer:
Heilongjiang Province Yimianpo Health Brewery China.

Importers:
Kim Sing Co. Pte Ltd. 54 Genting Lange #01-01 Singapore 349562.

164.   **Lumbar Waist Care (QianJin)**

Actions and Indications:
Strengthen ligaments. Relieve sciatica and lumbar muscular strain. Indicated with pain in the lower back or hip areas, limb pain or numbness, inflexible joint movement etc.

Ingredients:
Each 300 mg of capsule contains the following: *Fructus Chaenomelis* 40 mg, *Radix Angelicae Sinensis* 15 mg, *Rhizoma ChuanXiong* 30 mg, *Radix Angelicae Dahuricae* 20 mg, *Radix Clematidis* 25 mg, *Rhizoma Cibotii* 30 mg, *Radix Achyranthis Bidentatae* 30 mg, *Caulis Spatholobi* 25 mg, *Caulis Piperis Kadsurae* 25 mg, *Radix Ginseng* 20 mg, *Radix Angelicae Pubescentis* 20 mg, *Nodus Pini* 20 mg.

Dosage:
Oral administration: 4 capsules 3 times daily.

Safety considerations:
No known side effect. Not to be taken by pregnant woman; avoid taking cold food.

Price: 50 capsules — $7.50 (No PIL)

Manufacturer:
Kiat Ling Health Products & Trading Blk 3017 Bedok North St 5 #04-15 Singapore 486121 Tel: 674418668 Fax: 67435267.

165. **Maodongqing Compound Capsules (Mei Hua Brand)**

Description:
PIL: Meihua Brand Maodongqing compound capsules is made of maodongqing, Radix Salviae miltiorrhizae and Radix Notoginseng. It has the function to invigorate the circulation of blood. Lower the force of obstruction in the artery.

Actions:
To invigorate the circulation of blood, to improve the flow of blood in the coronary artery.

Ingredients:
Each capsule 300 mg contains: *Radix Ilicics Pubescentis* 180 mg, *Radix Salviae Miltiorrhizae* 60 mg, *Radix Notoginseng* 60 mg.

Dosage:
Four capsules to be taken 3 times a day.

Safety considerations:
Side effects not known (Not on packaging for 30 capsules but in PIL). For those who are allergic to certain herbal products or pregnant women. Please seek advice from medical professional before taking. (Not on packaging of 30 capsules but in PIL).

Price: 30 capsules — $ 7.80; 300 capsules — $68

Manufacturer:
Science Arts Co Pte Ltd 150 MacPherson Rd, Science Arts Building Singapore 348524.

166. **Mei Kuei Lu Chiew (Double Dog Brand)**

Details:
No information available

Ingredients:
Water, Sorghum, Ginseng, Sugar, Rose.

Dosage:
No information available

Price: 7, 05 for 150 ml

Manufacturer:
Asia Brewery (Xiamen) Ltd., Product of China.

Imported by:
ANGLEONG HUAT (PTE) LTD:, 330 Circuit Road, Singapore 379488.

167.   **Memore (Ocean Health)**

Description:
Specially formulated to help enhance optimal mental performance, concentration & alertness throughout the day. Features & Benefits — Ginkgo Biloba → enhance concentration and alertness. Korean Ginseng → enhance reflexes and reduce tiredness. Lecithin and fish oil → nourish the body and assist in thinking ability. Gurana Seed → maintain overall alertness, adding vitality and a general feeling of well-being.

Ingredients:
Ginkgo Biloba Dry Leaf 500 mg, Lecithin 210 mg, Korean Ginseng 50 mg, Fish Oil (DHA + EPA) 100 mg, Gurana Seed 100 mg (contains no added sugar, gluten, artificial flavors or preservatives).

Dosage:
Adults: Take 2 soft gels daily in the morning after meal, or as prescribed by your doctor.

Price: 60 capsules — $20.50 (Sealed)

Manufacturer:
21st Century HealthCare Inc., 2119 S. Wilson Street, Tempe, Arizona 85282-2034 USA.

Distributed by:
21st Century HealthCare Pte Ltd. 40, Jalan Pemimpin #03-02 Tat Ann Building Singapore 577185.

168.   **Men Tonic Capsule (Keyi)**

Actions:
To warm and invigorate kidney-yang, replenish qi and promote the production of body fluid, replenish essence and marrow, and reinforce the spleen to promote yang.

Indications:
It is indicated for syndrome of insufficient kidney-yang and decline of fire in gate of life, marked by kidney deficiency and mental fatigue from senility or protracted

diseases, soreness and weakness of the waist and knees, seminal emission, yang deficiency, urine dribbling after micturition, pale tongue with whitish fur, deep and feeble pulse and with above symptoms.

Ingredients:
Each capsule (400 mg) contains extracts equivalent to raw herbs: *Radix et Rhizoma Ginseng* 33.33 mg, *Rhizoma Curculiginis* 166.67 mg, *Herba Epimedii* 166.67 mg, *Cortex Cinnamomi* 16.67 mg, *Fructus Lycii* 166.67 mg, *Semen Cuscutae* 166.67 mg, *Fructus Rubi* 166.67 mg, *Fructus Schisandrae Chinensis* 166.67 mg, *Semen Plantaginis* 166.67 mg, *Bombyx Masculus* 33.33 mg.

Dosage:
Oral administration, 3 capsules each time, 2 times a day.

Safety considerations:
Side effects not known (only on the bottle of 300 capsules. Not indicated on the packaging of 60 capsules). Precaution: 1. Stop administration if symptom of dry throat occurs. 2. Be cautious about patient suffering from common cold. 3. Avoid pungent and irritant food. (Only on the bottle of 300 capsules).

Price: 60 capsules — $50.00 (sealed); 300 capsules — $210.00 (sealed)

Manufacturer:
Science Arts Co Pte Ltd. 150 MacPherson Rd, Science Arts Building, Singapore 348524.

169. **Meno Comfort Granules (Nature's Green)**

Actions:
Nourishes heart and kidney.

Indications:
Relieves the symptoms of insomnia, forgetfulness, palpitation, tinnitus, doubting and worry, hectic fever, excessive sweating, irritability, liability to anger, weakness and lumbago due to menopausal syndrome.

Ingredients:
Each dosage (5 g) contains extracts equivalent to raw herbs: *Herba Epimedii* 500 mg, *Radix Polygoni Multiflori Preparata* 500 mg, *Caulis Polygoni Multiflori* 500 mg, *Concha Ostreae* 500 mg, *Semen Juplandis* 250 mg, *Fructus Psoraleae* 250 mg, *Radix Dipsaci* 250 mg, *Fructus Mori* 250 mg, *Semen Plantaginis* 250 mg, *Radix Angelicae Sinensis* 250 mg, *Radix Paeoniae Alba* 250 mg, *Fructus Rosae Laevigatae* 170 mg, *Radix Achyranthis Bidentatae* 170 mg, *Radix Ginseng* 100 mg, *Radix Rehmanniae Preparata* 140 mg, *Colla Cornus Cervi* 100 mg, *Rhizoma Anemarrhenae* 100 mg, *Radix Scutellariae* 100 mg, *Radix Glycyrrhizae* 100 mg.

Dosage:

For oral administration, take 5 g with warm water, 3 times daily.

Safety considerations:

Side effects not known. Not suitable for those suffering from flu. Avoid greasy or spicy foods.

Price: 100 g — $12.50 (sealed bottle)

Manufacturer:

Tong Jum Chew Pte Ltd. 21 Alexandra Distripark Blk. 1. #08-15/17 Pasir Panjang Road Singapore 118478. Tel: 62781134 (3 Lines) Fax: 62781246 Manufacturer Licence No. MLCP: 0400040 Singapore CPM Product Reference No. 117138.

170. **Men's SeniorVite (with Saw Palmetto & Lycopene) (21st Century)**

Description:

Each tablet contains a complete range of vitamins, minerals, herbs and nutritional supplements especially formulated to maintain good health and for energy, for men over 50. A vitamin to Zinc formula.

Ingredients:

Vitamins: Vitamin A 2500 IU, Vitamin B1 10 mg, Vitamin B2 10 mg, Vitamin B3 10 mg, Vitamin B5 10 mg, Vitamin B6 10 mg, Vitamin B12 25 mcg, Vitamin C 100 mg, Vitamin D 200 IU, Natural Vitamin E 50 IU. Ginseng: Korean Ginseng 50 mg, American Ginseng 25 mg. Minerals: Manganese 1.5 mg, Chromium 200 mcg, Potassium 5 mg, Copper 1 mg, Calcium 82 mg, Zinc 7.5 mg, Magnesium 25 mg, Selenium 100 mcg, Molybdenum 25 mcg. Herbs: Garlic (25:1 extract 60 mg) 1500 mg, Ginkgo Biloba (50:1 extract 5 mg) 250 mg, Saw Palmetto (4:1 extract 10 mg) 100 mg, Gymnema (10:1 extract 10 mg) 100 mg, Bitter Melon (4:1 extract 12.5 mg) 50 mg. Other Supplements: PABA 15 mg, Biotin 150 mcg, Folic Acid 400 mcg, Iodine 15 mcg, Choline 50 mg, Inositol 50 mg, dl-Methionine 50 mg, Omega 3 (EPA/DHA 7.5%) 7.5 mg, Zeaxanthan 250 mcg, Lutein 50 mg, Lysine 5 mcg, Lycopene 250 mcg, Grape Seed Extract 10 mg. Saw Palmetto: For prostate health and improved urination. Bitter Melon: For reducing the absorption of sugar in the body. Lutein: For better eye health and improved night vision. Lycopene: Powerful antioxidant

Dosage:

Take 2 tablets daily. 1 tablet to be taken in the morning after breakfast and the second tablets to be taken not less than 6 hours before going to bed at night. If you are satisfied with your daily energy level, reduce dosage to one tablet daily. However, if you feel that your energy level is low, then return to taking 2 tablets daily.

Price: 30 tablets — $20.30 (sealed)

Manufacturer:

21st Century HealthCare Inc., 2119 S. Wilson Street, Tempe, Arizona 85282-2034 USA.

Distributed by:

21st Century HealthCare Pte Ltd. 40, Jalan Pemimpin #03-02 Tat Ann Building Singapore 577185.

171. **Mind Relaxing (Keyi)**

Actions:

To reinforce Qi and replenish Yin, regulate Qi and blood, clear heart-fire to anchor the mind.

Indications:

Used for symptoms of palpitation, caused by Qi and blood deficiency of heart and kidney, stasis blocking of Heart Meridian, disharmony between the Qi and blood, restlessness, which are manifested as paroxysmal palpitation, shortness of breath and lacking on strength, constriction and pain in the chest, poor sleep and dreamness, spontaneous perspiration, night sweat, dark reddened or reddened tongue with thin fur, petechia and ecchymosis.

Ingredients:

Each capsule (400 mg) contains extracts equivalent to raw herbs: *Radix et rhizoma Ginseng* 120 mg, *Radix Asparagi* 600 mg, *Radix Ophiopogonis* 400 mg, *Fructus Schisandrae Chinensis* 360 mg, *Herba Taxilli* 1200 mg, *Fructus Corni* 400 mg, *Radix et Rhizoma Salviae Miltiorrizae* 600 mg, *Radix Paeoniae Rubra* 400 mg, *Radix Angelicae Sinensis* 600 mg, *Radix et Rhizoma Nardostachyos* 600 mg, *Semen Ziziphi Spinosae* 600 mg, *Os Draconis Praeparata* 600 mg, *Plumula Nelumbinis* 120 mg, *Rhizoma Smilacis Glabrae* 600 mg.

Dosage:

Oral administration, 3 capsules each time, 2 times a day. 4–8 weeks for a course of treatment; after relief of symptoms, continuously take 2–3 courses of half dose for some patients, or consult physician.

Safety considerations:

Side effects not known. PIL: Warning: 1.Contraindicated for pregnant. 2.Precaution is warranted in patients with known sensitivity to the drug. 3.Contraindicated for the people with abnormal

Price: 60 capsules — $20.00

Manufacturer:

Science Arts Co. Pte Ltd. 150 MacPherson Rd, Science Arts Builidng Singapore 348524.

172.   **Mixture Ba Zhen [HJ-032] (Sanjiu Enterprise Group)**

Actions and Indications:

To replenish qi and blood, used for deficiency of both qi and blood with sallow complexion, anorexia, lack of strength.

Ingredients:

Each 6 g contain extracts equivalent to raw herbs: *Radix Ginseng* 3.5 g, *Rhizoma Atractylodis Macrocephalae* 3.5 g, *Poria* 3.5 g, *Radix Angelicae Sinensis* 3.5 g, *Rhizoma Chuanxiong* 3.5 g, *Radix Paeoniae Alba* 3.5 g, *Radix Rehmanniae Preparata* 3.5 g, *Radix Glycyrrhizae Preparata* 1.9 g, *Rhizoma Zingiberis Recens* 1.2 g, *Fructus Jujubae* 2.3 g.

Dosage:

2–3 times a day, 6 g each time or as prescribed by Herbalist.

Safety considerations:

Side effects and contraindications not known. Avoid cold and spicy foods.

Price: 100 g — $26.00 (sealed)

Manufacturer:

Sanjiu Medical & Pharmaceutical Co. Ltd. Shenzhen, Guangdong, China.

Importer:

Kinhong Pte. Ltd. No. 297 Kaki Bukit Ave 1, Shunli Industrial Park S416083. Tel: 67415561.

173.   **Mixture Bai Zhu [HJ-075] (Sanjiu Enterprise Group)**

Actions:

To reinforce the function of spleen and the stomach.

Indications:

Used for the diminished function of the spleen and the stomach marked by anorexia and loose bowels, accompanied by shortness of breath, and lassitude.

Ingredients:

Each 6 g contain extracts equivalent to raw herbs: *Radix Ginseng* 6.2 g, *Herba Agastaches* 11.6 g, *Rhizoma Atractylodis Macrocephalae* 11.6 g, *Radix Aucklandiae* 4.6 g, *Poria* 11.6 g, *Radix Puerariae* 11.6 g, *Radix Glycyrrhizae* 2.4 g.

Dosage:
2–3 times a day, 6 g each time or as prescribed by Herbalist.

Safety considerations:
Side effects and contraindications not known.

Price: 100 g — $29.00 (bottle is sealed)
Manufacturer:
Sanjiu Medical & Pharmaceutical Co., Ltd. Shenzhen, Guangdong, China.

Importer:
Kinhong Pte. Ltd. No. 297, Kaki Bukit Ave 1, Shunli Industrial Park S416083. Tel: 67415561.

174. **Mixture Bu Zhong Yi Qi [HJ-079) (Sanjiu Enterprise Group)**

Actions:
Reinforcing the middle, benefiting qi and elevating yang to raise qi sinking.

Indications:
Qi deficiency syndrome of the spleen and stomach manifested by fever with perspiration, thirst with desire of warm drink, short breath and disinclination to talk, lassitude of the extremities; or loss of appetite, pale complexion, deficient and weak pulse.

Ingredients:
Each 6 g contain extracts equivalent to raw herbs: *Radix Ginseng* 6 g, *Rhizoma Atractylodis Macrocephalae* 6 g, *Radix Astragali* 18 g, *Radix Glycyrrhizae* 9 g, *Radix Angelicae Sinensis* 6 g, *Pericarpium Citri Reticulatae* 6 g, *Rhizoma Cimicifugae* 6 g, *Radix Bupleuri* 6 g.

Dosage:
1–2 times a day, 6 g each time or as prescribed by Herbalist.

Safety considerations:
No known side effects. Contraindicated in use with indigenous heat due to yin deficiency contra-indicated.

Price: 100 g — $25.00 (sealed)
Manufacturer:
Sanjiu Medical & Pharmaceutical Co. Ltd. Shenzhen, Guangdong, China.

Importer: Kinhong Pte. Ltd. No. 297 Kaki Bukit Ave 1, Shunli Industrial Park S416083. Tel: 67415561

175.   **Mixture Du Huo Ji Sheng [HJ-047] (Sanjiu Enterprise Group)**

Actions:
Dispel wind and dampness, relieve pain, reinforce the liver and kidney, nourish Qi and blood.

Indications:
For the wind-cold Bi syndrome due to deficiency of the liver and kidney and deficiency of Qi and blood, marked by cold pain in lumbar region and knee, limited mobility, flaccidity, numbness of joints, aversion to cold and desire for warmth, palpitation, short breath, pale tongue with white coating, thready weak pulse.

Ingredients:
Each 6 g contain extracts equivalent to raw herbs: *Radix Angelicae Pubescentis* 3.1 g, *Cortex Cinnamomi* 1.0 g, *Herba Taxilli* 2.1 g, *Radix Saposhnikoviae* 2.1 g, *Cortex Eucommiae* 2.1 g, *Rhizoma Chuanxiong* 2.1 g, *Radix Achyranthis Bidentatae* 2.1 g, *Radix Ginseng* 2.1 g, *Radix Asari* 1.0 g, *Radix Glycyrrhizae* 1.0 g, *Radix Gentianae Macrophyllae* 2.1 g, *Radix Angelicae Sinensis* 2.1 g, *Poria* 3.1 g, *Radix Paeoniae Alba* 2.1 g, *Radix Rehmanniae* 2.1 g.

Dosage:
2–3 times a day, 6 g each time or as prescribed by Herbalist.

Safety considerations:
Side-effects not known. Avoid cold and spicy foods. Contraindication not known.

Price: 100 g — $28 (sealed)

Manufacturer:
Sanjiu Medical & Pharmaceutical Co. Ltd. Shenzhen, Guangdong, China.

Importer:
Kinhong Pte Ltd. No. 297 Kaki Bukit Ave 1, Shunli Industrial Park S416083. Tel: 67415561.

176.   **Mixture Gui Pi [HJ-026] (Sanjiu Enterprise Group)**

Actions:
To invigorate the spleen function, nourish blood and cause sedation.

Indications:
Used for the deficiency syndrome of both heart and spleen marked by shortness of breath, cardiac palpitation, insomnia, dreamed-disturbed sleep, dizziness, lassitude, anorexia, or hematochezia.

Ingredients:
Each 6 g contain extracts equivalent to raw herbs: *Rhizoma Atractylodis Macrocephalae* 2.7 g, *Radix Aucklandiae* 1.8 g, *Sclerotium Poriae Circum Radicem Pini* 2.7 g, *Radix Glycyrrhizae Preparata* 0.9 g, *Arillus Longan* 3.6 g, *Radix Angelicae Sinensis* 2.7 g, *Radix Astragali* 3.6 g, *Radix Polygalae* 2.7 g, *Semen Ziziphi Spinosae* 3.6 g, *Rhizoma Zingiberis Recens* 0.9 g, *Radix Ginseng* 2.7 g, *Fructus Jujubae* 1.8 g.

Dosage:
2–3 times a day, 6 g each time or as prescribed by Herbalist.

Safety considerations:
Side effects and contraindications not known.

Price: 100 g — $32.00 (bottle is sealed)

Manufacturer:
Sanjiu Medical & Pharmaceutical Co., Ltd. Shenzhen, Guangdong, China.

Importer:
Kinhong Pte. Ltd. No. 297, Kaki Bukit Ave 1, Shunli Industrial Park S416083. Tel: 67415561.

177. **Mixture Liu Jun Zi [HJ-112] (Sanjiu Enterprise Group)**

Actions:
Replenishing qi to invigorate the spleen. Strengthen the spleen and to stop vomiting.

Indications:
Use for qi deficiency of the spleen and stomach accompanied by symptoms of phlegm and damp, clincal manifestations are poor appetite, nausea, vomiting, stuffy chest and abdomen, loose stool, white sputum.

Ingredients:
Each 6 g contain extracts equivalent to raw herbs: *Radix Ginseng* 6 g, *Pericarpium Citri Reticulatae* 6 g, *Rhizoma Atractylodis Macrocephalae* 12 g, *Rhizoma Pinelliae Preparata* 9 g, *Poria* 6 g, *Fructus Jujubae* 1 g, *Radix Glycyrrhizae* 6 g, *Rhizoma Zingiberis Recens* 1 g.

Dosage:
2–3 times a day, 6 g each time or as prescribed by Herbalist.

Safety considerations:
Side effects and contraindications not known.

Price: 100 g — $26.00 (bottle is sealed)

Manufacturer:
Sanjiu Medical & Pharmaceutical Co., Ltd. Shenzhen, Guangdong, China.

Importer:
Kinhong Pte. Ltd. No. 297, Kaki Bukit Ave 1, Shunli Industrial Park S416083. Tel: 67415561.

178.   **Mixture Mai Men Dong [HJ-115] (Sanjiu Enterprise Group)**

Actions:
Nourishing the lung and stomach, lowering the rebelliou qi and harmonizing the middle.

Indications:
Insufficiency of the lung-yin marked by cough with sticky phlegm or frothy sputum, dry mouth and throat, feverish sensation of the palms and soles. Insufficiency of the stomach-yin marked by vomiting, thirst, dryness of throat.

Ingredients:
Each 6 g contain extracts equivalent to raw herbs: *Radix Ophiopogonis* 30 g, *Rhizoma Pinelliae Preparata* 10 g, *Radix Ginseng* 6 g, *Radix Glycyrrhizae* 6 g, *Semen Oryzae Sativae* 5 g, *Fructus Jujubae* 1 g.

Dosage:
2–3 times a day, 6 g each time or as prescribed by Herbalist.

Safety considerations:
Side effects and contraindications not known. Avoid cold and spicy foods.

Price: 100 g — $45

Manufacturer:
Sanjiu Medical & Pharmaceutical Co., Ltd. Shenzhen, Guangdong, China.

Importer:
Kinhong Pte. Ltd. No. 297, Kaki Bukit Ave 1, Shunli Industrial Park S416083. Tel: 67415561.

179.   **Mixture Qing Zao Jiu Fei [HJ-041] (Sanjiu Enterprise Group)**

Actions:
Clear away dryness and moisten the lungs.

Indications:
Damage of the lung by warm-dryness, marked by headache, fever, dry cough, dyspnea, dry throat and nose, thirst, stiffness in the chest, dry tongue with less coating, forceless, big and rapid pulse.

Ingredients:
Each 6 g contain extracts equivalent to raw herbs: *Folium Mori* 9 g, *Gypsum Fibrosum* 8 g, *Radix Ginseng* 2 g, *Radix Glycyrrhizae* 3 g, *Semen Sesami* 3 g, *Colla Corii Asini* 3 g, *Radix Ophiopogonis* 4 g, *Folium Eriobotryae* 3 g, *Semen Armeniacae Amarum* 2 g.

Dosage:
2–3 times a day, 6 g each time or as prescribed by Herbalist.

Safety considerations:
Side effects and contraindications not known.

Price: 100 g — $33 (sealed bottle)

Manufacturer:
Sanjiu Medical & Pharmaceutical Co., Ltd. Shenzhen, Guangdong, China.

Importer:
Kinhong Pte. Ltd. No. 297, Kaki Bukit Ave 1, Shunli Industrial Park S416083. Tel: 67415561.

180. **Mixture Ren Shen Yang Rong [HJ-022] (Sanjiu Enterprise Group)**

Actions and Indications:
Benefit qi, enriches the blood, nourishes the heart and calms the mind, is indicated for visceral impairment by overstrain, exhibiting shortness of breath, dyspnea upon exertion, palpitation, dry throat and tongue.

Ingredients:
Each 6 g contain extracts equivalent to raw herbs: *Radix Paeoniae Alba* 2.2 g, *Radix Angelicae Sinensis* 3.3 g, *Pericarpium Citri Reticulatae* 2.2 g, *Radix Astragali* 4.4 g, *Cortex Cinnamomi* 1.1 g, *Radix Ginseng* 2.2 g, *Rhizoma Atractylodis Macrocephalae* 2.2 g, *Radix Glycyrrhizae Preparata* 1.1 g, *Radix Rehmanniae Preparata* 3.3 g, *Fructus Schisandrae* 2.2 g, *Poria* 3.3 g, *Radix Polygalae* 2.2 g.

Dosage:
2–3 times a day, 6 g each time or as prescribed by Herbalist.

Safety considerations:
Side effects and contraindications not known.

Price: 100 g — $30.00 (Sealed)

Manufacturer:

Sanjiu Medical & Pharmaceutical Co. Ltd. Shenzhen, Guangdong, China.

Importer:

Kinhong Pte. Ltd. No. 297 Kaki Bukit Ave 1, Shunli Industrial Park S416083. Tel: 67415561.

181.   **Mixture San Bi [HJ-072] (Sanjiu Enterprise Group)**

Actions:

To boost qi and nourish blood.

Indications:

Used for stagnant of blood and qi, marked by hands and feet hypotonicity, wind impediment, etc.

Ingredients:

Each 5 g contains extract equivalent to raw herbs: *Radix Dipsaci* 0.9 g, *Radix Saposhnikoviae* 0.9 g, *Herba Asari* 0.9 g, *Poria* 0.9 g, *Radix Paeoniae Alba* 0.9 g, *Radix Achyranthis Bidentatae* 0.9 g, *Radix Gentianae Macrophyllae* 0.9 g, *Rhizoma Chuanxiong* 0.9 g, *Rhizoma Zingiberis Recens* 0.9 g, *Cortex Eucommiae* 0.9 g, *Cortex Cinnamomi* 0.9 g, *Radix Ginseng* 0.9 g, *Radix Angelicae Sinensis* 0.9 g, *Radix Astragali* 0.9 g, *Radix Glycyrrhizae* 0.9 g, *Radix Pubescentis* 0.9 g, *Fructus Jujubae* 0.9 g, *Radix Rehmanniae* 0.9 g.

Dosage:

2–3 times a day, 5 g each time or as prescribed by Herbalist.

Safety considerations:

Side-effect not known. Used with caution in pregnancy.

Price: 100 g — $28 (sealed)

Manufacturer:

Sanjiu Medical & Pharmaceutical Co. Ltd. Shenzhen, Guangdong, China.

Importer:

Kinhong Pte. Ltd. No. 297 Kaki Bukit Ave 1, Shunli Industrial Park S416083. Tel: 67415561.

182.   **Mixture Shen Ling Bai Zhu [HJ-037] (Sanjiu Enterprise Group)**

Actions:

To reinforce the function of spleen and the stomach and replenish qi of the lung.

Indications:
Used for the diminished function of the spleen and the stomach marked by anorexia and loose bowels, accompanied by shortness of breath, cough and lassitude.

Ingredients:
Each 6 g contain extracts equivalent to raw herbs: *Semen Nelumbinis* 3.8 g, *Semen Coicis* 5.1 g, *Fructus Amomi* 5.1 g, *Radix Platycodi* 1.5 g, *Semen Lablab Album* 3.8 g, *Poria* 2.6 g, *Radix Ginseng* 2.3 g, *Radix Glycyrrhizae Preparata* 0.8 g, *Rhizoma Atractylodis Macrocephalae* 2.3 g, *Rhizoma Dioscoreae* 2.6 g.

Dosage:
2–3 times a day, 6 g each time or as prescribed by Herbalist.

Safety considerations:
Side effects and contraindications not known. Avoid cold and spicy foods.

Price: 100 g — $35 (bottle is sealed)

Manufacturer:
Sanjiu Medical & Pharmaceutical Co., Ltd. Shenzhen, Guangdong, China.

Importer:
Kinhong Pte. Ltd. No. 297, Kaki Bukit Ave 1, Shunli Industrial Park S416083. Tel: 67415561.

183. **Mixture Sheng Mai [HJ-127] (Sanjiu Enterprise Group)**

Actions and Indications:
Replenishing qi, promoting generation of body fluid, astringing yin and ceasing sweating.

Ingredients:
Each 6 g contain extracts equivalent to raw herbs: *Radix Ginseng* 3 g, *Radix Ophiopogonis* 12 g, *Fructus Schisandrae Chinensis* 6 g.

Dosage:
2–3 times a day, 6 g each time or as prescribed by Herbalist.

Safety considerations:
Side effects and contraindications not known.

Price: 100 g — $45 (sealed bottle)

Manufacturer:
Sanjiu Medical & Pharmaceutical Co., Ltd. Shenzhen, Guangdong, China.

Importer:
Kinhong Pte. Ltd. No. 297, Kaki Bukit Ave 1, Shunli Industrial Park S416083. Tel: 67415561.

184.   **Mixture Si Jun Zi [HJ 132] (Sanjiu Enterprise Group)**

Actions and indications:
Replenishing qi to invigorate the spleen Qi deficienct syndrome of the spleen and stomach with symptoms such as yellow complexion, low and weak voice, lassitude of limbs, poor appetite, loose stool, pale tongue, soft and weak pulse.

Ingredients:
Each 6 g contain extracts equivalent to raw herbs: *Radix Ginseng* 9 g, *Rhizoma Atractylodis Macrocephalae* 9 g, *Pori*a 9 g, *Radix Glycyrrhizae* 6 g.

Dosage:
2–3 times a day, 6 g each time or as prescribed by Herbalist.

Safety considerations:
Side effects and contraindications not known.

Price: 100 g — $29.00 (bottle is sealed)

Manufacturer:
Sanjiu Medical & Pharmaceutical Co., Ltd. Shenzhen, Guangdong, China.

Importer:
Kinhong Pte. Ltd. No. 297, Kaki Bukit Ave 1, Shunli Industrial Park S416083. Tel: 67415561.

185.   **Mixture Wan Dai [HJ-045] (Sanjiu Enterprise Group)**

Actions:
Strengthen the spleen, promote the circulation of the liver Qi, resolve dampness and relieve leukorrhagia.

Indications:
Leukorrhagia due to spleen deficiency. Manifested as white or light yellow and thin leukorrhea without smell, fatigue, loose stool, pale complexion, pale tongue with white coating, soft and weak pulse.

Ingredients:
Each 6 g contain extracts equivalent to raw herbs: *Rhizoma Atractylodis Macrocephalae* 8.4 g, *Rhizoma Dioscoreae* 8.4 g, *Radix Ginseng* 1.7 g, *Radix Paconiae Alba* 4.2 g, *Semen Plantaginis* 2.5 g, *Rhizoma Atractylodis* 2.5 g, *Radix*

Glycyrrhizae 0.8 g, *Pericarpium Citri Reticulatae* 0.4 g, *Herba Schizonepetae* 0.4 g, *Radix Bupleuri* 0.5 g.

Dosage:
2–3 times a day, 6 g each time or as prescribed by Herbalist.

Safety considerations:
Side effects and contraindications not known. Avoid cold and spicy foods.

Price: 100 g — $27.00 (sealed)

Manufacturer:
Sanjiu Medical & Pharmaceutical Co. Ltd. Shenzhen, Guangdong, China.

Importer:
Kinhong Pte. Ltd. No. 297 Kaki Bukit Ave 1, Shunli Industrial Park S416083. Tel: 67415561.

186. **Mixture Xiang Sha Liu Jun Zi [HJ-012] (Sanjiu Enterprise Group)**

Actions:
To replenish qi, invigorates the function of the spleen and regulate the function of the stomach.

Indications:
Used for the diminished function of the spleen with the stagnation of qi marked by dyspepsia, belching, anorexia, epigastric and abdominal distension and loose bowels.

Ingredients:
Each 6 g contain extracts equivalent to raw herbs: *Radix Ginseng* 5.0 g, *Rhizoma Atractylodis Macrocephalae* 5.0 g, *Poria* 5.0 g, *Radix Glycyrrhizae* 2.5 g, *Pericarpium Citri Reticulatae* 2.5 g, *Rhizoma Pinelliae* 5.0 g, *Fructus Amomi* 2.5 g, *Radix Aucklandiae* 2.5 g.

Dosage:
2–3 times a day, 6 g each time or as prescribed by Herbalist.

Safety considerations:
No known side effects. Precaution: Incompatible with pungent and oil foods; use with caution during pregnancy. Not stated on package.

Price: 100 g — $29.00 (bottle is sealed)

Manufacturer:
Sanjiu Medical & Pharmaceutical Co., Ltd. Shenzhen, Guangdong, China.

Importer:
Kinhong Pte. Ltd. No. 297, Kaki Bukit Ave 1, Shunli Industrial Park S416083. Tel: 67415561.

187.   **Mixture Xiao Chai Hu [HJ-004] (Sanjiu Enterprise Group)**
Actions:
To eliminate pathogens from Shaoyang.

Indications:
Used for Shaoyang syndrome marked by alternating episodes of chills and fever, fullness in the chest and hypochrondrium, poor appetite, restlessness, vomiting, bitter-taste, dry throat, dizziness, thin white tongue coating, and taut pulse.

Ingredients:
Each 6 g contain extracts equivalent to raw herbs: *Radix Bupleuri* 6.1 g, *Radix Scutellariae* 4.6 g, *Rhizoma Pinelliae* 4.6 g, *Rhizoma Zingiberis Recens* 4.6 g, *Radix Ginseng* 3.1 g, *Fructus Jujubae* 4.6 g, *Radix Glycyrrhizae Preparata* 2.5 g.

Dosage:
2–3 times a day, 6 g each time or as prescribed by Herbalist.

Safety considerations:
Side effects and contraindications not known.

Price: 100 g — $31.00 (bottle is sealed)

Manufacturer:
Sanjiu Medical & Pharmaceutical Co., Ltd. Shenzhen, Guangdong, China.

Importer:
Kinhong Pte. Ltd. No. 297, Kaki Bukit Ave 1, Shunli Industrial Park S416083. Tel: 67415561.

188.   **Mixture Xuan Fu Dai Zhe [HJ-049] (Sanjiu Enterprise Group)**

Actions:
To descend adverse rising qi, eliminate phlegm, reinforce qi and regulate stomach.

Indications:
Use for the deficiency of the stomach and adverse rise of the stomach qi, manifested as epigastric fullness, belching, vomiting phlegm fluid with mucous, white and smooth tongue coating, wiry and weak pulse.

Ingredients:
Each 5 g contain extract equivalent to raw herbs: *Flos Inulae* 2.8 g, *Radix Ginseng* 1.9 g, *Rhizoma Zingiberis Recens* 3.1 g, *Haematitum* 2.8 g, *Radix Glycyrrhizae Preparata* 1.9 g, *Rhizoma Pinelliae Preparata* 2.8 g, *Fructus Jujubae* 1.9 g

Dosage:
2–3 times a day, 5 g each time or follow Herbalist's advice.

Safety considerations:
Side effects and contraindications not known. Avoid cold and spicy foods.

Price: 100 g — $32.00 (bottle is sealed)

Manufacturer:
Sanjiu Medical & Pharmaceutical Co., Ltd. Shenzhen, Guangdong, China.

Importer:
Kinhong Pte. Ltd. No. 297, Kaki Bukit Ave 1, Shunli Industrial Park S416083. Tel: 67415561.

189. **Mixture Zhu Ye Shi Gao [HJ-153] (Sanjiu Enterprise Group)**

Actions and Indications:
Clearing heat and promoting generation of body fluid, reinforcing qi and harmonizing stomach.

Ingredients:
Each 6 g contain extracts equivalent to raw herbs: *Herba Lophatheri* 3.2 g, *Gypsum Fibrosum* 10.7 g, *Rhizoma Pinelliae Preparata* 4.8 g, *Radix Ophiopogonis* 3.2 g, *Radix Ginseng* 3.2 g, *Radix Glycyrrhizae* 1.6 g, *Fructus Oryzae Sativae* 3.2 g.

Dosage:
1–2 times a day, 6 g each time or as prescribed by Herbalist.

Safety considerations:
No known side effect. Used with caution in pregnancy. Avoid cold and spicy foods.

Price: 100 g — $29.00 (sealed bottle)

Manufacturer:
Sanjiu Medical & Pharmaceutical Co., Ltd. Shenzhen, Guangdong, China.

Importer:
Kinhong Pte. Ltd. No. 297, Kaki Bukit Ave 1, Shunli Industrial Park S416083. Tel: 67415561.

190. **Multi energy & performance (Healtheries Men's)**

Description:
Healtheries Men's Multi is especially formulated to assist the general health and wellbeing of men. B Vitamins with added Zinc, Ginseng, and Selenium provide extra energy & fight fatigue.

Ingredients:
(per tablet) Thiamine Nitrate (B1) 35 mg, Riboflavin (B2) 30 mg, Nicotinamide 35 mg, Pantothenic Acid (B5) (as Calcium d-Pantothenate) 70 mg, Pyridoxine Hydrochloride (B6) 35 mg, Cyanocobalamin (B12) 40 mcg, Folic Acid 100 mcg, Ascorbic Acid (Vit. C) 100 mg, Betacarotene 2.5 mg, Cholecalciferol (Vit. D3 100IU) 2.5 mcg, dl-Alpha Tocopheryl Acetate (Vit. E 100IU) 100 mg, Calcium (as Amino Acid Chelate) 10 mg, Magnesium (as Oxide) 40 mg, Zinc (as Amino Acid Chelate) 15 mg, Iron (as Ferrous Fumarate) 1 mg, Manganese (as Amino Acid Chelate) 1 mg, Iodine (as Potassium Iodide) 50 mcg, Chromium (as Chloride) 50 mcg, Selenium (as Selenomethionine) 20 mcg. Extracts equiv. dry: *Panax ginseng* root 1.0 g, Milk Thistle fruit 2.0 g (equiv. flavanolignans as silybin 22.86 mg). Tabletting Aids, Colour- Natural, Flavour-Natural.

Dosage:
Adults: 1 tablet daily with food, or as directed by your healthcare practitioner.

Price: 60 capsules — $30.50 (sealed bottle)

Manufacturer:
Healtheries of New Zealand Ltd. Cnr Jordel Place and Accent Drive, Auckland, New Zealand. Made in New Zealand. Freephone: 0800 848 254.

191.   **Multi energy & vitality (Healtheries Women's)**

Description:
How it works: A high potency "one-a-day" formulation of essential nutrients including extra Iron, Calcium, Folic Acid and B Vitamins to help boost energy levels and maintain good health. Proud supporters of the New Zealand Breast Cancer Foundation.

Ingredients:
(per tablet) Betacarotene 240 mcg, Vit. B1 25 mg, Vit. B2 25 mg, Nicotinamide 50 mg, Vit. B5 30 mg, Vit. B6 35 mg, Vit. B12 50 mcg, Folic Acid 300 mcg, Biotin 50 mcg, Vit. C 100 mg, Vit. D3 (100IU) 2.5 mcg, Vit. E(100IU) 100 mg, Calcium (as Amino Acid Chelate) 40 mg, Potassium (as Amino Acid Chelate) 10 mg, Magnesium (as Oxide) 20 mg, Iron (as Ferrous Fumarate) 10 mg, Zinc (as Amino Acid Chelate) 6 mg, Selenium (as Amino Acid Chelate) 25 mcg, Manganese (as Amino Acid Chelate) 1 mg, Copper (as Amino Acid Chelate) 200 mcg, Chromium (as Amino Acid Chelate) 100 mcg, Iodine (as Potassium Iodide) 15 mcg. Extract equiv. to Siberian ginseng root 1.5 g, Spirulina powder 100 mg. Tabletting Aids, Colour-Natural, Flavour-Nature Identical

Dosage:
Adults: 1 tablet daily with food, or as directed by your healthcare practitioner.

Price: 60 capsules — $35.60 (sealed bottle)

Manufacturer:
Healtheries of New Zealand Ltd. Cnr Jordel Place and Accent Drive, Auckland, New Zealand. Made in New Zealand. Freephone: 0800 848 254

192. **Multi Herbs Cooling Tea (Min Feng)**

Details:
No information available

Ingredients:
Flos Chrysanthemi (2.25 g), Radix Glycyrrhizae (0.15 g), Radix Platycodi (0.25 g), Fructus Forsythiae (0.25 g), Herba Menthae (0.35 g), Flos Lonicerae (0.15 g), Folium Eriobotryae (0.25 g), Folium Mori (0.6 g), Radix Saposhnikoviae (0.25 g), Radix Panaxis Quinquefolii (0.5 g)

Dosage:
No information available

Price: 5 g — $1.24

Manufacturer:
No information available

193. **Muscle Relaxing Herbal Analgesic Oil (QianJin)**
Actions and Indications:
Injury, fall, pain in limbs & numbness in joints, due to the effect of wind, bruise & swelling, coldness and dampness & insect bites.

Ingredients:
Formula: Cinnamon Leaf Oil 4%, Cinnamon Oil 5%, Citronella Oil 2%, Turpentine Oil 22%, *Capsicum Oleoresin* 1%, *Sanguis Draconis* 0.3%, *Musk* 3%, Tian Qi 5%, Methyl Salicylateto 100%

Dosage:
No information available

Price: 60 ml — $6.30 (not sealed but no PIL)

Sole Agent:
Kiat Ling Heath Products Trading. Blk 3017 Bedok North St. 5 #04-15 Singapore 486121. Fax: 67435267.

194.   **851 Musk Tienchi Rheumatic Plaster (Mei Hua Brand)**

Indications:

Disperse swellings & bruises, activate blood circulation and relieve blood circulation and relieve rheumatic pain. It is used for rheumatism, arthritis, muscular aching, sciatica, wounds and sprain etc.

Ingredients:

Mastix 10%, *Myrrha* 8%, Menthol 4%, Cinnamomum Oil 15%, *Flos Cartiami* 8%, *Borneolum* 12%, *Rhizome of davallia* 13%, *Radix Pseudoginseng* 22%, *Cortex Acanthopanacis* 8%

Dosage:

No information available

Safety considerations:

Precautions: 1. It is not indicated for use on injured skin or dermatosis. 2. It is not indicated for use during pregnancy. 3. Use a new plaster every 24 hours. 4. Well-sealed and keep away from heat.

Price: 1 pack (5 plaster sheets) — $2.20

Sole Agent:

Science Arts Co Pte Ltd. 150 MacPherson Rd, Science Arts Building Singapore 348524.

195.   **MV 21G + Selenium (Apeton Essentials)**

Description:

21 vitamins, anti-oxidants, lipotropic substances and minerals with selenium and ginseng extract. Helps cognitive function, to combat fatigue, increase alertness for overall health.

Ingredients:

Each caplet contains: Vitamin A 2667 IU, Vitamin D 200 IU, Vitamin B1 1.5 mg, Vitamin B2 1.7 mg, Vitamin B6 2 mg, Vitamin B12 2 mcg, Vitamin C 60 mg, Pantothenic Acid 5 mg, Vitamin E 10 IU, Nicotinamide 19 mg, Folic Acid 0.2 mg, Selenium 55 mcg, Calcium 100 mg, Iron 5 mg, Potassium 4.98 mg, Copper 0.45 mg, Iodine 0.75 mcg, Magnesium 10 mg, Manganese 0.5 mg, Zinc 5 mg, Ginseng Extract (*Panax Ginseng*) 48 mg, Choline Bitartrate 30 mg, Inositol 15 mg

Dosage:

1 caplet daily, or more if necessary, as directed by physician. To be taken with food preferably at breakfast.

Safety considerations:
Safe use of ginseng in pregnant women, children and for long term use has not been established. Do not exceed the stated dose.

Price: 30 caplets — $52.64 (Sealed)

Manufacturer:
Kotra Pharma (M) Sdn. Bhd. (90082-V). No. 1, Jalan TTC 12, Cheng Industrial Estate, 75250 Melaka, Malaysia. Tel: + 606 336 2222 Fax: + 606 336 122 www. appeton.com.

196. **Nature's Cool JiaJia Herbal Tea (Jia Jia)**

Description:
No Preservative. No Flavouring. Awarded Healthier Choice Symbol. Best chilled before consumption. Refrigerate after opening.

Ingredients:
Water, Cane Sugar, Natural Extract of Herbs, Fructus momordicae, Chrysanthemum, Ginseng, Caramel Colour (E150d).

Dosage:
No information available

Price:
300 ml — $0.70

Manufacturer:
JJ DRINKS MANUFACTURING PTE LTD Member of JJ Group of Companies 12 Tuas West Road JJ Building Singapore 638378; Customer Hotline: 1800-8633679; Website: www.jjdrinks.com.sg; HAACP, ISO 9001: 2008; ISO 22000: 2005

197. **Nature's Cool JiaJia Herbal Tea-Less Sugar (Jia Jia)**

Description:
No Preservative. No Flavouring. Awarded Healthier Choice Symbol. Best chilled before consumption. Refrigerate after opening.

Ingredients:
Water, Cane Sugar, Natural Extract of Herbs, Fructus momordicae, Chrysanthemum, Ginseng, Caramel Colour.

Dosage:
No information available

Price: 300 ml — $0.70

Manufacturer:
JJ DRINKS MANUFACTURING PTE LTD Member of JJ Group of Companies 12 Tuas West Road JJ Building Singapore 638378; Customer Hotline: 1800-8633679; Website: www.jjdrinks.com.sg; HAACP, ISO 9001: 2008; ISO 22000: 2005.

198. **Naughty G Cola (Naughty G)**

Description:
Work Hard, Play Harder; ENERGY, STAMINA & PERFORMANCE SUPPLEMENT DRINK for him & her

Ingredients:
L-Arginine (1000 mg), Taurine (1000 mg), Glucuronolactone (600 mg), Horny Goat Weed Extract (20 mg), Tribulus Terrestris Extract (200 mg), Korean Ginseng Extract (200 mg), Gingko Biloba Extract (100 mg), Caffeine (80 mg), Niacin (Vitamin B3) (5 mg), Vitamin B6 (3 mg), Vitamin B12 (3 mcg); Other Ingredients: Water, Sugar, Acidifier Citric Acid, Carbon Dioxide, Colouring Sulphite Ammonia Caramel, Flavour: Caffeine, Stabilizer Gum Arabic, Flavour.

Dosage:
2 CANS MAX DAILY.; Lightly carbonated, serve chilled.

Safety considerations:
Not suitable for children, pregnant or lactating women, those who have suffered a heart attack or have a heart condition or those who are sensitive to Caffeine. This product is not intended to treat or prevent any disease or disorders.

Price: 250 ml — $1.95

Imported by:
Naughty G Pte. Ltd. 1 Claymore Drive #10-02 Orchard Towers Singapore 229594; Product of Austria.

199. **Naughty G Original (Naughty G)**

Description:
Work Hard, Play Harder; ENERGY, STAMINA & PERFORMANCE SUPPLEMENT DRINK for him & her.

Ingredients:
L-Arginine (400 mg), Taurine (400 mg), Glucuronolactone (240 mg), Horny Goat Weed Extract (80 mg), Tribulus Terrestris Extract (80 mg), Korean Ginseng Extract (80 mg), Gingko Biloba Extract (40 mg), Caffeine (32 mg), Niacin (Vitamin B3) (2 mg), Vitamin B6 (1.2 mg), Vitamin B12 (1.2 mcg); Other Ingredients: Water,

Sugar, Acidifier Citric Acid, Carbon Dioxide, Caramel-Sugar-Syrup, Flavour: Caffeine, Stabilizer Gum Arabic, Flavour. Concentrate (Hibiscus, Carrot).

Dosage:
2 CANS MAX DAILY.; Lightly carbonated, serve chilled

Safety considerations:
Not suitable for children, pregnant or lactating women, those who have suffered a heart attack or have a heart condition or those who are sensitive to Caffeine. This product is not intended to treat or prevent any disease or disorders.

Price: 250 ml — $1.95

Imported by:
Naughty G Pte. Ltd. 1 Claymore Drive #10-02 Orchard Towers Singapore 229594; Product of Austria.

Imported into Australia by:
Naughty Pty Ltd. Shop 1/10 Jacques Avenue Bondi Beach NSW 2026.

200. **Naugthy G sugar free (Naughty G)**

Description:
Work Hard, Play Harder; ENERGY, STAMINA & PERFORMANCE SUPPLEMENT DRINK for him & her

Ingredients:
L-Arginine (1000 mg), Taurine (1000 mg), Glucuronolactone (600 mg), Horny Goat Weed Extract (20 mg), Tribulus Terrestris Extract (200 mg), Korean Ginseng Extract (200 mg), Gingko Biloba Extract (100 mg), Caffeine (80 mg), Niacin (Vitamin B3) (5 mg), Vitamin B6 (3 mg), Vitamin B12 (3 mcg); Other Ingredients: Water, Acidifier, Citric Acid, Carbon Dioxide, Caramel-Sugar-Syrup, Sweetener, Sucralose, Flavour: Caffeine, Stabilizer Gum Arabic, Flavour. Concentrate (Hibiscus, Carrot).

Dosage:
2 CANS MAX DAILY.; Lightly carbonated, serve chilled.

Safety considerations:
Not suitable for children, pregnant or lactating women, those who have suffered a heart attack or have a heart condition or those who are sensitive to Caffeine. This product is not intended to treat or prevent any disease or disorders.

Price: 250 ml — $1.95

Imported by:
Naughty G Pte. Ltd. 1 Claymore Drive #10-02 Orchard Towers Singapore 229594;
Product of Austria.

201.   **Neck Pain Relief Granules (Nature's Green)**

Actions:
Promotes blood circulation and activates channels.

Indications:
Helps relieve the symptoms of neck or shoulder pain, poor blood flow to brain, neck
stiffness or numbness, dizzy and numbness of hands caused by cervical ailments.

Ingredients:
Each dosage (5 g) contains extracts equivalent to raw herbs: *Radix Notoginseng*
400 mg, *Radix Astragali* 800 mg, *Radix Salviae Miltiorrhizae* 800 mg, *Flos
Carthami* 200 mg, *Semen Persicae* 200 mg, *Rhizoma Chuanxiong* 500 mg, *Radix
Paeoniae Alba* 500 mg, *Radix Puerariae* 500 mg, *Radix Clematidis* 500 mg, *Rhizoma
et Radix Notopterygii* 500 mg, *Radix Gentianae Macrophyllae* 500 mg, *Semen
Vaccariae* 500 mg, *Radix Rehmanniae* 500 mg, *Radix Codonopsis* 500 mg, *Rhizoma
Atracylodis* 500 mg, *Eupolyphaga Seu Steleophaga* 300 mg, *Ophicalcitum
(Calcined)* 600 mg, *Concha Haliotidis* 600 mg, *Olibanum (Processed)* 300 mg,
Myrrha (Processed) 300 mg.

Dosage:
For oral administration, take 5 g with warm water, 3 times daily.

Safety considerations:
Side effects not known. Not to be taken by pregnant women. Use with caution for
the patients suffering from digestive tract ulcer and renal hypertension. Stop using
the medicine if the patients suffering from flu, fever and nose pharyngalgia.

Price: 100 g — $15.00 (sealed bottle)

Manufacturer:
Tong Jum Chew Pte Ltd. 21 Kaki Bukit View Tech Park II Singapore 415957. Tel:
62781134 Fax: 62781246. Singapore Manufacturer Licence No. MLCP 0400040
Singapore CPM Product Reference No.: 117097.

202.   **New BIO-Cleanse (Naturopath)**

Description:
Cleanse the digestive system, to improve overall well being and detoxify the system,
to strengthen the spleen and kidney, and keeps you energized and revitalized.

It draws out impurities, wastes and pollutants from every part of your body and eliminates them through your bowel. Good result can be experienced on the treatment of constipation, bloated feeling of the stomach. It helps lowers high cholesterol, triglycerides, uric acid, and fistulous disease. Promotes the digestive function of the intestines and help to achieve healthy complexion and skin.

Actions:
Improves overall well being, detoxifies your digestive system, boosts your immune system, keeps you energized and revitalized.

Ingredients:
600 mg per capsule. Main ingredients: *Panax Ginseng* 90 mg, *Polygonum Multiflorum Preparata* 90 mg, *Herba Cistanches* 90 mg, *Rheum Palmatum* 75 mg, *Rosa Rugosa* 75 mg, *Aloe Vera* 60 mg, *Ginkgo Biloba* 60 mg, *Fritillaria Cirrhose* 60 mg.

Dosage:
Adult: 3–4 capsules (maximum 8 capsules) once every evening, Children between 2–5 years, 0.5–1 capsule once every evening, those between 6–12 years, 2–3 capsules once every evening.

Safety considerations:
Not for pregnant woman.

Price: 50 capsules — $32.80

Product of:
Naturopath Health & Beauty Pte Ltd No. 7 Eunos Ave 8A, Eunos Industrial Estate Singapore 409460 Tel: 65-67350880. Fax: 65-67349939.

Licensee Manufacturers:
Union Chemical & Pharmaceutical Pte Ltd No. 113, Eunos Ave 3, #08-06/09, Gordon Industrial Building, Singapore 409838.

203. **Notoginseng injuries capsules (Nature's Green)**

Description:
PIL: There are many factors linked to trauma and injuries such as over-exercising, sprains, falls, blows, fractures, contusions and sports injuries. Nature's Green Notoginseng Injuries Capsules is derived from Chinese herbal remedy, and is made into capsules prepared by modern pharmaceutical technology. It helps to reduce muscle and joint pain and relieve swelling and stiffness caused by physical trauma.

Actions and Indications:
Suitable for traumatic injuries, obstruction of the blood stasis, painful of the joint, acute and chronic bruises, sprains, and swellings due to trauma.

Ingredients:
Each 450 mg capsule contains extracts equivalent to raw herbs: Radix Notoginseng 150 mg, Ramulus Sambuci 400 mg, Rhizoma Drynariae 250 mg, Radix Angelicae Sinensis 100 mg, Radix et Rhizoma Rhei 60 mg, Flos Carthami 60 mg, Radix Paeeoniae Rubra 60 mg, Eupolyphaga Seu Steleophaga 50 mg, Fructus Aurantii Immaturus 50 mg, Olibanum 40 mg, Myrrha 40 mg.

Dosage:
For oral administration, take 3 capsules, three times daily.

Safety considerations:
Side effects not known. Not suitable for pregnant women and patients with acute bleeding.

Price: 30 capsules — $8 (PIL available)

Manufacturer:
Tong Jum Chew Pte Ltd. 21 Kaki Bukit View Tech Park II Singapore 415957. Tel: 62781134 Fax: 62781246. Singapore Manufacturer No: MLCP 0400040 Singapore CPM product reference number: 113974. Singapore CPM Product Reference No: 112828.

204.   **Nourish Hair Capsules (Nature's Green)**

Description:
PIL: There are many factors linked to hair loss, such as Frequent or continuous stress and strains (physical or emotional) of modern life, anxiety, irregular life, stay up late, smoking, or Imbalanced Diet. Nourish Hair Capsule is made from highly concentrated selected Chinese herbs and produced in accordance to the traditional Chinese formula. It can help nourish thinning hair. It is suitable for people with: Graying hair in the early stage, Withered hair, Loss of hair.

Actions and Indications:
It helps for nourishment of hair, darkening hair, promotion of hair growth, and prevention of thinning and dropping hair.

Ingredients:
Each 300 mg capsule contains extracts equivalent to raw herbs: *Radix Polygoni Multiflori Preparata* 600 mg, *Radix Ginseng* 400 mg, *Radix Angelicae Sinensis* 200 mg, *Radix Achyranthis Bidentate* 200 mg, *Fructus Lycii* 200 mg, *Semen Cuscutae* 200 mg, *Poria* 200 mg, *Fructus Psoraleae* 100 mg.

Dosage:
For oral administration, take 2–4 capsules, twice daily.

Safety considerations:
PIL: side effects and contraindications not known.

Price: 30 cap-sules — $7.50 (not sealed)

Manufacturer:
Tong Jum Chew Pte Ltd. 21 Kaki Bukit View Tech Park II Singapore 415957 Tel: 62781134, Fax: 62781246. Singapore Manufacturer Licence No. MLCP 0400040. Singapore CPM Product Reference No. 112832.

205. **Nourish-Eyes Capsule (Science Arts)**

Description:
PIL: Science Arts Nourish-Eyes Capsule provides the healing properites of enrich-ing blood, encouraging production of body fluids, replenishing yin and nourishing kidney, reinforcing spleen and ling, dispelling wind, clear heats, daily care of eyes and having effects for eyes-related diseases.

Actions:
Soothing liver to subside interior wind, replenishing yin and improving eyesight.

Indications:
Used for blurred vision, eyes fatigue, dizziness, unbearable of light and easy to flood tears caused by deficiency of liver and kidney.

Ingredients:
(Each 0.3 g contains extract equivalent to raw herbs) *Herba Dendrobii* 18.00 mg, *Radix Ginseng* 72.75 mg, *Rhizoma Dioscoreae* 27.00 mg, *Poria* 72.75 mg, *Radix Glycyrrhizae* 18.00 mg, *Herba Cistanches* 18.00 mg, *Fructus Lycii* 27.00 mg, *Semen Cuscutae* 27.00 mg, *Radix Rehmanniae* 36.00 mg, *Radix Rehmanniae Preparata* 36.00 mg, *Fructus Schisandrae Chinensis* 18.00 mg, *Radix Asparagi* 73.50 mg, *Radix Ophiopogonis* 36.00 mg, *Semen Armeniacae Amarum* 27.00 mg, *Radix Saposhnikoviae* 18.00 mg, *Rhizoma Chuanxiong* 18.00 mg, *Fructus Aurantii* 18.00 mg, *Radix Gentianae* 18.00 mg, *Radix Achyranthis Bidentatae* 27.00 mg, *Flos Chrysanthemi* 27.00 mg, *Fructus Tribuli* 18.00 mg, *Semen Celosiae* 18.00 mg, *Semen Cassiae* 27.00 mg, *Cornu Bubali* 54.00 mg.

Dosage:
3 capsules each time, three times daily, take with warm water.

Safety considerations:
PIL: Side effects and contraindications not known.

Price: 30 capsules — $10. (not sealed with pil)

Manufacturer:
Science Arts Co. Pte Ltd. 150 MacPherson Rd, Science Arts Building Singapore 348524.

206. **Nutri Tea Herbal Tea (F&N)**

Description:
Reduced Sugar; No Preservatives: NutriTea Herbal Tea is a fresh brew of quality traditional ingredients that harvests the goodness of Chrysanthemum, Luo Han Guo and Ginseng. Refreshingly delicious, it's the perfect drink to cool you down in this tropical climate. With carefully selected ingredients, freshly brewed to perfection, it's the beverage of choice. Make drinking NutriTea Herbal Tea a daily enjoyment!

Ingredients:
Water, Sucrose, Freshly Brewes Herbal Extract, Luo Han Guo (Grosvenor momordica Fruit), Ginseng, Chrysanthemum Flower, Permitted Colouring, Permitted Food Additives of Non-Animal Origin (E500).

Dosage:
No information available

Price: 500 ml — $1.22

Packed by:
F&N Foods Pte Ltd. 214 Pandan Loop, Singapore 128405. Consumer Hotline: 6210 8200, Email/Feedback: customerfeedback@fnnfoods.com.

Imported by:
F&N Dairies (M) Sdn Bhd 70 Jalan Universiti, 46700 Petaling Jaya, Selangor, Malaysia: Under Licence from FRASER AND NEAVE, LIMITED.

207. **Osteo-porosis Capsules [Bone Strengthening] (Mei Hua Brand)**

Actions:
Reinforce the kidneys, replenish liver and spleen and strengthen bones and tendons.

Ingredients:
350 mg per capsule, contain extract equivalent to raw herbs: *Cortex Eucommiae* 42 mg, *Fructus Corni* 21 mg, *Rhizoma Dioscoreae* 63 mg, *Radix Morindae Officinalis* 31.5 mg, *Fructus Lycii* 31.5 mg, *Radix Angelicae Sinensis* 52.5 mg, *Radix Rehmanniae* (Prep) 42 mg, *Rhizoma Ligustici Chuanxiong* 21 mg, *Rhizoma Curculigins* 21 mg, *Radix Ginseng* 24.5 mg.

Safety considerations:
Product has no side effect or contraindication.

Dosage:
For curative purpose: Take 3 capsules three times daily with warm water for a course of one month. For health supplement: Take 2 capsules twice daily.

Price: 300 capsules — $120.

Manufacturer:
Science Arts Co. Pte Ltd. 150 MacPherson Rd, Science Arts Building Singapore 348524.

208. **Pain & swelling Relieving Capsules (Nature's Green)**

Description on PIL:
Pain & Swelling Relieving Capsules are made from 12 natural Chinese herbs and prepared by modern pharmaceuticak technology based on a herbal remedy recognized by Chinese health authorites. This product is the typical formulation that has satisfactory effect in removing any obstructions in the channels, dispelling pathogenic wind and dampness, activating blood circulation and dredging collaterals. The product is superior in relieving the symptoms of joint swelling, stiffness and pain. It is also useful for alleviating traumatic injuries, skin infection, ecezma and snakebite.

Actions and Indications:
Relieves swelling and pain. It helps relieve the symptoms of joint swelling, stiffness and pain, difficulty in extension and flexion of limbs caused by wind-phlegm blocking the channels and collaterals. It is also used for traumatic injuries, skin infection, ecezma and snakebite.

Ingredients:
Each 300 mg capsule contains extracts equivalent to raw herbs: *Radix Notoginseng* 30 mg, *Rhizoma Gastrodiae* 15 mg, *Cornu Saigae Tataricae* 15 mg, *Bombyx Batryticatus* 14 mg, *Pheretima* 20 mg, *Rhizoma Typhonii Praeparata* 168 mg, *Caulis Bambusae* in Taeniam 18 mg, *Radix Saposhnikoviae* 14 mg, *Flos Curthami* 20 mg, *Rhizoma Seu Radix Notopterygii* 14 mg, *Rhizoma Arisaematis Praeparata* 14 mg, *Radix Angelicae Dahuricae* 14 mg.

Dosage:
For oral administration, take 2 capsules, 3 times daily. For external use, clean the wound with saline solution, apply the powder onto it, or mix with vegetable oil before use.

Safety considerations:
Side effects not known (Not on packaging of 60 capsules but on PIL). Not to be taken by pregnant women (not on packaging for 60 capsules but on PIL).

Price: 60 capsules — $10.50, 300 capsules — $45

Manufacturer:
Tong Jum Chew Pte Ltd 21 Kaki Bukit View Tech Park II Singapore 415957 Tel: 62781134 Fax: 62781246 Singapore Manufacturer Licence No. MLCP: 04000400 Singapore CPM Product Reference No.: 117324.

209. **Panax Ginseng Capsules (Pine Brand Trade Mark)**

Description:
It is a health food, and it is mainly made of Radix Ginseng, Salad oil, phosphatide, palm oil, hydropalm oil and beewax etc. It can resist fatigue, which has been proved by experience.

Actions:
Resist fatigue.

Suitable for:
Fatigued people

Ingredients:
Major materials: *Radix Ginseng*, Salad oil, phosphatide, palm oil, hydropalm oil, beewax. Active ingredient and content: Contain Gensenoside (Re) 2.2 g per 100 g. Each capsule 0.55 g contains equivalent to 550 mg *Radix Ginseng*. *Radix Ginseng* Extractum 0.22 g.

Dosage:
Once a day, two capsules each.

Safety considerations:
Side effects not observed. Precaution on PIL: It can't take the place of a drug. Not suitable for teen-ager and children.

Price: 30 capsules — $6.20 (PIL available)

Manufacturer:
Tianjin Central Pharmaceutical Co Ltd., Tianjin, China. Address: No. 1 Fujin Road, Beichen District, Tianjin 300400, China. Telephone: 0086-22-26918008 Fax: 0086-22-26918028.

Imported by:
Winlykah Trading Blk 8, Lorong Bakar Batu #06-09, Singapore.

210. **Panax Ginseng Extractum Oral Liquid (Pine Brand Trade Mark (Song Shu Pai Trade Mark Pine Brand))**

Description:
Panax ginseng, the root of Araliacene is a precious natural product growing in China. It is good for relieving fatigue, poor appetite, palpitation, insomnia and amnesia.

Ingredients:
Each bottle 10 ml contains 1000 mg *Panax Ginseng*, 30 mg Sodium benzoate

Dosage:
Each time 10 ml, 3 times a day.

Safety considerations:
Side effects unknown. Precautions: Unfit for the person with excess and heat symptom.

Price: 10 vials — $5.50 (sealed package)

Manufacturer:
Tianjin Central Pharmaceutical Co. Ltd. Tianjin, China. Importer: Joo Hong Medical Hall. 270, River Valley Road, Singapore 238314. Yue Fong (M) SDN. BHD. (21993-A) 27 Jalan Hujan O.U.G. 58200 Kuala Lumpur.

211. **Panax Notoginseng & American Ginseng (Ren Xin Tang)**

Description:
Panax Notoginseng has been used in Chinese medicine for thousands of years. Widely hailed as "the miracle root for the preservation of health", Tian Qi has long been recognised as the Oriental's tonic herb for improving circulation and supporting the immune system for overall bidy well-being. The herb is used as a general tonic to tone and strengthen the entire body system in Traditional Chinese Medicine. Tian qi is believed to supportthe channels that contain the flow of Qi (life energy) in the body. Tian Qi is used as a general tonic to improve the immune system, provide benefits for the heart and circulatory system, relieve pain and enhance overall well-being.

Actions and Indications:
Activates blood circulation and disperses blood clots. Also used for twinge at chest and upper abdomen and accelerating the healthy development of children.

Ingredients:
Each capsule 250 mg contains: 125 mg of *Panax Notoginseng*, 125 mg of American Ginseng.

Dosage:
Take 2 capsules daily.

Safety considerations:
Not suitable for pregnant woman.

Price: 60 capsules — $59.90 (sealed)

Manufacturer:
Kang Sheng Chinese Medicine Manufacturer (GMP) Blk 2015 Bedok North St. 5 #06-22, Shimei East Kitchen, (s) 486350.

Wholesaler:
LIXR Enterprise #11-15, 9 Penang Road Singapore 238459.

212. **Panax Quinquefolium & Panax Notoginseng capsules (Jin Pai Trademark)**

Description on packaging:
Panax Quinquefolium & Panax Notoginseng are used for improving blood circulation. Panax Notoginseng is able to activating blood circulation to disspiate blood stasis and increase the blood flow in coronary arteries with Radix Salvia Miltiorrhizae, which is also capable to expand blood vessels. Panax Quinquefolium is medicinally nutritious in bolstering proper Qi in the body. With regular consumption per the recommended dosage, it can nourish the bidy, strengthen physical conditions and improve the blood circulation.

Ingredients:
Each capsule (450 mg) contains raw herbs: *Radix Panax Quinquefolium* 25 mg, *Radix Panax Notoginseng* 380 mg, *Radix Salviae Miltiorrhizae* 45 mg.

Dosage:
Adult: 2 capsules each time and twice daily.

Safety considerations:
Side effects not known. Avoid medication during pregnancy, influenza and colds. Continuous use exceeding 3 months is not advisable. It is advisable to stop dosage for short interval after continuous use exceeding 3 months.

Price: 200 capsules — $36 (sealed)

Assembler & importer:
Kinhong Pte Ltd 297 Kaki Bukit Avenue 1, Shun Li Industrial Park, Singapore 416083. Tel: 67415561 Fax: 67413705.

213. **Pao Shen Cong Cao Capsule (Cotton Plant)**

Actions:
Restore vitality, increase immunity, delay grow old.

Ingredients:
Each capsule contains raw herbs 420 mg as below: *Radix Panacis Quinquefolii* 168.00 mg, *Cordyplus Mycellia* 252.00 mg.

Dosage:
Take 2 capsules, 1–2 times daily.

Safety considerations:
No known side effect. No known contraindication.

Price: 120 capsules — $45.00 (sealed).

Manufacturer:
Yi Shi Yuan Pte Ltd (GMP Manufacturer) No. 20, Bukit Batok Crescent #13-11/12/13 Enterprise Centre Singapore 658080 Tel: 65670900 Fax: 65672256.

214. **Pao Shen Tian Qi (Cotton Plant)**

Actions:
Restore vitality, promote blood circulation and remove blood stasis, improve memory and immunity.

Ingredients:
Each capsule contains raw herbs 260 mg as below: *Radix Notoginseng* 78.00 mg, *Radix Panacis Quinquefolii* 182.00 mg.

Dosage:
Take 2 capsules, 1–2 times daily.

Safety considerations:
No known side effect. No known contraindication.

Price: 120 capsules — $45.00 (sealed)

Manufacturer:
Yi Shi Yuan Pte Ltd (GMP Manufacturer) No. 20, Bukit Batok Crescent #13-11/12/13 Enterprise Centre Singapore 658080 Tel: 65670900 Fax: 65672256.

215. **Pao Shen Tian Qi (Wellring)**

Actions:
Restore vitality, promote blood circulation and remove blood stasis, improve memory and immunity.

Ingredients:
Each capsule contains raw herbs 260 mg as below: *Radix Panacis Quinquefolii* 182.00 mg, *Radix Et Rhizoma Notoginseng* 78.00 mg.

Dosage:
Take 2 capsules, 1–2 times daily.

Safety considerations:
No known side effect. No known contraindication.

Price: 60 vegetarian capsules — $28.00 (sealed).

Sole Agent:
Hua Bao Agency Pte Ltd 105, Sims Avenue #06-10, Chancerlodge Complex Singapore 387429 Tel: 67490809 Fax: 67493662. Manufacturer (GMP): Yi Shi Yuan Pte Ltd 20, Bukit Batok Crescent, Singapore 658080 Tel: 56570900.

216. **Pharmaton Capsules with selenium (Pharmaton)**

Description:
A combination of the standardized GINSENG EXTRACT G115 with vitamins, minerals and lipotropic substances for health.

Indications:
As a dietary supplement for health.

Ingredients:
Standardised G115 Ginseng Extract (made from the roots of *Panax ginseng* C.A. Meyer, adjusted to 4% ginsenosides) 40.0 mg, Vitamin A 2667 IU, Vitamin D3 200 IU, Vitamin E 10.0 mg, Vitamin B1 1.4 mg, Vitamin B2 1.6 mg, Vitamin B6 2.0 mg, Vitamin B12 1.0 mcg, Biotin 150.0 mcg, Nicotinamide 18.0 mg, Vitamin C 60.0 mg, Folic Acid 0.1 mg, Copper 2.0 mg, Selenium 50.0 mcg, Manganese 2.5 mg, Magnesium 10.0 mg, Iron 10.0 mg, Zinc 1.0 mg, Calcium 100.0 mg, Lecithin 100.0 mg.

Dosage:
One capsule daily.

Price: 130 capsules — $59.50 (sealed)

Imported & distributed by:
DKSH (Singapore) Pte Ltd 34 Boon Leat Terrace, Pasir Panjang Road Singapore 119856. Product Licence Holder: Boehringer Ingelheim (Malaysia) Sdn. Bhd. Suite 15-5 Level 15, Wisma UOA Damansara II. No. 6 Jalan Changkat Semantan, Damansara Heights, 50490 Kuala Lumpur.

Manufacturer:

Swiss Caps, Kirchberg, Switzerland. Packed by: Ginsana SA, Via Mulini 6934 Bioggio/Switzerland.

217. **Pien Tze Huang Hemorrhoids Ointment Compositum (Pien Tze Huang)**

Actions and Indications:

Help relieve pain, reduce swelling, and stop bleeding due to hemorrhoidal symptom. Suitable for internal hemorrhoid, external hemorrhoid and hybrid hemorrhoid.

Ingredients:

Pien Tze Huang (*Moschus* 0.009 g, *Calculus Bovis* 0.015 g, Snake Gall 0.021 g, *Radix Et Rhizoma Notoginseng* 0.255 g), Powder of *Margarita* 0.2 g, *Amber* 0.4 g, *Borneolum Syntheticum* 0.16 g, Bases 8.94 g.

Dosage:

Usage and dosage: For external use, infuse or spread on the effected part, 2–3 times a day.

Safety considerations:

Adverse reactions: Not yet discovered. (On PIL). Not to be used by pregnant women.

Price: 10 g — $8.80 (package not sealed).

Manufacturer:

Zhangzhou Pien Tze Huang Pharmaceutical Co., Ltd. Shang street Zhangzhou Fujian. China. Post code: 363000. tel: 0596-2307998 2305453. fax: 0596-2302993.

Imported by:

Jing Tai Hong No. 1 Park Road #01-20 Singapore 059108. Approval no. Guo Yao Zhun Zi B20060001.

218. **Pien Tze Huang Unguentum Compositum (Pien Tze Huang)**

Actions and Indications:

Clearing away heat, Removing toxic substances, Relieving pain. It is used for herpes zoster, simples herpes, impetigo, hair follicle inflammationa and ache.

Ingredients:

Pien Tze Huang (Moschus 0.015 g, *Calculus Bovis* 0.025 g, Snake Gall 0.035 g, *Radix Et Rhizoma Notoginseng* 0.425 g), *Rhizoma Parids* 0.1 g, *Herb Lobeliae Chinensis* 0.07 g, Bases 9.33 g.

Dosage:
Usage and Dosage: for external use, spread on effected part, 2–3 times a day.

Safety considerations:
Side effects not known (PIL). PIL: 1. Not to take pungent or fat food, alcohol and smoke. 2. Not to be taken by pregnant women. 3. It ise only for external use, not oral. 4. Anybody whose part appears hypersensitive after using the medicine stops using it. 5. Children must use the medicine under the guardianship of the adult. 6. Refer to doctor or apothecary before using the medicine if you just take other medicines.

Price: 10 g — $8.80 (package not sealed)

Manufacturer:
Zhangzhou Pien Tze Huang Pharmaceutical Co., Ltd. Add: Shang Street, Zhangzhou Fujian. China.

Imported by:
Jing Tai Hong No. 1 Park Road #01-20 Singapore 059108. Approval no. Guo Yao Zhun Zi Z35020234.

219. **Premium Bai Feng Wan with Pearl (60 vegecaps) (Borsch Med)**

Description:
Borsch Med Premium Bai Feng Wan with Pearl is specially developed from various natural and precious herbs such as Pearl and Ginseng. It is effective in treating symptoms such as deficiency of qi and blood, irregular menstruation and abdominal pain during menstruation.

Actions:
This product helps to reinforce qi and nourish the blood, regulate mentruation and improve skin complexion.

Ingredients:
per capsule of 480 mg: *Radix Rehmanniae Praeparata* 64.50 mg, *Radix Codonopsis* 33.30 mg, *Radix Paeoniae Alba* 32.50 mg, *Radix Angelicae Sinensis* 32.40 mg, *Herba Leonuri* 32.40 mg, *Radix Astragali* 32.40 mg, *Rhizoma Cyperi* 25.80 mg, *Rhizoma Chuanxiong* 25.00 mg, *Radix Et Rhizoma Glycyrrhizae Praeparata Cum Melle* 25.00 mg, *Rhizoma Atractylodis Macrocephalae* 25.00 mg, *Radix Angelicae Dahuricae* 25.00 mg, *Radix Dipsaci* 25.00 mg, *Semen Trigonellae* 25.00 mg, *Radix Scutellariae* 25.00 mg, *Fructus Amomi* 19.10 mg, *Herba Taxilli* 17.50 mg, *Margarita* (Pearl) 8.40 mg, *Radix Et Rhizoma Ginseng* (*Panax Ginseng*) 6.80 mg.

Instruction:

For overall maintenance of health: 2–3 capsules to be taken each time with lukewarm water, once a day. For treatment of general body weakness: 2 capsules to be taken each time with lukewarm water, twice a day. For regulating menstrual ailments: 3 capsules to be taken each time with lukewarm water, twice a day.

Safety considerations:

Adverse-Reactions: There are no known side effects for Borsch Med Premium Bai Feng Wan with Pearl. Avoid consumption when suffering from influenza or fever. Not to be taken by pregnant women. If symptoms persist, consult a physician.

Price: 60 vegecaps — $39.80

Manufacturer:

Yi Shi Yuan Pte Ltd. 20, Bukit Batok Crescent #13-11/12/13, Enterprise Centre, Singapore 658080.

Distributed by:

Borsch Med Pte Ltd. 60 Alexandra Terrace #03-28, The Comtech, Singapore 118502. Borsch Med, Inc. Suite #300 PMB #1024, 2711 Centerville Road, Wilmington, DE 19808, USA.

220. **Premium Ginseng Ji Tang (Star-flower)**

Details:

No information available

Ingredients:

Ginseng, Astragalia, Fructus Lycii, Radix Tang Shen, Chinese Yam, Polygonatum, (Special Recipe).

Instruction:

Cooking Instrutions: (1) Prepare to boil 2 little (4 bowls) of water (2) Add 500 gm of chicken or meat with Ginseng Ji Tang Wao & Recipe (Do not open) (3) Simmer for approximately 2–3 hours until the meal is tender. Then serve.

Price: 90 gm — $6.50

Packed By:

Hong Seah Food Industries Pte. Ltd. 10, TUAS BAY WALK, #03-18, Singapore 637780 Tel: 626 59728: Fax: 62681143: Packed in Singapore. Website: http://www. hongseah.com.sg; E-mail: hongseah@cyberway.com.sg.

Distributor:

HUP HUAT NODDLES Pte. Ltd., No. 8, Wan Lee Rd, Singapore 627940; Tel: 62688335; 62688011, 62614044; Fax: 62661215; Hong Kong.

Importer:

ADDISON INDUSTRIAL (GROUP) LTD. Tel: (85) 24181016 Fax: (85) 24870244

221.   **Pure Raw Pseudoginseng Powder (Mei Hua Brand)**

Description:

Original known as San Qi, and also called Jin Bu Huan, Pseudo-ginseng is a special kind of precious medicinal herb, growing in Yunnan Province, and classified under the acanthopanax plant, the common family of ginseng. As pseudo-ginseng is effective in preventing bleeding, dispersing clot, activating blood and relieving pain, Chinese physicians over the centuries used in singly or supplementarily as a main ingredient to treat different types of hemopathy and traumatic cases.

Actions and Indications:

It can be used to treat different kinds of hamorraghic symptoms, eg., hemoptysis, nosebleed, hemofaeces, internal bleeding, falls, blows, injuries, abdominal pain and blood clot in post-partum, unknown pain and sore.

Ingredients:

Radix Notoginseng 100%

Dosage:

Take 3 g each time, 3 times daily. For serious cases take 5 g each time. (for instructions please refer to leaflet)

Safety considerations:

Stop taking orally during pregnancy.

Price: 40 g — $12

Manufacturer:

Yunnan Bai Yao Group Co. Ltd. Imported and Packed by: Science Arts Co. Pte Ltd. 150 MacPherson Rd, Science Arts Building Singapore 348524.

222.   **Pure Yunnan Raw Pseudo Ginseng Capsules (Mei Hua Brand)**

Actions and Indications:

It can activate blood, clear clots in the veins, relieve angina pectoris, lower hyper-cholesterol level, dilate coronary arteries, reduce oxygen consumption in the myocardium, improve blood deficiency in the myocardium prevent coronary illness increase physical strength and promote the growth of children.

Ingredients:

Each capsule weighted 350 mg. *Radix Notoginseng* 100%.

Dosage:
Take 2–3 capsules each time, three times daily, together with warm water.

Safety considerations:
Side effects not known. Caution: Stop taking orally during pregnancy.

Price: 300 capsules — $60 (sealed)

GMP Certified Manufacturer:
Science Arts Co Pte Ltd. 150 MacPherson Rd, Science Arts Building Singapore 348524.

223.   **Pure Yunnan Raw Pseudo Ginseng capsules (Mei Hua Brand)**

Description:
Original known as San Qi, and also called Jin Bu Huan, Pseudo-ginseng is a special kind of precious medicinal herb, growing in Yunnan Province, and classified under the acanthopanax plant, the common family of ginseng. As pseudo-ginseng is effective in preventing bleeding, dispersing clot, activating blood and relieving pain, Chinese physicians over the centuries used in singly or supplementarily as a main ingredient to treat different types of hemopathy and traumatic cases.

Actions and Indications:
It can be used to treat different kinds of hamorraghic symptoms, eg., nosebleed, hemofaeces, internal bleeding, falls, blows, injuries, abdominal pain and blood clot in post-partum, unknown pain and sore. It can activate blood, clear clots in the veins, relieve angina pectoris, lower hypercholesterol level, dilate coronary arteries, reduce oxygen consumption in the myocardium, improve blood deficiency in the myocardium, prevent coronary illness, increase physical strength and promote the growth of children.

Ingredients:
Each capsule weighted 350 mg. *Radix Notoginseng* 100%

Dosage:
Take 2~3 capsules each time, three times daily, together with warm water.

Safety considerations:
Side effects not known. Caution: Stop taking orally during pregnancy.

Price: 30 capsules — $6.80 PIL available

Manufacturer:
Science Arts Co Pte Ltd 150 MacPherson Rd, Science Arts Building Singapore 348524.

224.   **909 Qing Du Xiao Yan Capsules (SeaGull)**

Actions:

Having antiphloistic disingectant, analgesic actions and having function of accelerating the growth of flesh.

Ingredients:

Each 300 mg capsule contains extracts equivalent to raw herb: *Radix Helicteris Angustifoliae* 278 mg, *Herba Andrographitis* 220 mg, *Herba Violae* 100 mg, *Flos Rosae Laevigatae* 100 mg, *Wiktroemia Indica* 100 mg, *Herba Plantaginis* 100 mg, *Radix Notoginseng* 47 mg.

Dosage:

1 capsule 3 times daily or 2 capsules when required

Safety considerations:

Side effects not known. Not to be over dosage consume for a long period. Not to be taken by pregnant women. Radish and salted vegetable are forbidden in the course of administration.

Price: 20 capsules — $8.50 (package not sealed but doesn't have PIL), 300 capsules — $70.00 (sealed bottle)

Sole agent:

Sea Gull Trading Pte Ltd. Blk 217 Henderson Industrial Park, #03-05 Henderson Road, Singapore 159555. Tel: 62741033, Fax: 62724997. Email: sea_gull@pacific. net.sg.

225.   **Radix Ginseng [D1960] (Sanjiu Enterprise Group)**

Actions:

To reinforce qi, rescue collapse and restore the normal pulse, to benefit the spleen and lung, promote the production of body fluids.

Ingredients:

Each 1.5 g contains extracts equivalent to raw herb *Radix Ginseng* 5 g.

Dosage:

Take 1.5 — 3 g a day with warm water orally or as prescribed by Herbalist.

Safety considerations:

Side effects not known. Incompatible with Rhizoma et Radix Veratri.

Price: 100 g — $28 (sealed)

Manufacturer:

Sanjiu Medical & Pharmaceutical Co. Ltd, Shenzhen, China.

Importer:
Kinhong Pte, Ltd. No. 297 Kaki Bukit Ave. 1 Shunli Industrial Park, Singapore Tel 67415561 Fax: 67413705.

226. **Radix Notoginseng [D2020] (Sanjiu Enterprise Group)**

Actions:
To eliminate blood stasis, arrest bleeding, cause subsidence of swelling and alleviate pain.

Ingredients:
Each 2 g contains extract equivalent to raw herb *Radix Notoginseng* 1.5 g.

Dosage:
Take 2–4 g a day with warm water orally or as prescribed by Herbalist.

Safety considerations:
Side effects not known. Do not use during pregnancy

Price: 100 g — $61 (sealed)

Manufacturer:
Sanjiu Medical & Pharmaceutical Co. Ltd. Shenzhen, China.

Importer:
Kinhong Pte Ltd. No. 297 Kaki Bukit Ave 1, Shunli Industrial Park S416083. Tel: 67415561 Fax: 67413705.

227. **Radix Panacis Quinquefolii [D2470] (Sanjiu Enterprise Group)**

Actions:
To tonify qi and nourish yin, remove heat and promote the production of body fluids. Dry and thristy mouth and throat.

Ingredients:
Each 1.5 g contains extracts equivalent to raw herb *Radix Panacis Quinquefolii* 5 g.

Dosage:
Take 1.5 a day with warm water orally or as prescribed by Herbalist.

Safety considerations:
Side effects not known. Incompatible with Rhizoma et Radix Veratri.

Price: 100 g — $110 (sealed)

Manufacturer:
Sanjiu Medical and Pharmaceutical Co. Ltd, Shenzhen, China.

Importer:
Kinhong Pte, Ltd. No. 297 Kaki Bukit Ave. 1 Shunli Industrial Park, Singapore Tel 67415561 Fax: 67413705.

228.   **Raw pseudoginseng capsules (Nature's Green)**

Actions:
Promotes blood circulation to remove blood stasis, stops bleeding, relieves swelling ad alleviates pain.

Indications:
Used for various kinds of bleeding, swelling and pain due to trauma and blood-stasis syndrome.

Ingredients:
Each 505 mg capsule contains: *Radix Notoginseng* 500 mg

Dosage:
For oral administration, take 2–6 capsules, 3 times daily.

Safety considerations:
Side effects not known. Not to be taken by pregnant women. Used with caution for children. Contraindicated for patients with poor liver or kidney functions.

Price: 300 capsules — $70; 60 capsules — $16 (CI and SE not on packaging).

Manufacturer:
Tong Jum Chew Pte Ltd. 21 Alexandra Distripark Blk. 1. #08-15/17 Pasir Panjang Road Singapore 118478. Tel: 62781134 (3 lines) Fax: 62781246 Manufacturer Licence No. MLCP: 0400040 Singapore CPM Product Reference No. 112821.

229.   **Raw Pseudoginseng powder (Nature's Green)**

Actions:
Promotes blood circulation to remove blood stasis, stops bleeding, relieves swelling ad alleviates pain.

Indications:
Used for various kinds of bleeding, swelling and pain due to trauma and blood-stasis syndrome.

Ingredients:
Each bottle (200 g) contains *Radix Notoginseng* 200 g

Dosage:
For oral administration, take 1 to 3 g each time, 3 times daily.

Safety considerations:
Side effects not known. Not to be taken by pregnant women. Used with caution for children. Contraindicated for patients with poor liver or kidney functions.

Price: 200 g — $70 (sealed)

Manufacturer:
Tong Jum Chew Pte Ltd 21 Kaki Bukit View Tech Park II Singapore 415957 Tel: 62781134 Fax: 62781246. Singapore Manufacturer Licence No. MLCP 0400040. Singapore CPM Product Reference No. 113723.

230. **Raw Pseudoginseng Tablets (Nature's Green)**

Actions:
Promotes blood circulation to remove blood stasis, stops bleeding, relieves swelling ad alleviates pain.

Indications:
Used for various kinds of bleeding, swelling and pain due to trauma and blood-stasis syndrome.

Ingredients:
Each 550 mg tablet contains *Radix Notoginseng* 550 mg.

Dosage:
For oral administration, take 2–6 capsules, 3 times daily.

Price:
500 tablets — $70 (sealed)

Manufacturer:
Tong Jum Chew Pte Ltd. 21 Kaki Bukit View Tech Park II Singapore 415957 Tel: 62781134. Fax: 62781246. Singapore Manufacturer Licence No. MLCP 0400040 Singapore CPM Product Reference No. 113722.

231. **Raw Tienchi Ginseng Tablet (Mei Hua Brand)**

Description:
PIL: Original known as San Qi, Pseudo-Ginseng is a special kind of precious medicinal herb growing in Yunnan Province, and classified under the acanthopanax plant, the common family of ginseng. As pseudo-ginseng is effective in preventing bleeding, dispersing clot, activating blood and relieving pain, Chinese physicians over the centuries used in singly or supplementary as a main ingredient to treat different types of hemopathy and traumatic cases.

Actions:

To eliminate blood stasis, arrest bleeding, cause subsidence of swelling and alleviate pain.

Indications:

Traumatic bleeding, traumatic swelling and pain.

Ingredients:

Each tablet 0.55 g contains *Radix Notoginseng* 500 mg.

Dosage:

Oral administration 2~6 tablets 3 times daily.

Safety considerations:

Side effects not known. PIL: Warning: 1. Contraindicated for pregnant 2. Precaution is warranted in patients with known sensitivity to the drug 3. Contraindicated for the people with abnormal function in kidney liver 4. Used with caution by children.

Price: 1000 tablets — $90; 60 tablets — $8; 48 tablets — $6.50; 48 and 60 tablets→ SE, precaution and contraindication not stated.) PIL available.

Manufacturer:

Yunnan Baiyao Group Co Ltd Kunming, Yunnan, P.R. China.

Imported and Packed by:

Science Arts Co. Pte Ltd. 150 MacPherson Rd, Science Arts Building Singapore 348524.

232.   **Raw Tienchi Tablets (Camellia Brand)**

Actions:

Disperses blood clots, eliminates swelling, arrests hemorrhage and relieves pain.

Indications:

Indicated for traumatic bleeding, swelling and pain due to injuries.

Ingredients:

Each tablet (0.55 g) contains *Radix Notoginseng* 0.5 g.

Dosage:

For oral administration, take 2–6 capsules, 3 times daily.

Price: 60 tablets — $8 (sealed)

Manufacturer:

Yunnan Weihe Pharmaceutical Co. Ltd. Yunnan. China. Exported by: Yunnan Camellia pharmaceutical Import & Export Co., Ltd.

Imported by: Tong Jum Chew Pte Ltd, 21 Kaki Bukit Tech Park II Singapore 415957 Tel: 62781134 Fax: 62781246.

233. **Raw Tienchi Tablets (YF)**

Description:
PIL: Ash yellow or light brown tablet, taste bitter and slight sweet.

Actions:
PIL: To eliminate blood stasis, arrest bleeding, cause subsidence of swelling and alleviate pain.

Indications:
PIL: Traumatic bleeding, traumatic swelling and pain

Ingredients:
Each tablet (0.55 g) contains *Radix Notoginseng* 0.5 g

Dosage:
Oral administration: 2–6 tablets 3 times daily.

Safety considerations:
Side effects not known. Warnings: 1. Contraindicated for pregnancy. 2. Contraindicated for person with abnormal liver-kidney function. 3. Used with caution in children and person with known sensitivity to this product. 4. Precaution is warranted in hypersensitivity constitution. 5. It is not recommended to use when the description of the product is changed. 6. Use according to usage and dosage, the old or weak should use under the doctor's direction. 7. Keep out of reach of children. 8. Ask a doctor or pharmacist before use if you are taking other medicines.

Price: 36 tablets — $5 PIL available

Manufacturer:
Yunnan Baiyao Group Co., Ltd, Kunming, Yunnan, P.R. China.

Imported by:
Science Arts Co. Pte. Ltd. 150 MacPherson Rd, Science Arts Building Singapore 348524.

234. **Raw Tienchi Tablets (Camellia Brand)**

Details:
**Package is sealed. No other info available.

Ingredients:
Each tablet (0.55 g) contains *Radix Notoginseng* 0.5 g

Dosage:
Oral administration 2–6 tablets 3 times daily.

Price: 36 tablets — $5 (sealed)

Manufacturer:
Yunnan Weihe Pharmaceutical Co. Ltd. Add: Yuxi, Yunnan, China.

Exported by:
Yunnan Camellia Pharmaceutical Import & Export Co., Ltd. Imported by: Tong Jum Chew Pte Ltd, 21 Kaki Bukit Tech Park II Singapore 415957 Tel: 62781134 Fax: 62781246.

235. **Red Ginseng Candy Rennesse (Korean Ginseng Corp.)**

Details:
No information available

Ingredients:
White Sugar, Corn Syrup, Isomalto Oligosaccharides, 6-Year-Old Korean Red Ginseng Extract, Xylitol, Ginseng flavor, Ginseng distillation flavor, 6-Year-Old Korean Red Ginseng Powder, L-Menthol.

Dosage:
No information available

Price: Net WT. 4.23 OZ (120 g)/Box — $8.50

Manufacturer:
Korea Ginseng Corp. Daejun, Seo-Ku, Dunsan-Dong 926 (Customer Service: TEL 1588-2304). Made in Korea.

Sole Authorized Distributor:
Wing Joo Loong Ginseng Hong (S) Co Pte. Ltd 30 & 31 North Canal Road, Singapore 059286, Tel: 6538-3838 Fax: 6534-2800.

236. **Red Panax Ginseng Extractum (Wellring)**

Description:
The Panax Ginseng Extractum (oral) is made of Chinese Panax Ginseng by extract-ing all the above-mentioned compositions from this material and manufactured into liquid by scientific method. Its taste a little bitter. This preparation is a valuable tonic good for organs of the body.

Actions and indications:
It is remedy for stimulates blood circulation, neurasthenia, over-fatigue, poor appe-tite, indigestion, insomnia, poor memory.

Ingredients:
Each bottle (10 ml) contains extract equivalent to raw herbs: Red *Panax Ginseng* 1 g, Sodium Benzoate 0.03 g.

Dosage:
Oral, 1 bottle (10 ml) each time, 3 time a day.

Safety considerations:
Side effects not known. Not for patients with Sthenia-syndrome and Heat-syndrome.

Price: 10 bottles — $7.20 (sealed)

Manufacturer:
Jilin Province Fusong Pharmaceutical Co., Ltd Song Shan, China.

Importer/Assembler:
Hua Bao Agency Pte Ltd. 105, Sims Avenue #06-10 Chancerlodge Complex Singapore 387429. Tel: 67490809, Fax: 67493662.

237. **Red Sun 3 In 1 Ling Zhi Spores [Cracked] (Red Sun)**

Description:
[LingZhi] has been well-known for its rare medicinal plant and precious herb since ancient time. What is Lingzhi Spores? Spores are released from Lingzhi when maturity. They are very tiny, which cannot be seen with our naked eyes, they can only be seen through a microscope. Lingzhi Spores powder are formed by numerous spores. Each 0.6 gm of Lingzhi Spore is 75 times more effective than ordinary Lingzhi. Red Sun 3 in 1 Ling Zhi Spores is manufactured in Japan using the latest scientific technology and under strict quality control. Red Sun 3 in 1 Ling Zhi Spores is specially formulated with the combination of cracked Spores Powder, Ginseng and Grape Seed Extract to further enhance the body's well being. It also combine Vitamin C, B1, B2 and B6 to aid better absorption in gastrointestinal tract thus strengthen the efficacy of the Ling Zhi Spore. Red Sun 3 in 1 Ling Zhi Spores which protects health, increases stamina, assists blood circulation and improves the complexion is your ideal choice to preserve one's health.

Ingredients:
Active ingredients: Ling Zhi Spores 200 mg, Ginseng 20 mg, Vitamin B1 2 mg, Vitamin B6 2 mg, Grape Seed Extract 20 mg, Vitamin C 20 mg, Vitamin B2 2 mg.
Dosage:
For general well-being, take 1 capsule daily. For the weak, 1 to 2 capsules twice daily, preferably in morning and at night for a period of 3 months. After body's condition improved, just take 1 capsule a day.

Price: 90 capsules — $85

Manufacturer:

Made in Japan. Redsun Singapore Pte Ltd. 43 Kaki Bukit Place Singapore 416221. Tel: (65)- 63377133 Fax: (65)-68421810. Website: www.redsunproducts.com

238.   **Sanye Goodnite (Camellia Brand)**

Description:

Relief stress

Actions:

To boost "qi" and relive stress. To improve blood ciculation

Indications:

It is most suitable for persons suffering from effect of low 'qi', such as insomnia and palpitation.

Ingredients:

Each 50 mg tablet contains extract equivalent to 1250 mg of Leaf of *Radix Notoginseng.*

Dosage:

Oral use. 1–2 tablets/dose, 3 times per day. To be taken after meals.

Safety considerations:

No known side effects. Patients with hypertension, heart disease, diabetics, liver and kidney troubles, should take under physician's advice. Not suitable for patient suffering from flu/cold.

Price: 80 tablets — $7.60 (sealed); 500 tabs — $38.00 (sealed bottle)

Manufacturer:

Weihe Pharmaceutical Co., Ltd. Yuxi, Yunnan, China. Exporter: Yunnan Camellia Pharmaceutical I/E Co., Ltd.

Importer:

Hygeian Medical Supplies (Pte) Ltd. 203 Henderson Rd. #07-06 Henderson industrial Park, Singapore 159546. Tel: 62702993 Fax: 63395034.

239.   **Senior-Time Once a day "Nutritional Insurance" (Kordel's)**

Description:

A special daily supplement formulated to meet the special nutritional needs of middle age onwards, the prime time of life! At a time when the need for energy is decreasing. It's easy to skip meals and miss out on those important nutrients so important for the extra energy and vitality needed to enjoy this special time of life. Senior-Time's Special formula provides the important nutrients needed for good health and vitality, every day.

Ingredients:
Each tablet contains: Vitamins & other cofactors: Thiamine Hydrochloride (Vitamin B1) 15 mg, Riboflavin (Vitamin B2) 15 mg, Nicotinamide 12 mg, Calcium Panthothenate 25 mg equivalent Pantothenic Acid (Vitamin B5) 23 mg, Pyridoxine hydrochloride (Vitamin B6) 10 mg, Cyanocobalamin (Vitamin B12) 50 µg, Cholecalciferol (Vitamin D3 200 IU) 5 µg, d-alpha Tocopheryl Acid Succinate (Vitamin E 75 IU) 62 mg, Ascorbic Acid (Vitamin C) 250 mg, Betacarotene 2 mg, Biotin 50 µg, Folic Acid 300 µg, Inositol 16 mg, Choline Bitartrate 40 mg, Cysteine hydrochloride 15 mg, Bioflavonoids 50 mg, Lecithin 30 mg, Rutin 10 mg, Papaon 25 mg. Minerals: Chromium (as Chromic Chloride) 50 µg, Copper (as Cupric Ssulphate) 170 µg, Iron (as Ferrous Fumarate) 5 mg, Magnesium (as Magnesium Oxide) 75 mg, Manganese (as Manganese Sulphate) 1.3 mg, Iodine (as Potassium Iodide) 46 µg, Zinc (as Zinc Gluconate) 15 mg, Selenium (as Selenomethionine) 26 µg. Herbal Extracts Equiv. Dry: Eleutherococcus senticosus (SIBERIAN GINSENG) Root 100 mg, Ginkgo biloba (GINKGO) standardised extract equivalent to leaf dry 250 mg equiv. Ginkgo flavonglycosides 1.34 mg.

Directions:
Adults: Take one tablet daily, with breakfast, as a dietary supplement. Vitamin supplements should not replace a balance diet. DO NOT EXCEED THE STATED DOSE.

Price: 30 tablets — $21.65 (sealed); Kordel's is a trademark of Health Foods International.

Manufactured for:
Nutra-Life Health & Fitness (NZ) Ltd. Auckland, New Zealand. www.kordelproducts.co.nz. Australian Distributor- Nutra-Life Health & Fitness. Australia Pty Ltd. 5 Kaleski Street, Moorebank, NSW 2170 www.nutralife.com.au.

Singapore/Malaysia Agent:
Cambert (F.E.) Pte Ltd

240. **Shen Yu Jing with Cordyceps, Wild Ginseng & Radix Aatragali (Ferragold)**

Description:
This is a traditional health product that blends the best Cordyceps, Wild Ginseng and Radix Aatragali extracts without adding any preservatives, using the best traditional manufacturing method. It has high nutritional protein that is easily absorbed

by the human body. It aids in speeding up the recovery of wounds and relief of mild swelling. It can also be consume as indicated for general health to boosts immunity system of the body.

Ingredients:

Cordyceps extract (20%), Wild Ginseng extract (20%), Radix Aatragali extract (15%), Shen Yu extract (45%).

Dosage:

Adult — 1 bottle each time; 2 times a day; Children — 1/2 bottle each time, 2 times a day.

Price: 6 bottles × 75 ml — $20.80

Sole Agent:

Ferragold (S) Pte Ltd., Blk 3015A #05-07, Ubi Road 1 S'pore 408705; Tel: (65) 6744 6656.

241. **Sheng Mai Yin He Ji (QianJin)**

Actions:

Benefit qi and promote the production of body fluid.

Indications:

Indicated for deficiency of qi and yin, marked by lassitude, breathless, mental fatigue, dry throat or thirst, prolong cough with little but sticky phlegm etc.

Ingredients:

Each 30 ml of this product contains the following raw herbs: *Radix Et Rhizoma Ginseng* 6.8 g, *Radix Ophiopogonis* 6.8 g, *Fructus Schisandrae* 4.4 g.

Dosage:

30 ml each time, 2 times daily. Shake well before use.

Safety considerations:

No known side effect. No known contraindication

Price: 500 ml — $17.00 (Sealed)

Manufacturer:

Kiat Ling Health Products & Trading. Blk 3017 Bedok North St. 5 #04-15 Singapore 486121. Tel: 67441868. Fax: 67435267.

242. **Sheng Yu Jing (Zhong Ti)**

Description:

Sheng-yu Jing is made up of natural protein, vitamins and amino acid, prescribed with selected quality chinese herbs. It has the effects of repairing tissue, eliminating swells and bruises and health building. It is especially effective for body repair after operations and child-delivery.

Ingredients:
Sheng Yu (44%), Radix Astragali (15%), Arillus Longan (5%), Radix Et Rhizoma Rehmanniae (6%), Fructus Lycii (8%), Radix Codonopsitis (6%), American Ginseng (16%)

Dosage:
No information available

Price: 70 ml × 6 — $12.50

Manufacturer:
Chung Kuo Refined Chinese Medicine Dealers Ltd.; Manufactured Under Supervision of Huangshi Tiancheng Pharmeucutical Co. Ltd., China.

Imported By:
Chung Kuo Refined Chinese Medicine Dealers Ltd. 554 Havelock Road #09-00, Singapore 169639; Tel: 7224121

243. **Shexiang Shuhuo-jing (Win Brand)**

Description:
Treatment of muscular sprains and twist, all kinds of contusions, muscular fatigue, pains in the neck, shoulders, lumber region or legs, nonulcerous chilblains and prickly heat.

Ingredients:
Each 60 ml contains the following raw herbs: *Artificial Moschus* 0.001 g, *Radix Notoginseng* 0.03 g, *Flos Carthami* 0.05 g, *Resina Draconis* 0.01 g, *Radix Rehmanniae* 1.10 g, *Camphora* 1.72 g, *Borneolum Syntheticum* 1.03 g, *Herba Menthae* 0.38 g, Alcohol 51 ml.

Direction:
For external application, 2–3 times a day.

Safety considerations:
Warning: Not for oral consumption. Pregnant women use with caution.

Price: 60 ml — $8.00 (sealed)

Manufacturer:
Huangshi Feiyun Pharmaceutical Co. Ltd., Hubei China.

Imported by:
Wideway Pte Ltd. 2 kallang Ave #06-07 Kallang Bahru Complex, S'pore 339407. Tel: 62923618. Fax: 62966956. Import Licence No. CPMI 0003.

244.   **Shou Wu Chih with Cordyceps & Ginseng (QianJin)**

Description:

Shou Wu Chih with Cordyceps & Ginseng is refinedly manufactured by modern technology with specially selected high quality tonic herbs. This health product is possessed of its efficacies in nourishing hair while restoring hair and its natural colour. It also strengthens the body, promotes health and vitality and increases one's resistance to illness. A superior product of effectiveness.

Actions and indications:

Treatment of general weakness; Anemia; Blackening hair, maintaining youthfulness; Increasing stamina, nourishing blood; Restoring nutrients in hair-roots; Strengthening sinens and bones, enhancing pigment of beard and hair

Ingredients:

Each 20 ml of this preparation contains extracts equivalent to: FORMULA: Radix Polygoni Multiflori (1 g), Radix Panacis Quinquefolii (0.15 g), Cordyceps (0.1 g), Semen Sesami (0.1 g), Radix Angelicae Sinensis (0.2 g), Poria (0.1 g), Fructus Psoraleae (0.1 g), Rhizoma Polygonati (0.15 g), Rhizoma Gastrodiae (0.15 g), Radix Achyranthis Bidentatae (0.1 g), Fructus Lycii (0.2 g), Semen Cuscutae (0.1 g).

Dosage:

2 to 3 times daily. Adult: 15 ml each time (3 teaspoons); Children: 10 ml each time (2 teaspoons)

Price: 320 ml — $8.50

Manufacturer:

Kiat Ling Health Products & Trading, Blk 3017 Bedok North St. 5, #04-15 Singapore 486121; Fax: 67435267.

245.   **Shu Jin Lu [Easy Flex] (Nan San Brand)**

Indications:

Trauma, sprain, rheumatic pain, sgony of muscles, tendons, joints and bones, muscle spasm, numbness and tingling of extremities, fatigue, headache, common cold and abdominal pain. Sports Massage.

Ingredients:

Each 60 ml of preparation contains extracts equivalent to raw herbs: *Rhizoma Curcumae* 1.08 g, *Ramulus Cinnamomi* 0.78 g, *Rhizoma Homalomenae* 0.72 g, *Rhizoma Sparganii* 0.54 g, *Radix Notoginseng* 0.30 g, *Radix Angelicae Dahuricae* 0.24 g, *Lignum Sappan* 0.12 g, *Flos Carthami* 0.06 g, *Mentholum* 3.60 g.

Directions:
1. Massage the affected part after spraying the tincture on it. 2. Before sports, massage the muscles and joints after spraying of the tincture to prevent muscle spasm. After sports, apply to relieve fatigue. 3. Spray around the navel for relieving abdominal pain. 4. Spray the appropriate amount of tincture into hot water and take an immersed bath for common cold or fatigue of the whole body.

Safety considerations:
Attention: Keep out of eyes. Keep away from fire and high temperature. Not to be taken internally.

Price: 60 ml — $ 27.00 (sealed)

Sole Agent:
Made in Hong Kong. Tong Jum Chew Pte Ltd 21, Kaki Bukit View Tech Park II, Singapore 415957 Tel: 62781134 (3 lines) Fax: 62781246

246. **Siberian Ginseng Pure Root [410 mg per capsule for active lifestyle 100 capsules] (Greenlife)**

Description:
Siberian Ginseng supports individuals leading an active and demanding lifestyle that can create fatigue or reduce work capacity and concentration.

Ingredients:
Serving size 3 capsules. Serving per container 33. Amount per serving: Calories 5, Total Carbohydrate 1 g, Dietary Fiber less than 1 gram, Calcium 25 mg, Siberian Ginseng (root) 1.23 g (1230 mg).

Dosage:
Recommendation: Take 3 capsules three times daily, preferably with food. Use continuously for eight weeks, followed by a two week break.

Price: 100 capsules — $27.80

Manufacturer:
GreenLife by the Schwabe Group of Companies, USA

247. **Siberian Ginseng Root 500 mg (Ginsa Gold)**

Description:
Product Features: Each capsule contains 500 mg Siberian Ginseng Root Extract standardized to provide 0.02% Eleuthorsides (0.1 mg). Is a distant relative of American and Korean Ginseng, with some overlap in its uses. Provides assured intake of Eleu-

thorsides, responsible for Siberian Ginseng's efficacy. Suitable for vegetarian. Benefits: Traditionally used to support and restore vitality and overall well-being. Maintains mental alertness hence enable one to concentrate and maintain a sharp mind. Enhances physical stamina and increase muscle strength, which particularly benefits those who feel fatigue. Helps body to deal with stressful condition like bacteria & virus infection.

Ingredients:
Supplement Facts: Serving Size 1 capsules. Servings per container 90. Amount per serving %DV Siberian Ginseng Root Extract 500.00 mg** (*Eleutherococcus Senticosus*) (0.02% Eleutherosides = 0.10 mg)** Daily Value (DV) not established. Other Ingredients: Cellulose, Gelatin. No Sugar, No Starch, No Artificial Color, No Artificial Flavors, Sodium Free, No Wheat, No Gluten, No Corn, No Soy, No Dairy.

Safety considerations:
Warning: Consult your physician prior to using this product if you are pregnant, nursing or taking medication, or have a medical condition. Discontinue use two weeks prior to surgery.

Dosage:
As a dietary supplement, take one capsule daily.

Price: 90 vcaps — $28.95

Manufacturer:
No information available

248. **Skin Allergy Relief Capsules (AL)**

Actions and indications:
Clearing away heat and toxins, removing dampness and relieving itch. It is effective for all kinds of skin pruritus, ocute and chronic rashes, eczema, dermatitis, urticaria, and skin allergy due to food consumption (such as fish, prawn, crab, spicy food or alcohol causing macular eruption).

Ingredients:
Each capsule (0.35 g) contains extract equivalent to raw herbs: *Herba Robdosiae Rubescentis* 100 mg, *Fructus Xanthii* 200 mg, *Radix Ginseng* 50 mg, *Radix Sophorae Flavescentis* 150 mg, *Periostracum Cicadae* 100 mg, *Fructus Cnidii* 200 mg, *Bombyx Batryticatus* 120 mg, *Rhizoma Smilacis Glabrae* 140 mg, *Cortex Dictamni Radicis* 100 mg, *Radix Glycyrrhizae* 50 mg, *Borneolum Syntheticum* 0.3 mg.

Dosage:
Adult: 3–4 capsules each time, twice a day. Half dosage for children. Each course of medication lasts 15 days.

Safety considerations:
Side effects and contraindications not known.

Price: 30 capsules — $7.10 (sealed)

Manufacturer and sole distributor in Singapore:
ALL Link Medical & health products pte ltd. 10 Kaki Bukit Road 1, #03-27 K B Industrial Building, Singapore 416175. Tel: 68460337. Fax: 68460336.

249. **Standardized American White Ginseng (Ginsa Gold)**

Description:
Product Features: Each capsule contains 500 mg American Ginseng Root Extract standardized to provide 3% Ginsenosides (15 mg). Provides assured intake of Ginsenosides, for health benefits. Standardized formula which provides uniformity of 15 mg of Ginsenosides per capsule batch after batch. Ginsenosides is considered by science to be the key ingredient responsible for ginseng's efficacy. Suitable for vegetarian. Benefits: Traditionally used to support vitality and overall well-being. Promotes Yin energy to enhance Yin-Yang balance in our body. Increases body's ability to tolerate stressful situation. Calms the body thus promotes relaxing effect. Reduces digestive upset & ulcers caused by emotional stress.

Ingredients:
Supplement Facts: Serving Size 1 capsules. Servings per container 90. Amount per serving %DV American Ginseng Root Extract 500.00 mg** (*Panax quinquefolium*) (3% Ginsenosides = 15 mg)** Daily Value (DV) not established. Other Ingredients: Cellulose, Gelatin. No Sugar, No Starch, No Artificial Color, No Artificial Flavors, Sodium Free, No Wheat, No Gluten, No Corn, No Soy, No Dairy, Yeast Free.

Dosage:
As a dietary supplement, take one or two capsules daily.

Safety considerations:
Warning: Consult your physician prior to using this product if you are pregnant, nursing or taking medication, or have a medical condition. Discontinue use two weeks prior to surgery.

Price: 90 vcaps — $69.95

Manufacturer:
No information available

250. **Standardized Triple Ginseng Root (Ginsa Gold)**

Description:

Product Features: Each capsule contains 3 types of ginseng: Panax Ginseng root extract, American Ginseng root extract and Siberian Root extract with its standardized active ingredient respectively. Provides assured intake of Ginsenosides and Eleutherosides responsible for ginseng's efficacy. Suitable for vegetarian. Benefits: Promotes Yin-Yang energy balance in our body which ensures overall well-being. Maintains mental alertness hence enable one to concentrate and maintain a sharp mind. Enhances physical stamina and increases muscle strength, thus very beneficial for those who feel fatigue. Promotes immune health by increasing body's resistance to common infections.

Ingredients:

Supplement Facts: Serving Size: One capsule. Servings per container: 90/180. Amount per serving Korean White Ginseng Root and Powdered Extract 156 mg* (*Panax ginseng*) (Ginsenosides = 6 mg) American Ginseng Root 200 mg* (*Panax quinquefolium*) (Ginsenosides = 6 mg) Siberian Root and Powdered Extract 127 mg* (*Eleutherococcus senticosus*) (Eleutherosides = 0.04 mg)* Daily Value (DV) not established. Other Ingredients: Vegeatble Cellulose Capsule. No Sugar, No Starch, No Artificial Colours, No Artificial Flavors, No Wheat, No Gluten, No Corn, No Soy, No Dairy, Yeast Free.

Dosage:

As a dietary supplement, take one or two capsules daily.

Price: 90 capsules — $53.50. 180 capsules — $98.95

Manufacturer:

No information available

251. **Steam-boat Herbal Soup (Yew Chian Haw)**

Details:

No information available

Ingredients:

Cordyceps Sinensis, Panax Ginseng, Codonopsis Pilosula, Rhizoma Dioscorea Batatas, Polygonatum Odoratum

Instruction:

Method: Boil 300 ml (or 12 rice bowls) water, add in YEW CHIAN HAW 'Steamboat Herbal Soup' ingredients and 1 kg chicken bone (or any kind of meat) simmer for 30 minute, add in 1 teaspoon salt to taste. Serve with any kind of seafood, meat, mushroom and vegetable into steamboat.

Price: 2 × 25 g — $3.90

Made & Distributed by:
YEW CHIAN HAW (MALAYSIA) SDN. BHD., (Company No. 218632-A) 2, Lingtang Beringin 2, Jalan Permatang Damar Laut, 11960 Batu Maung, Penang, Malaysia. Tel: 604-626 2020 (8 lines): Fax: 604-626 1010, Email: ych@e-ych.com.

Distributed by:
YEW CHIAN HAW (SINGAPORE) PTE. LTD. (Company No. 199200237-N) Blk 158, Mei Ling Street # 01-90 Singapore 140158, Tel: 65-64729442, Fax: 65-64729441, Email: ych.sg@e-ych.com; YEW CHIAN HAW TAIWAN INTERNATIONAL PTE. LTD, (rest all in Chinese).

252. **Steamed Tienchi Tablets (Camellia Brand)**
Actions:
Regulates and enriches the blood.

Indications:
Used for nutritional anemia or anemia due to loss of blood and irregular menstruation.

Ingredients:
Each tablet (0.55 g) contains *Radix Notoginseng Preparata* 0.5 g

Dosage:
For oral administration, take 6–10 tablets, 3 times daily. Reduce the dosage for children. This product may be taken with milk, chicken or meat soup.

Safety considerations:
Side effects not known.

Price: 60 tablets — $8 (sealed)

Manufacturer:
Yunnan Weihe Pharmaceutical Co. Ltd. Yunnan. China. Exported by: Yunnan Camellia pharmaceutical.
Import & Export Co., Ltd. imported by:
Tong Jum Chew Pte Ltd, 21 Kaki Bukit Tech Park II Singapore 415957 Tel: 62781134 Fax: 62781246.

253. **Summer-Heat Clearing Tablets (Nature's green)**
Actions and indications:
For fever and dizziness, fatigue and lack of strength, spontaneous perspiration, irritability, dry mouth and thirst caused by summer-heat.

Ingredients:
Each 420 mg tablet contains extracts equivalent to raw herbs: *Radix Panacis Quinquefolii* 18 mg, *Radix Astragali* 75 mg, *Rhizoma Atractylodis Macrocephalae* 180 mg, *Rhizoma Atracylodis* 70 mg, *Radix Ophiopogonis* 35 mg, *Rhizoma Alismatis* 30 mg, *Fructus Schisandrae* 18 mg, *Radix Angelicae Sinensis* 24 mg, *Radix Scutellariae* 30 mg, *Radix Puerariae* 180 mg, *Pericarpium Citri Reticulatae Viride* 35 mg, *Pericarpium Citri Reticulatae* 35 mg, *Massa Fermentata Medicinalis* 40 mg, *Rhizoma Cimicifugae* 30 mg, *Radix Glycyrrhizae* 60 mg.

Dosage:
For oral administration, take 4 tablets, 3 times daily.

Safety considerations:
Side effects not known. Take with caution for pregnant women.

Price: 500 tablets — $33 (sealed bottle)

Manufacturer:
Tong Jum Chew Pte Ltd. 21 Kaki Bukit View Tech Park II Singapore 415957. Tel: 62781134 Fax: 62781246. Singapore Manufacturer Licence No. MLCP 0400040, Singapore CPM Product Reference No. 113565.

254.   **Super Vita-Vim (Nature's Essence)**

Description:
39 sustained release balanced vitamins, minerals, phytonutrients, prebiotics and probiotics. A comprehensive combination of 39 important nutrients in a balanced sustained release formula (over 3–4 hours) to promote optimal assimilation and convenience. Ganeden BC30 is a proprietary, shelf stable probiotic strain of Bacillus coagulans. This beneficial bacteria, is highly resilient and has a high survival rate through the body's hostile gastric environment than many other probiotics. Ganeden BC30 is prolific colonizer which reproduces adequate numbers of probiotic cells to provide health benefits for the digestive tract and immune system. Store between 10 °C–28 °C to maintain optimum potency and shelf life. Best kept refrigerated. Keep out of reach of children.

Ingredients:
Vitamin A (acetate) 2000 IU, Beta Carotene (Provitamin A) 1000 IU, Vitamin D3 (Cholecalciferol) 300 IU, Vitamin E (d-alpha-tocopherol) 50 IU, Vitamin C (ascorbic acid) 100 mg, Vitamin B5 (pantothenic acid) 30 mg, Vitamin B3 (niacinamide) 20 mg, Vitamin B1 (thiamine) 10 mg, Vitamin B2 (riboflavin) 10 mg, Vitamin B6 (pyridoxine HCl) 10 mg, Choline 10 mg, Inositol 10 mg, Folic acid 200 mcg, Biotin 100 mcg, Vitamin B12 (methylcobalamin) 20 mcg, Calcium (carbonate) 100 mg, Magnesium

(amino acid chelate) 40 mg, Potassium (amino acid chelate) 15 mg, Phosphorus (phosphate) 10 mg, Zinc (amino acid chelate) 10 mg, Iron (amino acid chelate) 2 mg, Copper (amino acid chelate) 1 mg, Manganese (amino acid chelate) 1 mg, Boron (amino acid chelate) 500 mcg, Iodine (atlantic kelp) 100 mcg, Chromium (polynicotinate) 20 mcg, Selenium (1-selenomethionine) 20 mcg, Molybdenum (amino acid chelate) 10 mcg, American Ginseng SE (5%) 20 mg, Spirulina 20 mg, Citrus Bioflavonoids 10 mg, Rutin 10 mg, Ginkgo Biloba SE (24%/6%)** 5 mg, Bioperine (95% piperine) 2 mg, Lutein 1 mg, Lycopene 1 mg, Rosemary Oil Extract 1 mg, Ganeden BC (Bacillus coagulans GBI-30 6086 viable cells) 0.3 bln, Inulin/FOS 100 mg.** ginkgoflavonglycoside-24%, terpenelactones-6%.

Dosage:
Suggested use: 1 caplet daily.

Price: 60 caplets — $35.55 (Sealed)

Manufactured in USA by:
FDA registered facility.

Imported & distributed by:
WIL Harrisons (I/E) & Associates. Raffles City P.O. Box 1159, Singapore 911739.

255. **Superfine Supreme Ginseng & Bird's Nest with Rock Sugar (Nature's Green)**
Details:
No information available

Ingredients:
Bird's Nest, Ginseng, Rock Sugar Solution

Instruction:
Serving Suggestion: This product can be consumed directly from the bottle either chilled or warmed, depending on individual preferences.

Price: 150 g — $29.00

Distributed by:
Tong Jum Chew Pte. Ltd., 21 Kaki Bukit View Teck Park II Singapore 415957; Tel: 6278 1134; Fax: 6278 1246.

256. **Superior Ginseng Royal Jelly (Zhongti)**
Description:
Superior Ginseng Royal Jelly is prepared from Ginsengs that are at least 8 years of age, found in the renowned Chang Bai Shan Mountain of north eastern China.

Together with concentrated Royal Jelly, it is a superior tonic and balanced health supplement and manufactured under advance technological environment. This product contains nutrients, amino acids, RNA-Polymerase, vitamins, proteins, etc. It maintains the complete cell structure of Ginseng andthe therapeutic properties of other ingredients. It is easily assimilated by the human body and has no known side effect. The superior Ginseng restores youthful energy. Royal Jelly is a complex mixture secreted by the hypopharyngeal glands of worker bees. The queen bees which feed on Royal Jelly are much bigger in size than the worker bees and have much longer life span. Royal Jelly contains amino acids, pantothenic acids, minerals, proteins and carbohydrates. It promotes cell metabolism, improves immunity, revitalizes old cells and retards the aging process, etc.

Indications:
Immunity adjustment, retards the aging process, improve immunity.

Ingredients:
Ginseng 200 mg, Royal Jelly 300 mg, Fructus Schisandrae 100 mg, Honey Base 7000 mg, Water to 10 ml.

Dosage:
One bottle to be taken daily before breakfast with warm boiled water and another before dinner when necessary.

Safety considerations:
No known side effect. Cautions: Not suitable for children. This product may be suitable for asthma and allergy suffers.

Price: 10 ampules — $3.90 (sealed)

Manufacturer:
Harbin Pharm Group Sanjing Pharmaceutical Co., Ltd, Heilongjiang Province, China.

Importer & Assembler:
Chung Kuo Refined Chinese Medicine Dealers Ltd 554 Havelock Road, #09-00, Ganges Centre, Singapore 169639. Tel: 67334121 Fax: 67342804.

257.   **Superior Sore Throat Powder (Nature's green)**

Description:
Superior Sore Throat Powder is finely made with watermelon frost as the main ingredient in combination with various precious Chinese medicinal materials such as pearl powder, thunberg fritillary bulb and cow-bezoar. It helps bring quick, soothing relief for oral and throat diseases, and is effective for reducing the pain of sore thoart,

allaying tongue inflammation, relieving painful swollen gums and stopping gingival bleeding.

Actions and indications:
Allays inflammation and relieves pain. Gives symptomatic relief for sore throat, oral ulceration, painful swelling or bleeding of the gums, pharyngolaryngitis, tonsillitis, stomatitis and thrush.

Ingredients:
Each bottle (2 g) contains raw herbs: *Pulvis Pericarpii Citrulli Preparatus* 500 mg, *Margarita* 160 mg, *Calculus Bovis Artifactus* 100 mg, *Bulbus Fritillariae Thunbergii* 200 mg, *Rhizoma Menispermi* 240 mg, *Radix Trichosanthis* 200 mg, *Radix Ginseng* 100 mg, *Rhizoma Belamcandae* 120 mg, *Mentholum* 80 mg, *Borneolum Syntheticum* 100 mg, *Radix Glycyrrhizae* 200 mg.

Instruction:
Spray some powder directly onto the affected parts, 3–4 times daily. In serious cases, taken 1–2 g orally simultaneously, 3 times daily.

Safety considerations:
Side effects not known. Avoid smoking, alcohol, fried or spicy foods, and seafood. Contraindicated in pregnant and nursing women.

Price: $5

Manufacturer:
Tong Jum Chew Pte Ltd 21 Kaki Bukit View Tech Park II Singapore 415957 Tel: 62781134 Fax 62781246. Licence No: MLCP 0400040 CPM Reference No: 113835.

258. **Superior White Phoenix Pills (Nature's Green)**

Description:
Superior White Phoenix Pills is prepared and refined with traditional method from purebred Black Cock with precious medicinal herbs. It enjoys high reputation throughout the world for its superior qualities. Medication: Activates blood circulation to eliminate blood stasis, relieve menstrual period pain, make you savour your lives with more energy. Nourishs blood and qi, makes you ruddy and healthy, improves the immune system. Raise the body's resistance to disease. Helps you to adapt to high work pressure.

Actions:
Invigorating Qi and and enriching the blood, regulating menstruation and stopping leukorrhea.

Indications:
It can be used for deficiency of both qi and blood, thin and weak body, lassitude in loins and lence, irregular menstruation.

Ingredients:
Each bolus (6 g) contains extracts equivalent to raw herbs: *Pullus cum Osse Nigro* 978 mg, *Colla Cornus Cervi* 196 mg, *Carapax Trionycis* 98 mg, *Concha Ostreae* 73 mg, *Ootheca Mantidis* 73 mg, *Radix Ginseng* 196 mg, *Radix Astragali* 49 mg, *Radix Angelicae Sinensis* 220 mg, *Radix Paeoniae Alba* 196 mg, *Radix Asparagi* 98 mg, *Rhizoma Cyperi* 196 mg, *Radix Glycyrrhizae* 49 mg, *Radix Rehmanniae* 390 mg, *Radix Rehmanniae Perparata* 390 mg, *Rhizoma Chuanxiong* 98 mg, *Radix Stellariae* 40 mg, *Radix Salviae Miltiorrhizae* 196 mg, *Rhizoma Dioscoreae* 196 mg, *Cornu Cervi Degelatinatum* 73 mg, *Semen Euryales* 98 mg, Honey 2097 mg.

Dosage:
Take 1 bolus (6 g) orally, twice daily.

Safety considerations:
Side effects and contraindications not known.

Price: 6 Bolus × 6 g × 2 boxes — $37.00 (sealed)

Manufacturer:
GuangZhou ChenliJi Pharmaceutical Factory. Guangzhou, China.

Imported/Repacked by:
Tong Jum Chew Pte Ltd 21 Kaki Bukit View Tech Park II Singapore 415957 Tel: 62781134 Fax: 62781246

259. **Tasly Compound Danshen Dripping Pills (Jin Pai Trademark)**

Description:
Jin Pai Tasly Compound Danshen Dripping Pill is a natural medicine. Its characteristics coupled with the ingredients' water solubility make Compound Danshen Dripping Pill easily absorbed into the blood directly and rapidly through oral mucosa. This enables the onset of actions within 3 to 5 minutes. Compound Danshen Dripping Pill is highly bio-available hence no gastrointestinal tract side effects. Properties: Compound Danshen Dripping Pill is of dark brown colour; small round fragrated pills with a bitter taste.

Actions and indications:
For preventing and treating angina pectoris. Functions: Rejuvenates the blood and eliminates blood clots; easy breathing; relief chest pain.

Pharmacological action:
Dilate the coronary artery and increasing blood flow of the coronary artery. Decreasing blood platelet aggregation and lowering blood viscosity.

Ingredients:
Each pill 27 mg contains extract equivalent to raw herbs: *Radix Salviae Miltiorrhizae* 90 mg, *Radix Notoginseng* 17.6 mg, *Borneol* 1 mg.

Dosage:
To be administered orally or sublingually (ie below the tongue) For treatment: 10 pills each dose 3 times daily for 4 weeks or as prescribed by doctor. For preventation: 10 pills each dose, 2 times daily.

Safety considerations:
Not suitable for pregnant women.

Price: 27 mg/pill × 100 pills × 2 bottles (200 pills) — $20 (sealed)

Manufacturer:
Tianjin Tasly Pharmaceutical Co. Ltd. Tianjin, China.

Assembler and Importer:
No. 297 Kaki Bukit Avenue 1 Shun Li Industrial Park Singapore 416083. Tel: (65) 67415561 Fax: (65) 67413605.

260. **TCM Huoluo Capsule (Keyi)**
Actions:
To expel wind and cold, eliminate dampness and resolve phlegm, promote blood circulation to activate meridian and collateral.

Indications:
It is indicated for numbness of the four limbs due to blockage by wind-phlegm. It is indicated for blockage syndromes due to blockage by cold-dampness, which manifested as muscular spasm, pains in the lower back and legs, or traumatic injury, inconvenient in walking and pain in the heart due to obstruction of qi in the chest. It is also indicated and rheumatic arthritis with above symptoms.

Ingredients:
Each capsule (400 mg) contains extracts euivalent to raw herbs: *Faeces Trogopterori* 40 mg, *Radix et Rhizoma Clematidis* 40 mg, *Rhizoma Gastrodiae* 40 mg, *Carapax et Plastrum Testudinis* 40 mg, *Radix Polygoni Multiflori Praeparata* 40 mg, *Herba Ephedrae* 40 mg, *Rhizoma et Radix Notopterygii* 40 mg, *Radix et Rhizoma Glycyrrhizae Praeparata cum Melle* 40 mg, *Herba Agastaches* 40 mg, *Ramulus Cinnamomi* 80 mg, *Radix et Rhizoma Rhei Praeparata* 40 mg, *Radix Linderae* 40 mg,

Lignum Aquilariae Resinatum 40 mg, *Radix Rehmanniae Praeparata* 40 mg, *Radix Paeoniae Rubra* 20 mg, *Radix Aucklandiae* 40 mg, *Flos Caryophylli* 20 mg, *Rhizoma ChuanXiong* 40 mg, *Pericarpium Citri Reticulatae Viride* 20 mg, *Myrrha* 20 mg, *Semen Amomi Rotundis* 20 mg, *Olibanum* 20 mg, *Poria* 20 mg, *Rhizoma Pinelliae Praeparatum* 20 mg, *Radix Scrophulariae* 20 mg, *Rhizoma Drynariae* 20 mg, *Radix Saposhnikoviae* 50 mg, *Benzoinum* 20 mg, *Sanguis Draconis* 14 mg, *Radix Scutellariae* 20 mg, *Colophonium* 10 mg, *Rhizoma Cyperi* 20 mg, *Borneolum Syntheticum* 3 mg, *Rhizoma Atractylodis Macrocephalae* 20 mg, *Pheretima* 10 mg, *Radix Puerariae Lobatae* 30 mg, *Radix et Rhizoma Ginseng* 60 mg, *Radix Angelicae Sinensis* 30 mg, *Eupolyphaga Seu Steleophaga* 20 mg.

Dosage:
Oral administration, 3 capsules each time, 3 times a day.

Price: 60 capsules — $24 (sealed)

Manufacturer:
Science Arts Co Pte Ltd. 150 MacPherson Road, Science Arts Building, Singapore 348524.

261.   **Tea Egg Spices Sachet (nil)**

Details:
No information available

Ingredients:
Cinnamon, Star Anise, Pepper, Ginseng Root, cumin, Clove, Cardamon.

Instruction:
Preparation: (1) 25–30 hard boiled eggs. Crack the egg shells but don't peel it. (2) Boil 3.5 L of water. Put al eggs into boiled water and put other ingredients including Tea Egg Herbal 1 sachet, Light Soy Sauce 200–250 ml, Dark Soy Sauce 2 spoons and Sugar 200 gm into the water too. Cook over medium heat for about 3 hours and enjoy it.* Caution: Water must cover over the eggs

Price: 40 gm — $2.80

Packed by:
Unita Enterprise No. 9 Jalan Saga 3, Taman Desa Cemerlang, 81800 Ulu Tiram, Johr, Malysia. H/P: 016-730 6256, 019-752 0501; Fax: 07-861 0288.

Singapore Distributor:
Hua Bao Agency Pte Ltd. 105, Sims Avenue #06-10, Chancelodge Complex Singapore 387429; Tel: 6749 0809, Fax: 6749 3662.

262. **Thirst Relieving Capsules (Nature's Green)**

Description:

PIL: Xiao-Ke, or "wasting and thirsting" is a common health problem. The patient's metabolism is disrupted and the body is unable to manage its food intake properly. Thirst Relieving Capsules are made from highly concentrated, specially selected, all-natural Chinese herbs and produced in accordance with traditional Chinese formula. It can relieve the symptoms of unusual thirst woth excessive drinking, frequent and profuse turbid urination, weight loss in spite of increased appetite and food intake, as well as weakness and fatigue caused by metabolic disorder.

Actions and indications:

This product helps adjust metabolic function and relieves the "wasting and thirsting" syndrome characterized by excessive eating, unusual thirst, frequent and profuse urination, fatigue, feeble limbs, and loss of weight.

Ingredients:

Each 350 mg capsule contains extracts equivalent to raw herbs: *Radix Ginseng* 32 mg, *Radix Astragali* 52 mg, *Radix Trichosanthis* 209 mg, *Rhizoma Dioscoreae* 209 mg, *Radix Rehmanniae* 52 mg, *Fructus Lycii* 32 mg, *Rhizoma Anemarrhenae* 32 mg, *Radix Asparagi* 16 mg, *Poria* 21 mg, *Fructus Corni* 21 mg, *Fructus Schisandrae* 16 mg, *Radix Puerariae* 21 mg, *Endothelium Corneum Gigeriae Galli* 21 mg.

Dosage:

For oral administration, take 4 capsules, 3 times daily before meals. The recommended first course of treatment is twenty days.

Safety considerations:

Side effects not known (On PIL). Contraindications/Caution: Avoid alcohol, cigarette, and any food containing sugar. (On PIL)

Price: 60 capsules — $15.00 (not sealed)

Manufacturer:

Tong Jum Chew Pte Ltd. 21 Kaki Bukit View Tech Park II Singapore 415957. Tel: 62781134 Fax: 62781246. Singapore Manufacturer Licence No. MLCP 0400040, Singapore CPM Product Reference No. 112879

263. **Tian Qi Bu Chiew (Kwei Feng Trade Mark)**

Description:

Tian Qi or Radix pseudo-ginseng is one of the valuable medicinal herbs found in Guangxi. Its functions have been mentioned in the Chinese traditional pharmacological works several hundred years ago. Radix pseudo-ginseng has long been regarded and used among the folks as a tonic for the weak, the sick and the old. Tian Qi Bu Chiew is prepared mainly from Radix pseudo-ginseng of Guangxi origin and blended with more than ten kinds of valuable herbs such as Radix Astragali, Radix Codonopsitis, Lycium Chinese, and Eucommia ulmoides, being infused in pure spirit of rice for years. It is distinguished for its fragrant flavour and is regarded as a nutrition. To drink everyday will keep you healthy. Caution: Not to be taken by pregnant women or those suffering from fever. If symptoms persist, please consult a doctor.

Ingredients:
No information available

Dosage:
No information available

Safety considerations:
Not to be taken by pregnant women or those suffering from fever. If symptoms persist, please consult a doctor.

Price: 300 ml; 33% (V/V) — $14.80

Manufacturer:
Lungshan Shan Distillery, Wuzhou, Guangxi.

Importer:
Wah Thong Co. Pte. Ltd, 346/346A King Georger's Avenue, Singapore 208577.

264.   **Tian Qi Bu Chiew Likeur (Kwei Feng Trade Mark)**

Description:
Tian Qi or Radix pseudo-ginseng is one of the valuable medicinal herbs found in Guangxi. Its functions have been mentioned in the Chinese traditional pharmacological works several hundred years ago. Radix pseudo-ginseng has long been regarded and used among the folks as a tonic for the weak, the sick and the old. Tian Qi Bu Chiew is prepared mainly from Radix pseudo-ginseng of Guangxi origin and blended with more than ten kinds of valuable herbs such as Radix Astragali, Radix Codonopsitis, Lycium Chinese, and Eucommia ulmoides, being infused in pure sprit of rice for years. It is distinguished for its fragrant flavour and is regarded as a nutrition. To drink everyday will keep you healthy. Caution: Not to be taken by pregnant women or those suffering from fever. If symptoms persist, please consult a doctor.

Ingredients:
Radix Pseudoginseng (6 mg), Radix Astragali (5 mg), Radix Codonopsis (5 mg), Fructus Cyci (4 mg), Cortex Eucommiae (4 mg), Arillus Longanae (7 mg), Rhizoma Polygoeati (5 mg)

Dosage:
No information available

Safety considerations:
Caution: Not to be taken by pregnant women or those suffering from fever. If symptoms persist, please consult a doctor.

Price: Alcoholic Volume: 550 ml; Alcoholic Content: 33% Vol. — $27.55

Manufacturer:
Lungshan Medicated Winery, Wuzhou, Guangxi 27, 2nd Xin Xiang Road, Wuzhou Guangxi, China.

Imported by:
Wah Thong Co. Pte. Ltd., 346 King George's Ave (S) 208577; Tel: 52993722.

265. **Tian Qi Capsule (Camellia Brand)**

Actions and indications:
Stop bleeding and remove blood stasis, relieve swelling and alleviate pain. For traumatic bleeding swelling and pain due to external injury. (Usage: OTC medication for acute and chromic sprain injury of soft tissue.)

Ingredients:
Each capsule contains 300 mg extracts equivalent to raw *Radix Notoginseng* 350 mg.

Dosage:
For oral administration, take 6–8 capsules 2 times daily.

Safety considerations:
No known side effects. Expectant women or elderly and young children should take under physician's advice. Not recommended for individulas with liver dysfunction.

Price: 80 capsules — $11.80, 300 capsules — $32 (sealed)

Manufacturer:
Weihe Pharmaceutical Co. Ltd. Yuxi, Yunnan. Exporter: Yunnan Camellia Pharmaceutical I/E Co. ltd.

Importer:
Hygeian Medical Supplies (Pte) Ltd 203 Henderson Road #07-06. Henderson Industrial Park, Singapore 159546 Tel: 62702993 Fax: 63395034.

266. **Tian Qi Rheumatic Plaster (Nature's Green)**

Actions:
Removing obstruction of meridians, promoting blood circulation and expelling wind to relieve pain.

Indications:
Joint pain, lumbago and back pain, sprain and topical pain due to rheumatism.

Ingredients:
Each piece of plaster (7 × 10 cm) contains extracts equivalent to raw herbs: *Radix Notoginseng* 0.02 g, *Radix Paeoniae Rubra* 0.02 g, *Rhizoma Et Radix Notopterygii* 0.02 g, *Radix Gentianae Macrophyllae* 0.02 g, *Herba Schizonepetae* 0.02 g, *Herba Asari* 0.02 g, *Flos Carthami* 0.01 g, *Radix Angelicae Pubescentis* 0.02 g, *Cortex Cinnamomi* 0.04 g, *Ramulus Cinnamomi* 0.04 g, *Capsicum Frutescens L.* 0.12 g, *Rhizoma Curcumae Longae* 0.04 g, *Radix Angelicae Sinensis* 0.01 g.

Instruction:
Place plaster on the affected area or follow doctor's order.

Price: 1 pack (5 plasters) — $2.00

Manufacturer:
Anhui Anke YuLiangQing Pharmaceutical Co. Ltd.

Sole Agent:
Tong Jum Chew Pte Ltd 21 Kaki Bukit View Tech Park II Singapore 415957 Tel: 62781134. Fax: 62781246.

267. **Tianqi Baji Jiu (nil)**

Details:
No information available

Ingredients:
Radix Notoginseng (0.85%), Radix Morindae Officinalis (0.90%), Radix Codonopsis (1.15%), Rhizoma Polygonati (1.15%), Fructus Chaenomelis (0.49%), Fructus Roase Laevigatae (0.98%), Fructus Lycii (0.80%), Radix Aucklandiae (0.16%), Radix Glyczyrrhizae (0.48%), Sugar Candy (2.50%), Rice Wine (90.80%).

Dosage:
No information available

Price: 300 ml; 29% Vol. — $14.90

Manufacturer:
Sin Wah Thong Liquor Co Pte Ltd., 63 Ubi Ave 1 * 03-06 Singapore 408937.

Sole agent:
Sin Wah Thong Liquor Co. Pte Ltd, No. 4 New Industrial Road. #05-05 Mainland Industrial Building Singapore 535198; Tel: 282-8953(3 Lines); Fax: (65)284-0231.

268. **Tianqi Lingzhi bu Jiu (nil)**

Details:
No information available

Ingredients:
Radix Pseudoginseng (0,60%), Ganoderma Japonicum (0,45%), Radix Morindae officinalis (0,45%), Cortex Eucommiae (0,35%), Ginseng (0,45%), Radix Astragali (0,25%), Rhizoma Polygoeat (0,25%), Fructus Lycii (0,35%), Rock Sugar (0,35%), Rice Wine (93,35%).

Dosage:
No information available

Price: 150 ml 29% alcohol content — $7.13

Manufacturer:
Produced by the People's Republic of China (Guangxi).

Imported:
Sin Wah Thong Liquor Co Pte. Ltd. 63 Ubi Ave 1, # 03-06 Singapore 408937

269. **Tianqi Rheumatism Ointment (Baiyunshan)**

Description:
PIL: Physical Propery: It is a brownish ointment with menthol fragrance. Functions: It is an OTC pharmaceutical product and for relief of pains in muscle and joints.

Actions and indications:
By invigorating blood circulation and removing blood stasis, it relaxes sinews and reduces swelling. It is suitable for sprains, rheumatic aches and pain or pulled muscles.

Ingredients:
Each 1000 g ointment Contains extract equivalent to raw herbs: *Herba Glechomae* 35 g, *Radix et Rhizoma Rhei* 35 g, *Flos Lonicerae Japonica* 35 g, *Radix et Rhizoma Glycyrrhizae* 35 g, *Rhizoma Drynariae* 69 g, *Camphora* 52 g, *Semen Persicae* 35 g, *Herba Lycopi* 35 g, *Fructus Chaenomelis* 35 g, *Herba Lycopodii* 35 g, *Mentholum* 69 g, *Lignum Sappan* 69 g, *Radix Notoginseng* 17 g, *Radix Angelicae Sinensis* 35 g, *Rhizoma et Radix Notopterygii* 35 g, *Herba Siegesbeckiae* 35 g, *Radix Saposhnikoviae* 35 g, *Cortex Erythrinae Orientalis* 35 g, *Radix Angelicae Pubescentis* 35 g, *Radix Dipsaci* 35 g, *Fructus Gardeniae* 35 g, *Cortex Acanthopanacis* 35 g, *Radix Angelicae Dahuricae* 69 g, *Radix Clematidis* 35 g.

Instruction:
Apply onto affected area and rub in thoroughly 2–3 times daily.

Price: 25 g — $3.80

Safety considerations:
Do not apply over open wounds. Elderly and children- consult physician's advice before application. Discontinue using in the event allergic reaction. Not suitable for pregnant women.

Manufacturer:
Guangzhou Baiyunshan Pharmaceutical Co. Ltd. Baiyunshan He Ji Gong Pharmaceutical Factory. Guangzhou Baiyun district, Tonghe Street, No. 6 Yuntai Road. Guangzhou, China.

Importer:
Hyegian Medical Supplies (Pte) Ltd. 203 Henderson Road, #07-06 Henderson Ind Park, Singapore 159546. Tel: (65) 6270 2993. Fax: (65) 63395034.

270.   **Tien-chi feng-shi die-da jing [An essence for rheumatism & die-da] (Medicking)**

Description:
PIL: Properties: It is a clear, brownish-red liquid (PIL: The essence gives prompt effects chiefly because of the appropriate combination of all medical staffs as shown below: Tien-chi is the best remedy for die-da (it means "stumble & hit"), and when combined with other Chinese herbs such as Acanthopanax, Adenosma, etc., it exerts dissipation of bruise, analgeisa, hemostasia, activation and relaxation of muscles, as well as improvement of circulation. The addition of Syzygium, Oleum menthae and Oleum eucalypti gives the "wind-expelling", "cold-dissipating" and preventive actions against the sequela of die-da, whereas the addition of Oleum gaultheriae, Dryobalanops and Cinnamomum camphora helps the penetration of all active principles deeply into the skin and muscle, thus producing the effects onto the affected part. All medical staffs contained in the essence are prepared and refined by the scientific process. Their effects are prompt and significant. Indeed, the essence is an ideal remedy for dwellers and travellers.)

Indications:
Indication: (also in PIL): Rheumatism, ostalgia, muscular pain, lumbago, shoulder and neck stiffness, rheumatic neuralgia, arthritis, sprain and contusion muscular tension and sprain due to over-exercise.

Ingredients:
Herba Adenosma Glutinosum Druce (2 g/60 ml), Caulis Trachelospermi (2.5 g/60 ml), Cortex Acanthopancis (2.7 g/60 ml), Rhizoma Homalomenae

(2.2 g/60 ml), Caulis Piperis kadsurae (2.2 g/60 ml), Olcum Menthae (0.8 g/60 ml), Radix Notoginseng (7 g/60 ml), Ramulus Mori (2.5 g/60 ml), Flos Caryopylli (0.3 g/60 ml), Semen Dryobalanops Aromatica (2 g/60 ml), Cinnamomum Camphora (0.8 g/60 ml), Olcum Eucalypti (0.5 g/60 ml), Olcum Gaultheriae (0.5 g/60 ml), Ramulus Zanthoxylum (2 g/60 ml), Alcohol (42 g/60 ml), Distillated Water (36 g/60 ml).

Instruction:
Apply sufficient quantity evenly on the affected part 2–3 times daily, or more when needed.

Safety considerations:
For external use.

Price: 60 ml — $4.00

Manufacturer:
Wuzhou Yunshan Pharmaceutical Factory Guangxi, China.

Imported by:
Winlykah Trading, Blk 8, Lorong Bakar Batu, #06-09 Singapore

271. **Tien-chi Powder Raw (Camellia Brand)**

Details:
** Indications, administrations and dosage: See inside leaflet for details. Note: Packaging is sealed.

Ingredients:
Radix Notoginseng 100%

Dosage:
No information available

Price: 40 g per bottle — $12 (sealed)

Manufacturer:
Yunnan Weihe Pharmaceutical Co. Ltd.

Exported by:
Yunnan Camellia Pharmaceutical Import & Export Co., Ltd.

Imported by:
Tong Jum Chew Pte Ltd, Alexandra Distripark Blk 1 #08-15/17 Pasir Panjang Road Singapore 118478 Tel: 62781134 (3 Lines) Fax: 62781246.

272.   Tien-chi Powder Steamed (Yunnan Baiyao)

Description:

Yunnan Province is China's nateral treasury of medicinical herbs. It abounds in various kinds of crude medicine. Some of which are precious and are, enjoying a good reputation as exclusively unique and genuine. Tienchi, or Radix pseudo-ginseng is just one of these medicines, which is well-known as a highly nourishing tonic of Yunnan origin. In Pentsao Kangmu, one of the classics of Chinese traditional medicine, tienchi is also called chinpuhuan, which implies that it is so precious that one would not swop it even for gold. As a result of the researches by modern medical scientists. It has been found that tienchi not only contains five kinds of triterpenoidal saponins, the aglycones of which constitutes both panaxadiol and panaxatriol, but is also rich in iron, calcium, protein, fat, sugar etc. When steamed, tienchi becomes a very efficacious blood tonic, strengthens the body, promotes growth and increases vitality with durable effect. If taken frequently, it is good for health and the prevention of diseases, especially hypercholesterolemia. It may be taken by all, at any time, irresepective of sex, age or season for the year.

Indications:

General debility weakness after illness or childbirth, loss of appetite, anemia with sensation of chill, neurasthenia, insomnia, amnesi, night sweat due to weakness, over fatigue, under development of children, hypercholesterolemia.

Ingredients:

Radix Pseudoginseng 100%

Instruction:

Adminstration: tienchi powdered steamed is to be stewed together with chicken. The usual dosage is to add 5–10 g for each adult partaking of the dish. It must be appropriately reduced for children. For those who are not accustomed to the sweet bitterness of tienchi, it is advisable not to add the powder until after the chicken has been done to a turn. In this way the meat will retain its original taste, although the soup maybe slightly bitter. In order to obtain a better flavour, it is recommended that an earthenware steam pot specially made in Yunnan be used for this purpose. Tienchi Powder Steamed may also be taken with soup or milk, each time 3–5 g.

Safety considerations:

Common cold and fever. After administration, no sour or cold food and drinks should be taken.

Price: $12

Manufacturer:
Yunnan Baiyao Group Co., Ltd, Kunming, Yunnan, P.R. China.
Imported by:
Science arts co. pte ltd. 150 MacPherson Rd, Science Arts building Singapore 348524.

273. **Tienchi-Ginseng Tea (Yulin)**

Description:
Tienchi-Ginseng Tea is made from the finest selected Tienchi-Ginseng and is prepared scientifically to retain the efficacious ingredients of panaxosides. It is a natural health drink for both sexes of all ages and in all seasons.

Ingredients:
Notoginseng radix 2000 mg

Price: 20 bags 3 gm. Each; Netto: 60 g — $7.70

Importer:
Kinhong (Pte) Ltd., 297 Kaki Bukit Ave 1; Shun Li Industrial Park Singapore 416068.

274. **Tongkat Ali Capsules (Nature's Green)**

Description:
Eurycoma Longifolia, commonly known as Tongkat Ali, is a shrub-free found growing wild in the rainforest of Southeast Asia. Tongkat Ali has an ancient reputation in Malaysia and Indonesis and used traditionally to increase energy levels, endurance and stamina, and to enhance overall physical and sensual performance. Nature's Green Tongkat Ali Capsule contains a blend of pure quality raw Eurycoma powder from Malaysia and 6 other natural herbal extracts and prepared by modern pharmaceutical technology. The product's enhancing energy and stamina properties help support physical wellness and vitality in men, and make man stronger.

Actions:
Strengthens organic functions, restores and maintains vitality, energizes spirit, increases stamina, and improves physical endurances.

Ingredients:
Amount per serving (serving size: 2 Capsule 800 mg): Tongkat Ali Powder 560 mg, Maca (root) 100 mg, American Ginseng Extract 50 mg, *Epimedium* Herb Extract 50 mg, *Tribulus Terrestris* (fruit) Extract 40 mg.

Dosage:
for oral administration, take 2 capsules, 2 times daily before meals.

Price: 60 capsules — $42.00. 2 × 60 capsules — $73.00 (Sealed)

Manufacturer:
Tong Jum Chew Pte Ltd. 21 Kaki Bukit View Tech Park II Singapore 415957. Tel: 62781134 Fax: 62781246.

275. **Tongren Niuhuang Qingxin Wan (Tong Ren Tang)**

Actions:
To nourish qi and blood, to transquilize and allay excitement, to resolve phlegm and calm the endogenous wind.

Indications:
Heat stagnated in the chest, palpitation and fidgets due to deficiency, dizziness and accumulation and obstruction of the sputum caused by deficiency of qi and blood, phlegm-heat attacking upwards.

Ingredients:
Each pill weight 3 g contains raw herbs: *Calculus Bovis, Cornu Bubali, Cortex Cinnamomi, Massa Medicata Fermentata, Pollen Typhae Carbonisatum, Radix Ampelopsis, Radix Bupleuri, Radix Glycyrrhizae, Radix Paeoniae Alba, Radix Saposhnikoviae, Rhizoma Atractylodis Macrocephalae Preparata, Rhizoma Chuanxiong, Rhizoma Zingiberis, Semen Armeniacae Amarum Preparata, Semen Glycines Siccus, Colla Corii Asini, Cornu Saigae Tataricae, Fructus Jujubae, Moschus, Poria, Radix Angelicae Sinensis, Radix Ginseng, Radix Ophiopogonis, Radix Platycodi, Radix Scutellariae, Rhizoma Dioscoreae, Borneolum syntheticum*
**All the ingredients are written in Capitals and no strength is given.

Dosage:
1–2 pills, twice a day, appropraite reduction of the dosage for children.

Safety considerations:
Precaution: Used with caution in pregnancy. Notice: Remove the waxen shell, plastic shell and cellophane before being taken; Not to swallow in whole pill.

Price: $30 (packaging is sealed)

Manufacturer:
Beijing Tongrentang Co. Ltd Tongrengtang Pharmaceutical Factory Beijing, China. Imported by: Science Arts Co. Pte Ltd. 150 MacPherson Rd, Science Arts Building Singapore 348524.

276. **Tou Gu Jing Bone And Muscle Liniment (Nature's Green)**

Actions and indication:
Invigorate the circulation of blood, reduce swelling, abate pain, relax muscles and joints. For use in sports injuries, muscle pulls, sprains and contusion, aching back and leg.

Ingredients:
60 ml of this preparation contains extracts equivalent to raw herbs: *Moschus (syntheic)* 0.51 mg, *Radix Notoginseng* 25.56 mg, *Flos Carthami* 51.12 mg, *Resina Dracinis* 25.56 mg, *Radix Rehmanniae* 1097.28 mg, *Camphora* 1716 mg, *Borneolum Syntheticum* 1026 mg, *Mentholum* 384 mg.

Instruction:
Spread or spray on the affected parts, three times a day. For external use only, immediate effect is noticeable.

Safety considerations:
Side effects not known. Not to be used by pregnant woman.

Price: 60 ml — $5.50 (sealed)

Manufacturer:
Huangshi Fy Pharmaceutical Co. Ltd Hubei, China. Importer: Tong Jum Chew Pte Ltd 21, Kaki Bukit View Tech Park II, Singapore 415957 Tel: 62781134 (3 lines) Fax: 62781246

277. **8 Treasure Health Tea (Fei Fah Hall)**

Details:
No information available

Ingredients:
Green Tea, Chrysanthemum, The fruit of Chinese wolfberries, American, Ginseng, Longan, Jujube, Bud of Lotus seed, Grape, Rock sugar.

Instruction:
Empty one sachet of "8 Treasure Health Tea" into a tea cup or mug. Add boiling water and allow to infuse for 8 minutes before serving.

Price: 20 g × 10 — $8.50

Manufacturer:
Fei Fah Medical Mfg Pte Ltd (Singapore), No. 61 Kaki Bukit Ave 1 #02-29 Shun Li Industrial Park, Singapore 417943; Tel: (65)8440208; Fax: (65)8440209; email: feifah@mbox5.singnet.com.sg; Fei Fah Medibalm (HK) Co.; RM 1803 Nam Wo

Hong Bldg., 148 Wing Lok St., Sheung Wan, Hong Kongg; Tel: (852)2117 4638; Fax: (852)2119 0926; email: feifahmed@etimail3.com; Made in China; With Quality control by Hong Kong; This is a natural dry food. No artifical additives; Vaccum packets sachets.

278.   **Tri-improve capsule for men (QianJin)**

Description:

A great health supplement tonic for men well-being

Indications:

Revitalizes and invigorates body system. Supports vitality and stamina. Supports alertness and concentration. Supports cardiovascular health.

Ingredients:

Each capsule (350 mg) certains Tongkat Ali (*Eurycomo Longifolia Jack*) 200 mg, American Ginseng 50 mg, *Radix Monodae Officinalis* 50 mg, *Cordyceps* 50 mg.

Dosage:

Oral administration, 2 capsules each time, 2 times daily.

Price: 50 capsules — $28.00(sealed)

Quality Assurance by:

Kiat Ling Health Products & Trading. Blk 3017, Bedok North ST. 5, #04-15 Singapore 486121. Tel: 67441868 Fax: 67435267.

279.   **Tzepao Sanpien Jiu (Changyu Pioneer Wine Co.)**

Actions:

Nutrious and strengthening waist, promoting the brain and recovering memory and for general debility

Indication:

General weakness, untimely senility, neurasthenia, sores in waists and backs, over-burdens of the brain, dizziness, poor memory, involumtary perspiration, insomnia, pale faces, poor appetite.

Ingredients:

Penis Cervi (5%), Penis Otariae (1%), Penis Canitis (1%), Radix Ginseng (7%), Cornn Cervi Pantotrichum (5%), Radix Astragli (10%), Radix angelicae Sinensis (6%)

Instruction:

To be taken at any time according to drinker's capacity for liquor.

Price:
250 ml; 35% Alc. Vol. — $14.00

Imported by:
Wah Thong Co. Pte. Ltd., 346 King George's Ave (S) 208577; Tel: 52993722.
Changyu Pioneer Wine Company Limited Yantai China.

280. **Urinary Maintenance Tablets (Nature's Green)**

Actions and indications:
Astringes spontaneous urination and arrests enuresis. Relieves the symptoms of frequent urination, enuresis or urinary incontinence.

Ingredients:
Each 350 mg tablet contains extracts equivalent to raw herbs: *Ootheca Mantidis* 200 mg, *Os Draconis* 200 mg, *Carapax et Plastrum Testudinis* 200 mg, *Rhizoma Acori Talarinowii* 200 mg, *Radix Polygalae* 200 mg, *Radix Ginseng* 200 mg, *Sclerotium Poriae Circum Radicem Pini* 200 mg, *Radix Angelicae Sinensis* 200 mg.

Dosage:
For oral administration, take 5 tablets, 3 times daily. The recommended treatment course is 15 days.

Safety considerations:
Side effects and contraindications not known (only on the bottle of 500 tablets).

Price: 60 tablets — $9.50 (not sealed but no PIL); 500 tablets — $50.00 (sealed bottle)

Manufacturer:
Tong Jum Chew Pte Ltd. 21 Kaki Bukit View Tech Park II Singapore 415957. Tel: 62781134 Fax: 62781246. Singapore Manufacturer Licence No. MLCP: 0400040 Singapore CPM Product Reference No. 114072.

281. **Vegetarian White-Phoenix Tablets (Nature's Green)**

Actions and indications:
Regulates menstruation and arrests leukorrhea. Use for emaciation and general feebleness, aching, weakness and limpness of loins and knees, irregular menstruation with abnormal leukorrhea, fatigue, lassitude, and weakness after delivery.

Ingredients:
Each 380 mg tablet contains extracts equivalent to raw herbs: *Cordyceps* 50 mg, *Margarita* 35 mg, *Cordyceps Sinensis* (Fermented) 50 mg, *Ganoderma Lucidum* 100 mg, *Radix Panacis Quinquefolii* 75 mg, *Radix Astragali* 20 mg, *Radix Anglica Sinensis* 85 mg, *Radix Paeoniae Alba* 75 mg, *Rhizoma Cyperi* 75 mg, *Radix Asparagi*

40 mg, *Radix Rehmanniae* 150 mg, *Radix Rehmanniae Preparata* 150 mg, *Rhizoma Chuanxiong* 40 mg, *Radix Stellariae* 15 mg, *Radix Salviae Miltiorrhiae* 75 mg, *Flos Carthami* 65 mg, *Rhizoma Dioscoreae* 75 mg, *Radix Aucklandiae* 50 mg, *Concha Ostreae Preparata* 30 mg, *Semen Eutyales* 40 mg, *Radix Glycyrrhizae* 20 mg.

Dosage:
For oral administration, take 3 tablets, 2 times daily.

Price: 60 tablets — $25.00 (sealed)

Manufacturer:
Tong Jum Chew Pte Ltd 21 Kaki Bukit View Tech Park II Singapore 415957 Tel: 62781134 Fax: 62781246 Singapore Manufacturer Licence No.: MLCP 0400040 Singapore CPM Product Reference No. 114594.

282. **Vigorous walking Tablets (Nature's Green)**

Actions and indications:
Strengthens the muscles and bones. Relieves symptoms of weakness and soreness of back and knees, vertigo, flaccidity and weakness of the lower limbs, difficulty in walking caused by deficiency of kidney and liver.

Ingredients:
Cortex Eucommiae Preparata 50 mg, *Radix Notoginseng* 100 mg, *Radix Dipsaci* 100 mg, *Radix Achyranthis Bidentatae* 100 mg, *Fructus Psoraleae Preparata* 50 mg, *Carapax et Plastrum Testudinis Preparata* 50 mg, *Radix Fleminglae Philippinensis* 50 mg, *Radix Millettiae Speciosae* 50 mg, *Fructus Chaenomelis* 100 mg, *Radix Angelicae Pubescentis* 50 mg, *Radix Gentianae Macrophyllae* 50 mg, *Radix Saposhnikoviae* 50 mg, *Eupolyphaga Seu Steleophaga* 30 mg, *Radix Ginseng* 7.5 mg, *Radix Astragali* 50 mg, *Fructus Lycii* 100 mg, *Radix Rehmanniae Preparata* 50 mg, *Radix Angelicae Sinensis* 50 mg, *Semen Cuscutae* 50 mg, *Poria* 50 mg, *Herba Cynomorii* 50 mg, *Rhizoma Anemarrhenae* 50 mg, *Rhizoma Atractylodis Macrocephalae Preparata* 50 mg.

Dosage:
For oral administration, take 3 tablets, 2–3 times daily.

Safety considerations:
Side effects not known. Not to be taken by pregnant women.

Price: 500 tablets — $46 (sealed)

Manufacturer:
Tong Jum Chew Pte Ltd. 21 Kaki Bukit View Tech Park II Singapore 415957. Tel: 62781134. Fax: 62781246. Singapore Manufacturer No: MLCP 0400040 Singapore CPM product reference number: 113566.

283. **Vision Care Eye Capsules (QianJin)**

Actions and indications:
Nourish kidney and improve vision. Relieves vision discomforts and supports the health and care of the eyes.

Ingredients:
Each 300 mg of capsule contains the following: *cornu bubali* 9 mg, *cornu saigae tataricae* 15 mg, *flos chrysanthemi* 12 mg, *fructus aurantii praeparata* 6 mg, *fructus lycii* 18 mg, *fructus schisandrae* 9 mg, *fructus tribuli praeparata* 12 mg, *herba cistanches* 9 mg, *herba dendrobii* 24 mg, *poria* 15 mg, *radix achyranthis bidentate* 9 mg, *radix asparagi* 15 mg, *radix et rhizome glycyrrhizae* 9 mg, *radix ginseng* 12 mg, *radix ophiopogonis* 15 mg, *radix ophiopogonis* 15 mg, *radix rehmanniae* 15 mg, *radix rehmanniae praeparata* 15 mg, *radix saposhnikoviae* 6 mg, *radix scutellariae* 9 mg, *rhizoma chuanxiong* 6 mg, *rhizoma dioscoreae* 15 mg, *semen armeniacae amarum* 6 mg, *semen cassiae* 15 mg, *semen celosiae* 15 mg, *semen cuscutae* 9 mg.

Dosage:
Oral administration, 3 capsules 3 times daily.

Safety considerations:
Side effects not known. Pregnancy use with care.

Price: 50 capsules — $7.50.

Manufacturer:
Kiat Ling Health Products & Trading Blk 3017, Bedok North St 5, #04-15 Singapore 486121 Tel: 67441868 Fax: 67435267.

284. **Vision with Lutein & Bilberry (60Vcaps) (Greenlife)**

Description:
Vision formula is a synergistic blend of vitamins, minerals and herbal nutrients. This product is free of common food allergens. It contains no yeast, milk, lactose, wheat, sugar or corn.

Ingredients:
Serving size 2 capsules. Serving per container 30. Total Carbohydrate 1 g, Vitamin A (as retinol palmitate) 2000 IU, Vitamin E (as d-alpha tocopheryl succinate) 80 IU, Riboflavin (Vitamin B2) 8 mg, Niacin (as niacinamide) 20 mg, Biotin (as biotin-triturate) 40 mcg, Zinc (Zinc amino acid chelate) 16 mg, Copper (as Copper amino acid chelate (soy)) 1 mg, Citrus Bioflavonoids 10% 150 mg, Taurine 150 mg, Cayenne Pepper (fruit) 100 mg, Bilberry extract (fruit), 25% anthocyanins 50 mg, Siberian Eleuthero (root) 50 mg, Grape Seed extract (Tru-OPCs) 20 mg, Lutein 6 mg. Other ingredients: Millet, Plant-derived capsule, Magnesium Stearate.

Dosage:

Recommendation: Take 2 capsules daily, preferably with food.

Price: 60 vegecaps — $51.35

Manufacturer:

Manufactured for Green Life by NWP, Inc., Springville, UT 84663 USA.

285. **Vitaton Gold [100 softgels] (Vita Health)**

Description:

A premium multivitamin-mineral formulation fortified with exotic herbal ingredients, amino acids and new-age antioxidants.

Ingredients:

Each softgel contains: Betacarotene 1.4 mg, Vitamin C (ascorbic acid) 60 mg, Vitamin D2 200 IU, Vitamin E (d-alpha Tocopherol) 50 IU, Vitamin B1 (thiamin) 1.5 mg, Vitamin B2 (riboflavin) 1.7 mg, Vitamin B6 (pyridoxine) 2 mg, Folic Acid 50 mcg, Vitamin B12 (cyanocobalamin) 6 mcg, Nicotinamide 10 mg, Biotin 100 mcg, Calcium Pantothenate 7.5 mg, Elemental Calcium (From Calcium Amino Acid Chelate 50 mg) 10 mg, Elemental Magnesium (From Magnesium Amino Acid Chelate 12.5 mg) 2.5 mg, Iron 5 mg, Copper 100 mcg, Iodine 50 mcg, Selenium 26 mcg, Elemental Zinc (From Zinc Amino Acid Chelate 12.5 mg) 2.5 mg, Cysteine 10 mg, Lysine Hydrochloride 10 mg, Chromium 50 mcg. Herbal Extracts: Ginkgo Biloba 20 mg, *Panax Ginseng* 50 mg, Lycopene 1 mg, Lutein 500 mcg.

Dosage:

Adults: 1 softgel daily or as recommended by physician.

Price: No information available

Manufacturer:

Made in Australia under licence from Vita Health Laboratories (Aust) Pty. Ltd. 102 Bath Road, Kirrawee NSW 2232, Australia.

Imported by:

VitaHealth Asia Pacific (S) Pte Ltd Block 26 Kallang Place #05-04 Kallang Basin Industrial Estate Singapore 339157.

286. **Wellman [Co-Q10, L-Carnitine, Siberian Ginseng, Vitamins, Minerals, Amino Acids] (Vitabio-tics)**

Description:

It is to help maintain health, vitality, energy release for men of all ages. Wellman has been developed to help maintain health in men of all ages. It is ideal for those with a hectic lifestyle and is used by professional sportmen to help them maintain optimal nutrient levels during training. Unlike a general multivitamin the nutrient levels have been specifically formulated for men, often providing MORE THAN 100% of the Recommended Daily Allowance. Sport & Exercise: Vitamins C and E help protect against free radicals generated during exercise, plus amino acids and ginseng for all-round support. Hectic Lifestyle: L-Carnitine, Magnesium and Vitamin B complex for the effecient release of energy from food.

Ingredients:

Vitamin A (2500 IU) 750 μg [av.per tablet], Vitamin D (200 IU) [5 μg], vitamin E (natural source) [20 mg -TE], Vitamin C [60 mg], Thiamin (Vitamin B1) [12 mg], Riboflavin (Vitamin B2) [5 mg], Niacin (Vitamin B3) [20 mg NE], Vitamin B6 [9 mg], Folacin (as folic acid) [500 μg], Vitamin B12 [9 μg], Biotin [0.05 mg], Pantothenic Acid [10 mg], Iron [6 mg], Magnesium [50 mg], Zinc [15 mg], Iodine [150 μg], Manganese [3 mg], Copper [1 mg], Chromium [50 μg], Selenium [150 μg], Silicon [10 mg], Arginine [20 mg], Methionine [20 mg], Beta carotene [2 mg], P.A.B.A [20 mg], Siberian Ginseng [20 mg], Bioflavonoids [10 mg], Co-enzyme Q10 [2 mg], L-Carnitine [30 mg]

Dosage:

One tablet per day with your main meal. Swallow with a glass of water or a cold drink. Not to be chewed. Do not exceed the recommended intake. Wellman should only be taken on a full stomach.

Safety considerations:

Do not take while on warfarin therapy without medical advice.

Price: 30 tablets — $19.26

Manufacturer:

Neogetic International Pte Ltd Blk 1026 Tai Seng Avenue #06-3534 Tai Seng Ind. Estate Singapore 534413 RCB No: 200415355N.

287. **Wild Lingzhi Capsules (AL)**

Description:

"Wild Lingzhi Capsules" are the refined products made from extracts of strictly selected, natural, wild Ganoderma Lucidum and ginseng from China, using scientific extract technology. As such, it has the effects of Ganoderma being tranquilizing, expectorant, anti-asthmatic, anti-allergic & protects the lives. It also has the effects of ginseng in being a great energy tonic that can strengthen the spleen & heart. Combined together, each enhances the other to upgrade the overall potency. Daily dosage can enhance the different functions of the organs, soothe and regulate the activity of the central nervous system, improve circulation, strengthen the physique, enhance the memory, upgrade body immunity, promote longevity & good health.

Ingredients:
Each capsule (300 mg) contains extract equivalent to raw herbs: *Ganoderma Lucidum* 2000 mg, *Radix Ginseng* 120 mg.

Dosage:
1–2 capsules each time, twice a day, morning and evening.

Price: 60 capsules — $33.60 (sealed)

Manufacturer and Sole Distributor in Singapore:
All Link Medical & Health Products Pte Ltd. 10 Kaki Bukit Road 1, #03-27 K B Industrial Building, Singapore 416175. Tel: 68460337, Fax: 68460336.

288. **Win Brand Porous Capsicum Plaster [Strong Transdermal Plaster] (Win Brand)**

Actions:
Relieve Osteoarthritis Pain for 12 hours.

Indications:
Body aches and pains, rheumatic pain, arthralgia, lumbago, neuralgia, muscular aches, sprain, contusion etc.

Ingredients:
Pientzehuang 0.65% (combined of *Musk* 3%, *Calculus Bovis* 5%, *Radix Notoginseng* 85%, Snake Bile 7%), *Extractum Evodia Compositus* 45.30%, Menthol 17.25%, Camphor 12.90%, *Borneol* 12.90%, Wintergreen Oil 11.0%.

Instruction:
Wash affected area with soap and dry well. Cut appropriate size or whole piece of plaster and stick onto affected area. One plaster a day with maximum use of 12 hours. Ten days per therapeutic course. Hot compress and massage may improve curative effect.

Safety considerations:
Precaution: If the skin area is red and itchy, reduce the length of application. Series allergic patient, pregnant women and patient with skin problems should use with caution or seek doctor's advice.
Price: 1 box (5 plasters) — $2.20

Manufacturer:
Anhui Anke Yu Liang Qing Pharmaceutical Factory, Anhui, China.

Imported by:
Wideway Pte Ltd. 2 Kallang Ave #06-07 Kallang Bahru Complex, Singapore 339407 Tel: 62923618 Fax: 62966956.

289. **Woman's Harmony Tablets (Nature's Green)**

Actions and indications:
Nourishes heart and kidney. Relieves the symptoms of insomnia, forgetfulness, palpitation, tinnitus, doubting and worry, hectic fever, excessive sweating, irritability, liability to anger, weakness and lumbago due to menopausal syndrome.

Ingredients:
Each 400 mg tablet contains extracts equivalent to raw herbs: *Herba Epimedii* 125 mg, *Radix Polygoni Multiflori Preparata* 125 mg, *Caulis Polygoni Multiflori* 125 mg, *Concha Ostreae* 125 mg, *Semen Juplandis* 62.5 mg, *Fructus Psoraleae* 62.5 mg, *Radix Dipsaci* 62.5 mg, *Fructus Mori* 62.5 mg, *Semen Plantaginis* 62.5 mg, *Radix Angelicae Sinensis* 62.5 mg, *Radix Paeoniae Alba* 62.5 mg, *Fructus Rosae Laevigatae* 42 mg, *Radix Achyranthis Bidentatae* 42 mg, *Radix Ginseng* 25 mg, *Radix Rehmanniae Preparata* 35 mg, *Colla Cornus Cervi* 25 mg, *Rhizoma Anemarrhenae* 25 mg, *Radix Scutellariae* 25 mg, *Radix Glycyrrhizae* 25 mg.

Dosage:
For oral administration, take 4 tablets, 3 times daily.

Safety considerations:
Side effects not known. Not suitable for those suffering from flu. Avoid greasy or spicy foods.

Price: 500 tablets — $46.00 (sealed)

Manufacturer:
Tong Jum Chew Pte Ltd. 21 Alexandra Distripark Blk. 1. #08-15/17 Pasir Panjang Road Singapore 118478. Tel: 62781134 (3 Lines) Fax: 62781246 Manufacturer Licence No. MLCP: 0400040 Singapore CPM Product Reference No. 114416.

290. **Women's multi energy & vitality (Healtheries)**

Description:
How it works — A high potency "one-a-day" formulation of essential nutrients including extra iron, calcium, folic acid and B vitamins to help boost energy levels and maintain good health.

Ingredients:
(per tablet): Betacarotene 240 mcg, Vitamin B1 25 mg, Vitamin B2 25 mg, Nicotinamide 50 mg, Vitamin B5 30 mg, Vitamin B6 35 mg, Vitamin B12 50 mcg,

Folic Acid 300 mcg, Biotin 50 mcg, Vitamin C 100 mg, Vitamin D3 (100 IU) 2.5 mcg, Vitamin E (100 IU) 100 mg, Calcium (as amino acid chelate) 40 mg, Potassium (as amino acid chelate) 10 mg, Magnesium (as oxide) 20 mg, Iron (as ferrous fumarate) 10 mg, Zinc (as amino acid chelate) 6 mg, Selenium (as amino acid chelate) 25 mcg, Manganese (as amino acid chelate) 1 mg, copper (as amino acid chelate) 200 mcg, chromium (as amino acid chelate) 100 mcg, iodine (as potassium iodide) 15 mcg, Extract equivalent to Siberian ginseng root 1.5 g Spirulina powder 100 mg.

Dosage:
Adults: 1 tablet daily with food, or as directed by your healthcare practitioner.

Price: 60 tablets — $46.90 (sealed)

Manufacturer:
Made in New Zealand contact: For a personalised assessment and product information, visit us at www.healtheries.co.nz. Healtheries of New Zealand Ltd. Chr Kordel Place and Accent Drive. Auckland, New Zealand. Freephone: 0800848254.

Distributed by:
Medic Marketing Pte Ltd. 71 Tannery Lane #06-01/04 City Industrial Building Singapore 347807. email: enquiries@medic.com.sg.

291. **Women's Multivite (21st Century)**

Details:
No information available

Ingredients:
Each tablet contains: Vitamin E (natural) 50 IU, Vitamin D 200 IU, Calcium Ascorbate 100 mg, Beta Carotene (for Vitamin A) 5000 IU, Elemental Zinc 15 mg, Elemental Magnesium 50 mg, Elemental Iron 10 mg, Elemental Chromium 50 mcg, Vitamin B1 (Thiamine HCL) 30 mg, Vitamn B2 (Riboflavine) 30 mg, Vitamin B3 (Nicotinamide) 30 mg, Calcium Panthothenate (B5) 22 mg, Cyanocobalamin (B12) 75 mcg, Folic Acid 200 mcg, Biotin 40 mcg, Korean Ginseng (3:1 Extract) 17 mg, Bioflavonoids 30 mg, Royal Jelly 50 mg, Evening Primrose oil 50 mg.

Dosage:
Take one tablet daily after any meal or as prescribed by a physician.

Safety considerations:
Royal Jelly may cause allergic reactions for asthma patients and to those who suffer from allergy problems.

Price: 30 tablets — $17.95 (sealed)

Manufacturer:
21st Century HealthCare Inc., 2119 S. Wilson Street, Tempe, Arizona 85282-2034 USA.

Distributed by:
21st Century HealthCare Pte Ltd. 40, Jalan Pemimpin #03-02 Tat Ann Building Singapore 577185.

292. **Women's Senior-Vite [with lutein & Soy Isoflavones] (21st Century)**

Description:
Each tablet contains a complete range of vitamins, minerals, herbs and nutritional supplements especially formulated to maintain good health and for energy, for women over 50. Including special nutrients for women: Bitter Melon- for reducing the absorption of sugar in the body. Horse Chestnut- for improving blood circulation and reducing variscose veins. Lutein- for better eye health and improved night vision. Soy Isoflavones- for menopausal symptoms and conditions.

Ingredients:
Vitamins: Vitamin A 2500 IU, Vitamin B1 12.5 mg, Vitamin B2 12.5 mg, Vitamin B3 12.5 mg, Vitamin B5 12.5 mg, Vitamin B6 22.5 mg, Vitamin B12 25 mcg, Vitamin C 100 mg, Vitamin D 200 IU, Natural Vitamin E 50 IU. Ginseng: American ginseng 25 mg, Korean Ginseng 50 mg. Minerals: Calcium 100 mg, Magnesium 25 mg, Zinc 5 mg, Selenium 100 mcg, Copper 1 mg, Manganese 1.5 mg, Chromium 200 mcg, Potassium 5 mg. Herbs: Garlic (25:1 extract 60 mg) 1500 mg, Ginkgo Biloba (50:1 extract 5 mg) 1500 mg, Soy Isoflavones Extract 10 mg, Horse Chestnut (5:1 extract 40 mg) 200 mg, Gymnema (10:1 extract 10 mg) 100 mg, Bitter Melon (4:1 extract 25 mg) 100 mg, Red Clover 50 mg. Other supplements: PABA 7.5 mg, Biotin 150 mcg, Folic Acid 400 mg, Iodine 15 mcg, Choline 50 mg, Inositol 50 mg, dl-Methionine 50 mg, Zeaxanthan 250 mcg, Lutein 250 mcg.

Dosage:
Take 2 tablets daily. One tablet to be taken in the morning after breakfast and the second tablet to be taken not less than 6 hours before going to bed at night.

Price: 30 tablets — $20.30 (sealed)

Manufacturer:
21st Century HealthCare Inc., 2119 S. Wilson Street, Tempe, Arizona 85282-2034 USA.

Distributed by:
21st Century HealthCare Pte Ltd. 40, Jalan Pemimpin #03-02 Tat Ann Building Singapore 577185.

293.   **Women's Tonic Capsules (Nature's Green)**

Actions and indications:

Regulating menstruation and arresting leukorrhea. Use for irregular menstruation with leukorrhea, and abdominal pain during menstruation or after delivery.

Ingredients:

Each 300 mg capsule contains extracts equivalent to raw herbs: *Cordyceps* 40 mg, *Margarita* 20 mg, *Colla Corii Asini* 25 mg, *Radix Ginseng* 58 mg, *Foetus Cervi* 2.5 mg, *Radix Stellariae* 65 mg, *Cortex Moutan* 65 mg, *Lignum Aquilariae Resinatrm* 32 mg, *Fructus Evodiae* 15 mg, *Cortex Cinnamomi* 50 mg, *Radix Aucklandiae* 50 mg, *Rhizoma Cyperi* 82 mg, *Radix Anglica Sinensis* 100 mg, *Os Sepiae* 50 mg, *Pericarpium Citri Reticulatae Viride* 50 mg, *Herba Schizonepetae Carbonaria* 82 mg, *Rhizoma Zingiberis* 50 mg, *Radix Salviae Miltiorrhiae* 65 mg, *Rhizoma Alismatis* 50 mg, *Radix Glycyrrhizae Carbonaria* 32 mg, *Semen Persicae* 65 mg, *Cortex Eucommiae* 15 mg, *Radix Achyranthis Bidentatae* 50 mg, *Flos Carthami* 125 mg, *Rhizoma Chuanxiong* 82 mg, *Fructrs Amomi Rotundus* 25 mg, *Cornu Cervi Pantotrichum* 15 mg, *Poria* 65 mg, *Young Deer* 80 mg, *Fructus Amomi* 25 mg, *Rhizoma Atractylodis Macrocephalae* 65 mg, *Pericarpium Citri Reticulatae* 82 mg, *Caraoax et Plastrum Testudinis* 15 mg, *Resina Toxicodendri Carbonaria* 15 mg, *Semen Arecae Preparata* 50 mg, *Carapax Trionycis* 15 mg, *Radix Rehmanniae Preparata* 82 mg, *Rhizoma Curcumae* 32 mg, *Cortex Magnoliae Officinalis* 50 mg, *Fructus Foeniculi* 65 mg, *Radix Paeoniae Alba* 82 mg, *Pollen Typhae Carbonaria* 50 mg, Radix Paeoniae Rubra 50 mg, *Petiolus Trachycarpi Carbonaria* 15 mg, *Rhizoma Sparganii* 32 mg.

Dosage:

For oral administration, take 1–2 capsules, 3 times daily.

Price: 30 capsules — $35.00. 60 capsules (2 boxes) — $62.00 (sealed).

Manufacturer:

Tong Jum Chew Pte Ltd. 21 Kaki Bukit View Tech Park II Singapore 415957. Tel: 62781134 Fax: 62781246. Singapore Manufacturer Licence No. MLCP: 0400040 Singapore CPM Product Reference No. 113489.

294.   **Women's Vitality Multi (Blackmores)**

Description:

An energy-boosting multi specifically formulated to provide support for women's hectic, active lifestyles. It helps to provide an optimum intake of vitamins, minerals and herbs including a potent dose of Siberian ginseng to help boost energy levels. Helps to boost energy levels and help support normal cognition and balanced mood.

Ingredients:

Betacarotene (from Dunaliella Salina extract equivalent to fresh cell 37.5 mg) 1.5 mg, Vitamin B1 (thiamine nitrate) 25 mg, Vitamin B2 (Riboflavin) 12 mg, Nicotinamide 50 mg, Vitamin B5 (Pantothenic acid from calcium pantothenate 30 mg) 27.5 mg, vitamin B6 (pyridoxine hydrochloride) 25 mg, vitamin B12 (cyanocobalamin) 50 µg, vitamin C (asccorbic acid) 100 mg, vitamin D3 (cholecalciferol 5 µg) 200 IU, Natural vitamin E (d-alpha-tocopheryl acid succinate 20.7 mg) 25 IU, vitamin H (Biotin) 50 µg, calcium hydrogen phosphate anhydrous (calcium 50 mg) 170 mg, Folic acid 300 µg, magnesium oxide-heavy (magnesium 67.5 mg) 121.7 mg, ferrous fumarate (iron 5 mg) 16 mg, Manganese amino acid chelate (manganese 2 mg) 20 mg, potassium iodid (iodine 150 µg) 196 µg, Cupric sulphate pentahydrate (copper 600 µg) 2.4 mg, Chromic chloride (chromium 100 µg) 513 µg, Selenomethionine (selenium 26 µg) 64.6 µg, Silybum marianum (milk thistle) extract equivalent to dry fruit 4 g (4000 mg), Eleutherococcus senticosus (siberian ginseng) extract equivalent to dry root 2 g(2000 mg)

Dosage:

Adults: Take 1 tablet a day with a meal, or as professionally prescribed.

Safety considerations:

Not recommended for children under 15 years.

Price: 50 tablets — $38.00

Manufacturer:

Free advice from Blackmores naturopath: Call 0508757473 or cisit www.blackmoresnz.co.nz. Blackmores Ltd Auckland New Zealand

295. **Wu Ji Bai Feng Wan (Jin Pai Trademark)**

Description:

Jin Pai Wu Ji Bai Feng Wan is prepared from an ancient Chinese proven formula. This formula were used long before the Song Dynasty and is very accepted by women due to its efficacy on gynecological disorders, youth-preserving and rejuvenating effects. This product can help overcome anemia, postpartum (ie a few days after childbirth) weakness due to blood loss, improve one's qi (ie energy) and promotes the circulation of blood. This product is suitable for women of all ages. The manufacturer, Maanshan Shenlu Kerui Pharmaceutical Co., Ltd. has reputable history manufacturing this product and the herbs used are carefully selected. Product quality is maintained by using the latest scientific technology in the manufacturing process.

Indications:

This product is used to overcome lack of energy, anemia, postpartum weakness due to blood loss, menstrual problems.

Actions:
Revitalizing and nourishing blood.

Ingredients:
Each 6 g contains: *Pullus Cum Osse Nigro* 1203 mg, *Colla Cornus Cervi* 241 mg, *Carapax Trionycis Praeparata* 120 mg, *Concha Ostreae Praeparata* 90 mg, *Ootheca Mantidis* 90 mg, *Radix Ginseng* 241 mg, *Radix Astragali* 60 mg, *Radix Angelicae Sinensis* 271 mg, *Radix Paeoniae Alba* 241 mg, *Rhizoma Cyperi* 241 mg, *Radix Asparagi* 120 mg, *Radix et Rhizoma Glycyrrhizae* 60 mg, *Radix Rehmanniae* 481 mg, *Radix Rehmanniae Praeparata* 481 mg, *Rhizoma Chuanxiong* 120 mg, *Radix Stellariae* 49 mg, *Radix Salviae Miltiorrhizae* 241 mg, *Rhizoma Dioscoreae* 241 mg, *Semen Euryales* 120 mg, *Cornu Cervi Degelatinatum* 90 mg.

Instruction:
One bottle daily to be taken after menstruation before sleep preferably with warm water. If heat or feverish occurs we recommend that your daily intake of water can be increased, alternatively to reduce dosage to one bottle every alternate day. (Stop dosage during menstruation and resume dosage after menstruation)

Safety considerations:
No known side-effect. Do not use during pregnancy; shoud be used with caution in kidney disease and high blood pressure. Use with caution during cold and hyper-menorrhea. Cannot be taken together with medicine with Fructus Gleditsiae, Faeces Trogopterori.

Price: 6 g × 8 bottles — $24.00 (sealed)

Manufacturer:
Maanshan Shenlu Kerui Pharmaceutical Co. Ltd. Maanshan, Anhui, China. Assembler and importer: Kinhong Pte Ltd No. 297 Kaki Buki Avenue 1 Shun Li Industrial Park Singapore 416083 Tel: (65)67415561 Fax: (65) 67413705.

296.   **Wuji Bai Feng Wan (AL)**

Description:
Dark-brown to black water-honeyed pills, sweet in taste with slight bitterness.

Actions and indications:
Reinforces qi, nourishes blood, invigorates vital energy, regulates menstruation and leucorrhea. For recovery from emacination, puerperal debility, weakness and aching in the lower back and kness, as well as to regulate irregular menstruation, minimize dysmenorrhoea (menstrual cramps) and relieve leucorrhea due to a deficiency of qi, vital energy and blood.

Ingredients:
Each 6 gm pills contains raw herb as follows: *Pullus cum Osse Nigro* (Preparata) 1052 mg, *Colla Cornus Cervi* 211 mg, *Carapax Trionycis* (Preparata) 105 mg, *Concha Ostreae* (Preparata) 79 mg, *Ootheca Mantidis* 79 mg, *Radix et Rhizoma Ginseng* 211 mg, *Radix Astragali* 53 mg, *Radix Angelicae Sinensis* 237 mg, *Radix Paeoniae Alba* 211 mg, *Rhizoma Cyperi* (Preparata) 211 mg, *Radix Asparagi* 105 mg, *Radix et Rhizoma Glycyrrhizae* 53 mg, *Radix Rehmanniae* 421 mg, *Radix Rehmanniae Praeparata* 421 mg, *Rhizoma Chuanxiong* 105 mg, *Radix Stellariae* 43 mg, *Radix et Rhizoma salviae Miltiorrhizae* 211 mg, *Rhizoma Dioscoreae* 211 mg, *Semen Euryales* (Preparata) 105 mg, *Cornu Cervi Degelatinatum* 79 mg.

Instruction:
Compress wax ball to retrieve small plastic ball within. Remove cap to retrieve all the pills (6 g). Swallow pills with warm water once a day, or once every 2 days.

Safety considerations:
Side effects not known. Precaution: Refer booklet inside the box.

Price: 3 wax balls × 6 g — $10.00 (sealed)

Manufacturer:
Nanjing TonRenTang Pharmaceutical Co. Ltd China.

Imported by:
AL. 10 Kaki Bukit Road 1 #03-27 KB Industrial Building Singapore 416175 Tel: 65-68460337 Fax: 65-68460336.

297. **Wuji Baifeng Wan (Tong Zhi Tang)**

Actions:
Invigorating vital energy, nourishing the blood, regulating menstruation and relieving leukorrhagia.

Indications:
Cases with deficiency of both vital energy and blood, general debility, lumbago and weakness of kness, irregular menstruation, and leukorrhagia.

Ingredients:
Each 6 g contains: *Pullus Cum Osse Nigro* 1113.72 mg, *Colla Cornus Cervi* 223.10 mg, *Carapax Triongcis* 111.55 mg, *Concha Ostreae* 83.55 mg, *Ootheca Mantidis* 83.55 mg, *Radix Ginseng* 223.00 mg, *Radix Astragali* 56.00 mg, *Radix Angelicae Sinensis* 250.65 mg, *Radix Paeoniae Alba* 223.10 mg, *Rhizoma Cyperi* 223.10 mg, *Radix Asparagi* 111.55 mg, *Radix Glycyrrhizae* 56.00 mg, *Radix Rehmanniae* 445.75 mg, *Radix Rehmanniae Preparata* 445.75 mg, *Rhizoma*

Chuanxiong 111.55 mg, *Radix Stellariae* 45.33 mg, *Radix Salviae Miltiorrhizae* 223.10 mg, *Rhizoma Dioscoreae* 223.10 mg, *Semen Euryales* 111.55 mg, *Cornu Cervi Degelatinatum* 83.55 mg.

Dosage:
One bolus 1–2 times daily, taken with warm water.

Safety considerations:
Side effects not observed. For those with common cold and fever and avoid to take raw and cold foods during administration.

Price: 10 pills × 6 g — $11.00 (sealed)

Manufacturer:
Guangzhou Chenliji Pharmaceutical Factory P.R. China.

Imported by:
Winlykah Trading, Block 8, Lorong Bakar Batu #06-09, Singapore 348743.

298.   **Wuji Baifeng Wan Women Supplement (Tong Ren Tang)**

Actions:
To invigorate the vital energy, nourish the blood, regulate the menstruation and stop leukorrhea.

Indications:
Irregular menstruation, dysmenotthea, cold pain of the lower abdomen, general debility, feeling weak, lassitude of loins and legs, puerperal debility, night sweat due to the deficiency of the refined material in the viscera, these caused by deficiency of both vital energy and blood.

Ingredients:
Each 6 gms contains raw herbs: *Pullus Curn Osse Nigro* (Preparata) 1113.7 mg, *Colla Cornus Cervi* 222.7 mg, *Carapax Trionycis* (Preparata) 111.4 mg, *Concha Ostreae* (Preparata) 83.5 mg, *Ootheca Mantidis* 83.5 mg, *Radix Ginseng* 222.7 mg, *Radix Astragali* 55.7 mg, *Radix Angelicae Sinensis* 250.6 mg, *Radix Paeoniae Alba* 222.7 mg, *Rhizoma Cyperi* (Preparata) 222.7 mg, *Radix Asparagi* 111.4 mg, *Radix Glycyrrhizae* 55.7 mg, *Radix Rehmanniae* 445.5 mg, *Radix Rehmanniae* (Preparata) 445.5 mg, *Rhizoma Chuanxiong* 111.4 mg, *Radix Stellariae* 45.2 mg, *Radix Salviae Miltiorrhizae* 222.7 mg, *Rhizoma Dioscoreae* 222.7 mg, *Semen Euryales* (Preparata) 111.4 mg, *Cornu Cervi Degelatinatum* 83.5 mg.

Dosage:
Twice daily, all the water-honeyed pills (6 g) in one wax ball each time.

Method of administration:
Take out the wax ball, squeeze the wax ball to open, take out the inner plastic capsule, open the inner plastic capsule and take the pills.

Price: 6 g × 10 waxballs (2 boxes) — $36 (sealed), 1 box — $20.00.

Manufacturer:
Beijing Tongrentang Co. Ltd. Tongrentang Pharmaceutical Factory Beijing China.

Imported by:
Science Arts Co. Pte Ltd. 150 MacPherson Rd, Science Arts Building Singapore 348524.

299. **Xin Pi Fu Zhi Yang Wan (Ferragold)**

Actions and indications:
Expel pathogenic wind promote blood flow, remove heat from blood, remove blood stasis and relieve dampness, relieve itching, use for ezema.

Ingredients:
Rhizoma seu Radix Notopterygii (7%), Radix Angelicae Dahuricae (7%), Radix Notoginseng (10%), Fructus Gardeniae (6%), Rhizoma Ligustici Chuanxiong (7%), Fructus Xanthii (7%), Semen Lepidii seu Descurainiae (8%), Rhizoma Atractylodis Macrocephalae (7%), Aloe (10%), Flos Sophorae (10%), Radix Linderae (7%), Radix Aconiti (6%), Herba Salviae Chinensis (4%), Rhizoma Pinelliae (4%); Each capsule weight 319 mg.

Dosage:
Take 3–4 capsules 2 times daily.

Price: 30 capsules

Sole Agent:
Ferragold Trading Enterprise, 32, Defu Lane 10, #04-08 Singapore 539213; Tel: (65)383 4091, Fax: (65)383 4092; Email: bihmedco@singnet.com.sg.

Manufacturer:
Yi Shi Yuan Pte Ltd.

300. **Yao shan gong ting (Chwee Song)**

Actions and indications:
Ginseng helps to improve immunity and body resistence. It also helps to improve blood circulation especially good for those who has just recovered from illness.

Ingredients:

Astragalus Memranaceus 10 gm, Boxthorn Fruit (20 gm), Codonopsis Pilosula (15 gm), Dioscorea Opposita (11 gm), Polygonatum Odoratum (25 g), Ginseng (14 gm), Nelumbo Nucifera (15 gm).

Instruction:

Cook all the ingredients for half an hour, then place them into the chicken body. Wrap the whole chicken with aluminium foil. Steam it for about 2 1/2 hours and ready to serve.

Price: 110 gm — $6.40

Packed by:

Chwee Song Supplies Pte. Ltd. Blk 5, Ang Mo Kio Industrial Park 2A Tech II, #07-14 to 16 Singapore 567760; e-mail: sales@chweesong.com.sg; Internet: www. chweesong.com.sg; Tel: (65) 6482 3935, 6482 3386 Fax: (65) 6778 5028 Product of China.

301. **Yizhi Cong Ming Tang (Chwee Song)**

Actions and indication:

Enhance memory and quick recovery from illnesses. Helps relieve stress, increase stamina and prevent fatigue.

Ingredients:

Agaricus Brazei Murri Mushroom (5 gm), Astragalus Membarraceus (10 gm), Ginseng (10 gm), Glossy Ganoderma (5 gm), Disocorea Opposita (20 gm), Porras Cocos (15 gm), Paeoria Lactiflora (15 gm), Glycyrrhiza uralensis (10 gm), Boxthorn fruit (10 gm).

Instruction:

Cooking information: Cook or double boil ingredients with 300 g of meat in 1500 ml of water for 1 to 2 hours.

Price: 100 gm — $5.35

Packed by:

Chwee Song Supplies Pte. Ltd. Blk 5, Ang Mo Kio Industrial Park 2A Tech II, #07-14 to 16 Singapore 567760; e-mail: sales@chweesong.com.sg; Internet: www. chweesong.com.sg; Tel: (65) 6482 3935, 6482 3386 Fax: (65) 6778 5028 Product of China.

302. **Yomeishu Herbal Health Tonic (Yomeishu)**

Description:

Yomeishu is a herbal health tonic first produced in Japan in 1602, and its excellent effects have been experienced by millions of people. The principal ingredients used in Yomeishu are fourteen kinds of medicinal herbs widely known in the Orient for their effects, and are extracted by a tradition-based unique formula. Therefore, Yomeishu has a unique flavour, and when taken, it gives a pleasant feeling that refreshes the body and mind. Yomeishu is absorbable even by weak digestive systems, and it spreads quickly throughout the body organs, promoting the natural activities of the body, and it displays efficacy in regulating physical and mental functions to maintan health.

Actions and indications:

Yomeishu, as a health tonic, is taken for the improvement of the following symptoms: poor appetite, gastroenteric weakness, poor blood circulation, chills, fatigue, weak constitution, and weakness after disease.

Ingredients:

Per 60 ml: Cinnamomi Cortex (J.P.) (270 mg), Carthami Flos (J.P.) (12 mg), Rehmanniae Radix (J.P.) (60 mg), Caryophylli Flos (J.P.) (24 mg), Ginseng Radix (J.P.) (60 mg), Saposhnikoviae Radix (J.P.) (96 mg), Curcumae Rhizoma (36 mg), Leonuri Herba (48 mg), Epimedii Herba (114 mg), Linderae Umbellatae Ramus (594 mg), Eucommiae Cortex (18 mg), Cistanchis Herba (48 mg), Agkistrodan Japonicae (12 mg); Yomeishu is an extracted preparation of the above natural medicinal ingredients through the process of tincture preparation method prescribed in Japanese Pharmacopoeia. Glucose (13 g), Ethanol (alcohol) 14% vol.

Instruction:

Adults: Take 1 cup each time (20 ml), 3 times daily before meals and/or at bedtime. Dosage can be slightly increased or decreased depending on the body condition. However, overdosage should be avoided. Avoid taking it in the case of profuse bleeding of ulcers or outer injuries, since Yomeishu has a promoting action on blood circulation; Always cap the bottle tightly and avoid direct sunlight)

Safety considerations:

Avoid taking it in the case of profuse bleeding of ulcers or outer injuries, since Yomeishu has a promoting action on blood circulation.

Price: 700 ml — $39.60

Manufacturer:

Yomeishu Seizo Co., Ltd, Tokyo, Japan.

Imported By:
Letat Agencies (Private) Limited 61 Yishun Industrial Park A #04-01 Singapore 768767; Product of Japan.

303.   **Youth and Beauty Capsules (AL)**

Actions and indications:
Facilitating bowel movement and clearing away toxins, replenishing the vital essence and preserving youth. It is effective for constipation, halitosis, anorexia pallor, insomnia, pimples and acne caused by heat and wase accumulation inside the body, which help to reduce illness and promote health and skin beauty.

Ingredients:
Each capsule (0.35 g) contains extract equivalent to raw herbs: *Radix Quinquefolium* 100 mg, *Radix Rehmanniae* 200 mg, *Radix Scrophulariae* 300 mg, *Radix Salviae Miltiorizae* 100 mg, *Rhizoma Bistortae* 200 mg, *Radix Polygoni Multiflori* 400 mg, *Cordyceps* 60 mg, *Margarita* 50 mg, *Rhizoma Atractylodis Macrocephalae* 200 mg, *Radix et Rhizoma Rhei*

Dosage:
Adult with constipation 3–4 capsules each time, twice a day, morning and evening. For health maintenance: Take 2 capsules each time, once a day, or adjust the dosage according to stool condition to keep 1–2 motions every day.

Safety considerations:
Side effects not known. Note: At the first application it may happen to have bowels, but after a few times of application the excrement will be loose and soft. Do not eact fried, spicy and oily food. Not recommended for pregnant women.

Price: 60 capsules — $22 (sealed)

Manufacturer and sole distributor in singapore:
ALL Link Medical & Health Products Pte Ltd. 10 Kaki Bukit Road 1, #03-27 K B Industrial Building, Singapore 416175. Tel: 68460337. Fax: 68460336.

304.   **Yunnan Baiyao Capsules (Yunnan Baiyao)**

Actions and indications:
Dispersing blood stasis and hemostasis, activating blood circulation and alleviating pain, detoxification and promoting subsidence of swelling, used in treatment for traumatic injury, stagnated blood and tumefaction pain, spitting blood, hemoptysis, hematochezia, hemorrhoid hemorrhage, suppurative infection on body surface and pyogenic infections, contusion of soft tissue, closed fracture, hemoptysis of bronchiectasis and hemorrhage of peptic ulcer and infection diseases of skin.

Ingredients:

No information available

Dosage:

Administer orally, 0.25–0.5 g one time, 4 times daily (for children aged 2–5 years will be given 1/4 dose for adults; 6–12 years 1/2 dose for adults). PIL: Administration and Dosage: Knife, bullet wounds, traumatic injury, no matter how light or severe, Yunnan Baiyao is administered with lukewarm boiled water for bleeding patients, for patients of stagnated blood and oncotic pain but no bleeding administer with wine. For initial supprative infection on body surface and pyogenic infection, one capsule (0.25 g) is given orally, and another portion drug powder is mixed with wine homogeneously and applied on affected part, for pyosis affected part administer orally only. For other diseases of hemorrhage administer orally. Administer orally, 1–2 capsules one time, four times daily (for children aged 2–5 years will be given 1/4 dose for adults; 6–12 years 1/2 dose for adults). For the patient of serious traumatic one red safety pill may be taken at first which need not administering for light trauma and other diseases.

Safety considerations:

Broad beans, fish, sour or cold food should not be taken within 24 hours after administration. PIL: Caution: Yunnan Baiyao capsules should not be taken during pregnancy.

Price: 6 capsules — $6.60

Manufacturer:

Yunnan Baiyao Group Co. Ltd. Address: 222 Erhuan Xi Road, Kunming, Yunnan, P.R. China. Tel: +86-871-8327398. Fax: +86-871-8325455.

Imported by:

Science Arts Co. Pte Ltd. 150 MacPherson Rd, Science Arts Building Singapore 348524.

305. **Yunnan Baiyao Powder (Yunnan Baiyao)**

Actions and indications:

Activating blood circulation and arresting pain perception, counteracting toxin and eliminating swelling.

Ingredients:

4 g contains extract equivalent to raw herbs: *Radix Notoginseng* 1.6 g, *Borneolum Syntheticum* 0.6 g, *Ajuga Forrestii Diels* 0.68 g, *Herba Inulae Cappae* 0.2 g, *Rhizoma Dioscoreae Nipponicae* 0.4 g, *Rhizoma Dioscoreae* 0.532 g, *Dioscoreae Parviflora Ting* 0.24 g, *Herba Geranii & Herba Erodii* 0.288 g.

Dosage:
No information available

Price: 4 g — $5 (sealed)

Manufacturer:
Yunnan Baiyao Group Co. Ltd. 51 Xiba Road Kunming Yunnan China.

Importer:
Science Arts Co. Pte Ltd. 150 MacPherson Road Singapore 348524.

306.   **Yunnan Baiyao Powder (Yunnan Baiyao)**

Actions and indications:
Traditionally used for improving blood circulation.

Ingredients:
4 g contains extract equivalent to raw herbs: *Radix Notoginseng* 1.6 g, *Borneolum Syntheticum* 0.6 g, *Ajuga Forrestii* 0.68 g, *Herba Inulae Cappae* 0.2 g, *Rhizoma Dioscoreae Nipponicae* 0.4 g, *Rhizoma Dioscoreae Opposita* 0.532 g, *Dioscorea Parviflora* 0.24 g, *Herba Erodii Seu Geranii* 0.288 g.

Dosage:
**Refer enclosed leaflet for details. Packaging is sealed.

Price: 4 g × 6 — $30.00 (sealed)

Manufacturer:
Yunnan Baiyao Group Co. Ltd Yunnan China. Importer: Science Arts Co. Pte Ltd. 150 MacPherson Road Singapore 348524.

307.   **Yunnan Baiyao Tincture (Yunnan Baiyao)**

Actions and indications:
Traditionally used for symptomatic relief of joint and muscle pains; PIL: Bruises, contusions, injuries, wounds, swelling and pain due to blood stagnation, rhumatism and numbness, pains in bones, muscles and sinew; pain due to arthritis, etc.

Ingredients:
30 ml contains extract equivalent to raw herbs: Ingredient; In English: Radix Notoginseng (1.2 g), Borneolum Syntheticum (0.045 g), Ajuga forrestii Diels (0.15 g), Herba Inulae Cappae (0.15 g), Rhizoma Dioscoreae Nippponicae (0.75 g), Rhizoma Dioscoreae (0.3999 g), Dioscoreae parviflora Ting (0.18 g), Herba Geranii & Herba Erodii (0.126 g).

Dosage:
Orally taken: 3–5 ml each time, 3 times a day. The dosage limit is 10 ml per time. External application: massage the affected part 3 minutes each time and 3–5 times daily. PIL: Oral Administration: 3 times a day and 3–5 ml each time. The dosage limit is 10 ml. Dosage for children should be reduced adequately according to doctor's directions. External Application: Turn bottle upside down and wet the sponge head with liquid and rub onto affected area. 3 times daily.

Safety considerations:
Broad beans, fish, sour or cold food should not be taken within 24 hours after administration. It is prohibited for pregnant women. No use for individuals with an allergic reaction to alcohol.

Price: 30 ml — $4.00

Imported by:
Science Arts Co. Pte. Ltd, 150, Mac Pherson Road, Science Arts Building, Singapore 348524

308. **Zest for men [with Damiana Aphrodisiaca, Ginseng and Zinc] (Kordel's)**

Description:
It is a special high-potency nutritional supplement formulated for men to counteract flagging energy and stamina associated with stress and poor diet. Zest for Men includes Zinc, an essential trace mineral for men. Plus … Nature's own power and energy releasers Siberian Ginseng, and Turnera herb (Damiana aphrodisiaca), plus Vitamin E, to put back the zest, you thought you'd lost!

Ingredients:
Each tablet provides Vitamins: Cyanocobalamin 50 mcg, Thiamine Hydrochloride 10 mg, Riboflavine 10 mg, Nicotinic Acid 50 mg, Calcium Pantothenate 10 mg, Pyridoxine Hydrochloride 10 mg, d-alpha tocopheryl acid succinate (VIT E-100IU) 84 mg, Betacarotene 3 mg, Calcium Ascorbate providing Vitamin C 150mg. Minerals: Zinc sulphate providing zinc 15 mg, Ferrous fumarate providing iron 10 mg, Magnesium oxide providing Magnesium 95 mg. Herbal Extracts & Energisers: Smilax officinalis (SARSAPARILLA) Root 100 mg, Serenoa serrulata (SAW PALMETTO) Fruit 100 mg, Eleutherococcus senticosus (GINSENG SIBERIAN) Root 250 mg, Turnera diffusa (DAMIANA) Herb 250 mg, Capsicum frutescens (CAYENNE) Fruit Powder 50 mg.

Dosage:
Adults: Take one tablet daily, with a meal, as a dietary supplement.

Safety considerations:
Contains Nicotinic Acid which may cause transient flushing in some individuals.

Price: 30 tablets — $29.30 (Sealed) Kordel's is a trademark of Health Foods International.

Manufactured for:
Nutra-Life Health & Fitness (NZ) Ltd. Auckland, New Zealand. www.nutralife.co.nz.

Australian Distributor:
Nutra-Life Health & Fitness. Australia Pty Ltd. 5 Kaleski Street, Moorebank, NSW 2170 www.nutralife.com.au. Singapore/Malaysia Agent: Cambert (F.E.) Pte Ltd.

309. **Zhen Huang Wan (Yulin)**

Description:
Our Company specially selects important medicine good for anti-inflammation, antidote, antipyretic, anodyne and extracts their essence for making into "Zhen Huang Wan" which is efficacious for all kinds of inflammation, carbuncles and anonymous swelling boil. This medicine can be taken internally and rubbed externally. Better result will be obtained if using it in both ways simultaneously. It is packed in capsules convenient for using and is really good medicine to be kept always in household and on travelling.

Indications:
Throat swelling and pain, boil, carbuncle.

Ingredients:
Each Capsule (200 mg) contains: *Radix Notoginseng* 71.10 mg, *Radix Scutellariae* 55.60 mg, *Fel Suillus* 44.40 mg, *Calculus Bovis* (Synthetic) 35.50 mg, *Margarita* 8.80 mg, *Borneolum Syntheticum* 2.20 mg.

Dosage:
Internally: For adults, 3 times a day, 2 capsule a time. For children, reducing adequately. Externally: Open the covers of few capsules and pour out the powder. Mix the powder with cold boiled water or vinegar into paste and then spread the paste on the swelling.

Safety considerations:
Side effects not known. It is prohibition to be taken internally by the pregnant women. Stop spreading when the pus bursts out from reddish swelling or the abscess is broken and rotten.

Price: 30 capsules — $5.80

Manufacturer:

Guangxi Yulin Pharmaceutical Co., Ltd. Yulin Guangxi China.

Assembler and Importer:

Kinhong (pte) ltd 297 Kaki Bukit Ave 1, Shun Li Industrial Park, Singapore 416083.

Index

www.ingramcontent.com/pod-product-compliance
Lightning Source LLC
Chambersburg PA
CBHW051947270326
41929CB00015B/2564